Dental ⑪ Materials

FOUNDATIONS AND APPLICATIONS

JOHN M. POWERS, PhD

Senior Vice President and Senior Editor, The Dental Advisor,
Dental Consultants, Inc., Ann Arbor, Michigan
Clinical Professor of Oral Biomaterials,
Department of Restorative Dentistry and Biomaterials,
University of Texas School of Dentistry at Houston,
Houston, Texas

JOHN C. WATAHA, DMD, PhD

Professor of Dentistry, Department of Restorative Dentistry,
School of Dentistry, University of Washington,
Seattle, Washington

Contributing Editor

YEN-WEI CHEN, DDS, MSD

Assistant Professor
Department of Restorative Dentistry
School of Dentistry
University of Washington
Seattle, Washington

ELSEVIER

ELSEVIER

3251 Riverport Lane
St. Louis, Missouri 63043

DENTAL MATERIALS: FOUNDATIONS AND APPLICATIONS, ELEVENTH EDITION

ISBN: 978-0-323-31637-8

Notices

Knowledge and best practice in this field are constantly changing. As new research and experience broaden our understanding, changes in research methods, professional practices, or medical treatment may become necessary.

Practitioners and researchers must always rely on their own experience and knowledge in evaluating and using any information, methods, compounds, or experiments described herein. In using such information or methods, they should be mindful of their own safety and the safety of others, including parties for whom they have a professional responsibility.

With respect to any drug or pharmaceutical products identified, readers are advised to check the most current information provided (i) on procedures featured or (ii) by the manufacturer of each product to be administered, to verify the recommended dose or formula, the method and duration of administration, and contraindications. It is the responsibility of practitioners, relying on their own experience and knowledge of their patients, to make diagnoses, to determine dosages and the best treatment for each individual patient, and to take all appropriate safety precautions.

To the fullest extent of the law, neither the Publisher nor the authors, contributors, or editors, assume any liability for any injury and/or damage to persons or property as a matter of products liability, negligence or otherwise, or from any use or operation of any methods, products, instructions, or ideas contained in the material herein.

Library of Congress Cataloging-in-Publication Data

Names: Powers, John M., 1946- , author. | Wataha, John C., author.
Title: Dental materials : foundations and applications / John M. Powers, John C. Wataha.
Description: Eleventh edition. | St. Louis, Missouri : Elsevier, [2017] |
    Includes bibliographical references and index.
Identifiers: LCCN 2015039912 | ISBN 9780323316378 (pbk. : alk. paper)
Subjects: | MESH: Dental Materials.
Classification: LCC RK652.5 | NLM WU 190 | DDC 617.6/95–dc23 LC record available at http://lccn.loc.gov/2015039912

Content Strategist: Kristin Wilhelm
Content Development Specialist: Diane Chatman
Publishing Services Manager: Hemamalini Rajendrababu
Project Manager: Manchu Mohan
Designer: Christian Bilbow

Printed in the United States of America.

Last digit is the print number: 9 8 7 6 5 4

 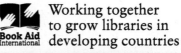

Working together
to grow libraries in
developing countries

www.elsevier.com • www.bookaid.org

Dental Materials: Foundations and Applications presents contemporary information about clinical and laboratory dental materials used throughout all dimensions of dental care.

BACKGROUND

Now in its eleventh edition, this textbook was edited for over 30 years until 2003 by Dr. Robert G. Craig. Dr. Craig contributed to the education of literally thousands of health profession students, using his research knowledge and inherent teaching skills to promote an understanding of dental materials. This text continues to honor Dr. Craig's commitment to the dissemination of accurate, current knowledge about dental materials in clinical practice. We continue to follow his philosophy of teaching students and clinicians the "hows & whys" of the materials they use to treat their patients.

AUDIENCE

This textbook is intended for students in dental, dental assisting, and dental hygiene programs. It also is an excellent resource for dental technology programs or programs training midlevel providers and will serve as a comprehensive, contemporary reference for any practicing dentist or dental professional. Finally, it is a good resource for those in need of a thorough review of dental materials for general or specialty board examinations.

ORGANIZATION

Our goal with *Dental Materials: Foundations and Applications,* 11th Edition, is to provide a comprehensive source of information about dental materials. Following a discussion of the nature of materials, the book provides an overview about how materials are used to treat or prevent disease and trauma. The book then covers important properties of materials, followed by all preventive and direct restorative materials used in contemporary dental practice. Later chapters focus on materials used to fabricate indirect restorations that are critically important to the restoration of a patient's oral health and are important to the dentist or dental professional because of the need to communicate expectations accurately to the patient or laboratory technician.

In this edition, all chapters have been revised, but chapters on ceramics, implants, impression materials, and polymers have been completely redone to present up-to-date information at an appropriate level. We have added over 60 new clinical photos to help students understand the applications of materials in dental practice and help teachers convey the same. We have added information throughout about the rapidly emerging area of "digital dentistry." We have also added

an introductory section on the nature of materials to give readers a solid foundation to understand how different materials are, or are not, related.

Key terminology is set in bold type, critical statements are italicized, unusual words are defined in brief text boxes, and quick review or summary statements are placed at the ends of chapters or major sections. Finally, a glossary of terms is placed at the end of the textbook. In addition, a companion website created just for this book (http://evolve.elsevier.com/Powers/dentalmaterials) contains a variety of resources designed to enhance both education and study (see listing below).

KEY FEATURES

- *Comprehensive, Focused Coverage:* Fifteen chapters plus an introductory section present detailed information about dental materials used in the dental office and laboratory and all the materials relevant to day-to-day practice for dentists, dental hygienists, and dental assistants.
- *Cutting-Edge Content:* The latest materials used in dental practice are discussed, including those used in esthetic dentistry, digital dentistry, and preventive dentistry, and new advanced technologies in laboratory practice.
- *Art Program:* More than 500 full-color illustrations and photographs liberally supplement the text descriptions to help students learn to recognize the differences among the many types of dental materials and thoroughly comprehend their appropriate clinical manipulation. Dozens of intraoral photos show how materials are used, step-by-step, in many cases.
- *Consistent Presentation:* Each material presentation begins with a study of the properties and uses of that material before moving on to the specific manipulations and applications in dentistry, providing a logical framework for comparison among materials.
- *Review Questions:* Each chapter ends with 20 to 30 self-test questions, the answers to which are provided in the online instructor's materials, as a student study and assessment tool.
- *Quick Review Boxes:* Each chapter wraps up with a brief narrative summarizing the content to recap key concepts and help students assess their readiness to progress onto the next topic.
- *Note Boxes:* Interspersed throughout the text, these notes highlight key points and important terminology to help students build the foundational information necessary for clinical competence.
- *Summary Tables and Boxes:* Chapters summarize concepts and procedures within boxes and tables throughout the text for easy-to-read summaries of text discussions for reference and study.
- *Vocabulary Resources:* Bolded upon their initial text mention within the chapter, and defined in a back-of-book

glossary to help students master the language of dental materials.

- *Learning Objectives:* Each chapter begins with a detailed list of student outcomes that serve as study tools and checkpoints for student comprehension.
- *Supplemental Readings:* Chapters include listings of contemporary texts and journal articles that supply further information on the topic at hand to promote evidence-based practice and provide students with sources of in-depth study on specific topics.
- *Conversion Factors:* The inside back cover includes listings of common metric conversions as a handy reference for students.
- *Evolve Website:* A companion site provides resources to ease both instruction and learning.

NEW TO THIS EDITION

- *New Content:* Expanded and updated discussions are included for particularly dynamic areas such as esthetics, CAD/CAM technology, cements, ceramics, dental implants, and impressions (including digital impressions) to keep up with changes and advances in dental materials and associated technology.
- *Full Color:* This text is in full color, improving the clarity of images and helping students understand complex processes and sequences, and differentiate among the numerous types of dental materials, particularly.
- *New Artwork:* More than 70 new illustrations and photographs have been added, including images that show materials being mixed and used, making this often-difficult subject matter easier to grasp. Many intraoral photos are included to give the reader a sense of how the materials are used in sometimes complex sequences.

- *Appendices:* Several chapters include appendices that set apart from the text discussion and describe dental materials (e.g., agar impression material and zinc phosphate cement) that are less commonly used in modern dental practices.
- *New Ancillary Materials:* A color image collection, expanded test bank, and the addition of case studies are added to the instructor materials, whereas students benefit from access to instant-feedback assessment questions and interactive exercises to reinforce glossary terms.

COMPANION WEBSITE

An Evolve website has been created specifically for this text and is accessible via http://evolve.elsevier.com/Powers/dentalmaterials. Assets on this site include the following:

STUDENT RESOURCES

- Self-Assessment Practice Quizzes
- Instructional Videos
- Vocabulary Flashcards

INSTRUCTOR RESOURCES

- Test Bank (approximately 650 questions)
- Case Studies (including critical thinking questions)
- PowerPoint Presentations
- Image Collection
- Answers to Textbook Self-Test Questions
- Performance Skills Checklists

John M. Powers
John C. Wataha

ACKNOWLEDGMENTS

We gratefully acknowledge the donations of photographs for the previous editions by Dr. Regina Messer of Georgia Regent's University and Drs. Kavita Shor, Ricardo Schwedhelm, Richard D. Tucker, Mats Kronström, J. Martin Anderson, Xavier Lepe, Ariel Raigrodski, James Johnson, Brandon Seto, Mr. Richard Lee, Sr., and Mr. Andreas Saltzer, all from the University of Washington School of Dentistry, greatly enhance the learning and understanding of the reader, and we thank these individuals for contributing them.

In addition, we especially thank Dr. Yen-Wei Chen from the University of Washington School of Dentistry for his perspective and expertise as we constructed the eleventh edition. We also acknowledge his donation of many clinical photographs. As a practicing prosthodontist, teacher of predoctoral dental and graduate prosthodontic students, and academician, his extensive knowledge about how restorative materials are used in contemporary dental practice has added immense value to the book for readers and instructors alike. We are grateful for his many contributions.

Introduction: The Building Blocks of Restorative Dental Materials

OBJECTIVES

After reading this chapter, the student should be able to:

1. Describe the importance of the atomic number and the periodic table of the elements.
2. Compare and contrast ionic, covalent, and metallic bonds and their role in restorative dental materials.
3. Describe the differences between molecules and lattices and cite which restorative materials occur in which arrangement along with examples of materials using each arrangement.
4. List the four major classes of restorative dental materials and explain how each is unique and how the atomic structure of each leads to its macroscopic and clinical properties.

What makes up the materials in the world around us? What makes materials different from one another in color, strength, flexibility, conductivity, or weight? And why can we use some materials to restore teeth but not others? Why are some materials best suited for oral impressions, others for fillings, still others for implants? The answers to these questions are based on the way the most basic units of matter are arranged and interact. In the current preview, we will briefly explore the world of matter and materials as an introduction to restorative dental materials.

The oral environment is harsh and diverse, and the materials we use in that environment must survive many challenges. This environment experiences remarkable changes in temperature, substantial mechanical forces, adhesion of communities of microorganisms on every exposed surface, and chemical attacks from foods and from the body, with all these occurring over years to decades. Is it any wonder, then, that the materials needed to function in this environment are themselves diverse and complicated? Even more remarkable is that the roles we ask these materials to play. We have asked materials to act as surrogates for missing oral structures for thousands of years. But today, we increasingly ask materials to also serve as therapeutics or to adapt automatically to changing oral conditions.

The world of restorative dental materials is complex, exciting, and evolving. In this preview, we will introduce materials from the most basic perspective of the atom and explore how atoms interact to form the classes of materials we use every day in the treatment of oral disease. In the end, understanding these basic ideas is the key to understanding and predicting whether our everyday clinical treatments with dental materials will succeed or fail.

ATOMS: THE BUILDING BLOCKS OF DENTAL MATERIALS

The basic building block of all restorative dental materials is the atom. Atoms combine various ways via bonding; the bonding between atoms is a key feature of what makes dental materials behave the way they do. Beyond atom-to-atom bonding, atoms are arranged at a higher level into molecules or crystals that ultimately give dental materials their familiar clinical properties. It is these arrangements of atoms and the nature of the bonds among them that allows metals to conduct electricity, ceramics to have translucence, and elastomers to stretch. We will briefly discuss these ideas further in the following sections.

> **! ALERT**
>
> Atoms are the basic building block of all dental materials. The interactions between atoms are the key difference among materials.

Atoms

Every atom consists of a nucleus of protons and neutrons and electrons in cloudlike areas around the nucleus (Figure 0-1). The numbers of protons (the atomic number) determines the identity of the atom—whether it is copper, gold, or carbon, etc. We call atoms with different numbers of protons different elements. The components of atoms have a property known as charge: protons are positively charged, neutrons have no charge, and electrons are negatively charged. In their native state, all atoms have equal numbers of protons and electrons and therefore have no net charge.

The number of protons in the nucleus of an atom determines the number and arrangement of the electrons and electron clouds around it. These clouds are technically referred to as atomic orbitals; the complex shapes and properties of these orbitals are well beyond the focus of this chapter. For our purposes, it is sufficient to understand that these clouds of electrons are the basis by which atoms interact with each other and that electron numbers and properties are determined by the number of protons.

The atoms in our universe are arranged into a sophisticated table called the periodic table of the elements (Figure 0-2); this table is arranged in rows (periods) according

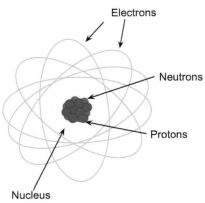

FIG 0-1 The atom is the basic building block of all restorative dental materials. Every atom consists of a nucleus of protons (positively charged) and neutrons (no charge) surrounded by clouds of electrons (negatively charged). In its native state, every atom is electrically neutral, having an equal number of positive and negative charges. The number of protons determines the identity of the atom in the periodic table of elements (see Figure 0-2) and is known as the atomic number. Thus, the atomic number determines the element. The number of electrons and their configuration around the nucleus largely determines how the element bonds with other elements to form the materials we use in clinical practice.

to the number of protons in the nucleus of the elements. Complex chemical rules dictate the number of elements in each row. Each element has a one- or two-letter symbol; the first letter is always capitalized. If there is a second letter, it is lower case. Remarkably, from this table, we can predict the physical and chemical behavior of an element and general ways of how it will interact with other elements. For example,

the periodic table is divided roughly into metals and non-metals. Metals tend to donate their electrons to other elements; nonmetals tend to accept electrons. There are currently about 109 elements in the periodic table, but the dental materials we use every day are comprised of only about 40 or so of these. Common examples in dental materials are oxygen (O), palladium (Pd), tin (Sn), titanium (Ti), aluminum (Al), silicon (Si), carbon (C), copper (Cu), and gold (Au).

Bonds between Atoms

Atoms form various types of bonds with one another, and it is these bonds that, in large part, determine the physical and chemical properties of dental materials. It is the electrons of atoms and the configurations of atomic electron clouds that govern bonding between atoms. The electrons of the elements interact in several basic ways (Figure 0-3). In this introductory discussion, we will only touch upon the most basic types of bonds.

> **! ALERT**
>
> It is the electrons of atoms and the configurations of atomic electron clouds that govern bonding between atoms and ultimately the clinical behavior of restorative dental materials.

Ionic bonds are formed when an electron from one element is given completely to another in return for forming the bond (Figure 0-3, *upper diagram*). In dental materials, ionic bonds are often formed between electron-donating elements and oxygen. Ionic bonds are common in dental ceramics and are among the strongest type of bond. Ionic bonds also are very directional, tolerating little movement of the atoms that they bind. One unique aspect of an ionic bond is that it leaves the

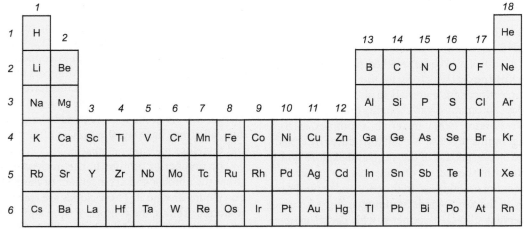

FIG 0-2 The periodic table of the elements is the tabulation of all elements in the known universe, currently numbering about 109 (not all are shown here). The rows of the table (called periods) determine the nature of the electron configuration of the elements; complex rules dictate the number of elements in each row or period. Each element has a two-letter symbol. For example, gold is "Au." The position of an element in the table is predictive of its electron configuration and its bonding, chemical behavior, and clinical properties. For example, metallic elements (those that tend to release some of their electrons) are generally situated toward the left of the table, whereas nonmetallic elements (those that tend to accept electrons) are toward the right. At the extreme right (column 18) sits the inert elements helium (He) through radon (Rn). These gases do not either release or accept electrons and are often referred to as the inert gases. Restorative dental materials are comprised of about 40 or so of elements, both metals and nonmetals.

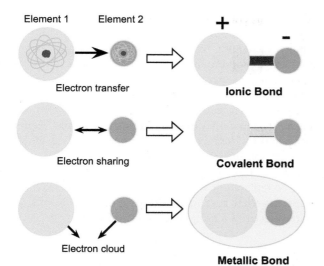

FIG 0-3 Bonding between elements (atoms) is determined largely by the number and configuration of the electrons of the elements involved. If one element transfers an electron to another *(upper diagram)*, an ionic bond is formed and the donating element assumes a positive charge, with the recipient element becoming negatively charged. If the elements share electrons *(middle diagram)*, a covalent bond is formed with no net transfer of charge. If elements (two or more) donate electrons to an electron cloud *(lower diagram)*, a metallic bond is formed, with the electrons associated with the elements but belonging to neither. The types of bonds formed between atoms are a major determinant of the properties of different restorative dental materials.

donor of the electron positively charged and in a state we call "oxidized." The recipient of the electron becomes negatively charged and is said to be reduced. Furthermore, an atom can form multiple ionic bonds with other atoms; this allows the formation of arrays of atoms (see next sections).

Covalent bonds form when atoms share electrons to form a bond (Figure 0-3, *middle diagram*). Direct esthetic materials (Chapter 4) are in part the product of these types of bonds. Similar to ionic bonds, covalent bonds are relatively strong and directional; also atoms may form multiple covalent bonds with other atoms, similar to the atoms forming ionic bonds. But the palette of elements that form covalent bonds is much broader than that which forms ionic bonds. In addition, atoms linked by covalent bonds do not exchange or disrupt charge. Covalent bonds occur in a variety of subtypes not known with ionic bonds. It is these subtypes that give covalently bonded atoms a great diversity in properties, but the reader is referred to an organic chemistry text for more detail.

Metallic bonds result when electrons are shared among many atoms (Figure 0-3, *lower diagram*). In the metallic bond, all of the atoms of the material donate electrons to form a "community" electron cloud. The cloud provides a strong bond among the atoms, but unlike covalent and ionic bonds, metallic bonds are not as directional and the electrons in the cloud do not "belong" to any one atom in material. This attribute gives the material unique properties, which will be discussed in the next section.

There are a number of other types of bonds between atoms, but their discussion is beyond the scope of this introduction. Thus, the three most important and strongest bonds between atoms are ionic, covalent, and metallic bonds. It is important to understand that it is primarily the type and number of bonds among the atoms of a material that give it the properties we know and use for our clinical treatment. We will discuss this idea more in the next section.

> **! ALERT**
>
> The type of bonding among atoms in restorative dental materials largely determines their physical, chemical, and clinical properties.

Molecules and Crystals

Atoms bond together into various larger-scale units. It is these larger units that make up dental materials. Two of the most basic and important larger-scale atomic arrangements are molecules and crystals.

Molecules are formed when several different elements bond together into a discrete unit, usually via covalent bonds (Figure 0-4). Molecules may contain only two atoms or many thousands, but they are a defined entity with definite spatial boundaries and a specific inventory of atoms (number and type) in each molecule. Therefore, we say that every molecule has a discrete, definable **molecular weight**, which is the sum of the mass of its component atoms. Molecules have other

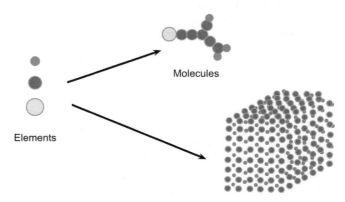

FIG 0-4 Elements are arranged in fundamentally different ways that have profound effects on the properties of restorative dental materials. Elements may combine into discrete units called molecules; each molecule may contain from only two to over 100,000 atoms and one to a dozen types of elements. Molecules have a defined mass (the molecular weight) and a defined three-dimensional structure, and are generally bonded through covalent bonding. On the other hand, elements may combine to form crystalline lattices, which are vast repeating arrays of elements bonded to one another. Crystals generally contain fewer types of elements than molecules and have no defined boundaries or mass. The atoms in a crystal are generally bonded by ionic or metallic bonds and each element is generally bonded to several others around it.

unique properties that result from a specific three-dimensional structure and the nature of the covalent bonds between the elements. Molecules generally have no net charge. Dental composite resins are comprised partly of long molecular chains called polymers (see next section).

Crystals are vast repeating arrays of bonded elements (Figure 0-4). Generally, the arrays of atoms in a crystal involve fewer types of elements than in a molecule, but extend in all directions with a repeated pattern called a unit cell. Unlike molecules, crystalline arrays have no definitive spatial boundaries; the unit cell represents the repeating unit, not a discrete atomic structure. Thus, unlike molecules, crystals have no definable mass or "molecular weight".

Metallic bonds and ionic bonds are most common in crystalline arrays. There are a number of specific types of crystals, each involving differences in angles and lengths of bonds among the components of the crystal; however, a more specific definition is beyond the scope of this book. In dental materials, ceramics and alloys (discussed in the next section) commonly form crystals rather than molecules. Additionally, molecules often arrange themselves into crystalline arrays; in this latter case, the molecule itself is the unit cell of the crystalline array.

BASIC TYPES OF DENTAL MATERIALS

Through covalent, metallic, or ionic bonding into either molecules or crystalline arrays, elements in the periodic table form the materials we use in restorative dentistry. There are three major classes of materials that result from these combinations of elements: alloys, ceramics, and polymers (Figure 0-5). Composite materials result when at least two of these three classes occur together in a material. We will discuss each of these in more detail.

Metals and Alloys

Metals are comprised of elements that donate their electrons toward formation of metallic bonds (Figure 0-5). The metal atoms (e.g., copper) form a repeating crystalline array, held together by these metallic bonds. The metallic bonds and resulting electron cloud are in large part responsible for the properties we associate with metals such as ductility, strength, shininess, and conduction of heat or electricity. If the element in a metal has a high number in the periodic table (see Figure 0-2, large atomic number), then the metal will be dense and heavy, as with gold (atomic #79) for example. If the atomic number is lower, then the metal will be lighter and less dense, as with aluminum (atomic #13). One rather unique consequence of the metallic bond is the relative freedom that the atoms in the array have for movement. Because the electrons in the cloud do not belong to any particular atom in the array, movement of the atoms does not disrupt the integrity of the material. This freedom translates to the malleability and ductility of metals to which we are accustomed in everyday life. On the other hand, the tendency of the electron cloud to scatter light makes metals opaque.

When different elements bond together in the same metallic array, we refer to the material as an alloy. Alloys may be simple, containing only two elements in the array, or complex, containing over a dozen elements. The crystalline arrays may be simple or complex, forming various types of crystal unit cells that are beyond the scope of the discussion here. Alloys are prevalent in dental restorative materials (Figure 0-5) and are discussed in more detail in Chapters 5, 11, 12, and 15. Dental materials rely on the strength, ductility, conductivity, and hardness of metals and alloys to serve successfully in the oral cavity, particularly when missing teeth must be replaced. It is instructive to remember that all these properties relate back to the nature of the metallic bonds and shared electrons among the atoms in the alloy.

Ceramics

Ceramics are a second major class of dental restorative material (Figure 0-5). Ceramics are collections of metallic elements, such as aluminum, and nonmetallic elements such as oxygen, held together by ionic bonds in crystalline arrays. The strong directional nature of the ionic bonds gives ceramics their strength, brittleness, rigidness, and relatively high melting temperatures. The lack of electron mobility in the ionic bonds gives ceramics their insulating properties. The repeating nature of the unit cell within the crystal allows visible light to be refracted predictably, giving ceramics their optical properties such as transparency or translucency. Similar to alloys, ceramics may be relatively simple, combining one metallic element with oxygen, or may be exceptionally complex, containing several different metallic elements and other nonmetals in addition to oxygen. Also similar to alloys, ceramic crystalline arrays can take on a variety of geometries and unit cells that are beyond the scope of this discussion.

Ceramics play major roles in the restoration of teeth. The optical properties of ceramics are especially useful for mimicking lost tooth structure; thus, ceramics are important to the esthetic aspects of dental restorations (see Chapter 14). However, the strength and hardness of ceramics allows them to play more subtle, if equally important, roles. Ceramics are used to abrade other materials (see Chapter 6), as containers for molten materials during casting or soldering (see Chapter 12), and as fillers to add strength to dental composites (see Chapter 4) and prosthodontic polymers (see Chapter 13). Ceramics play many other roles in dentistry (see Chapters 7 and 9) and are probably the most rapidly growing type of material used for dental restorations.

As with alloys, it is instructive to remember that the nature of the ionic bond between atoms is the fundamental basis for how ceramics behave and the way they are used in restorative dentistry.

> **! ALERT**
>
> Polymers are the most diverse class of restorative dental materials.

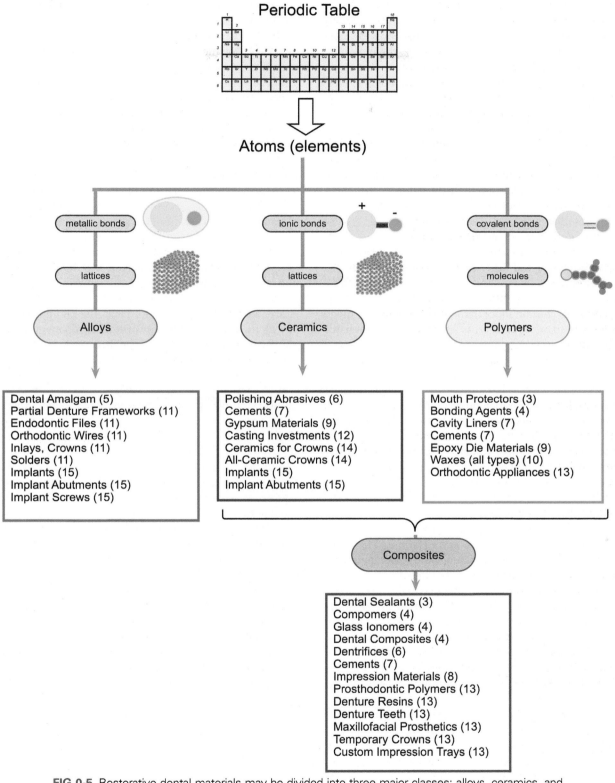

FIG 0-5 Restorative dental materials may be divided into three major classes: alloys, ceramics, and polymers. Elements in alloys are bonded by metallic bonds into crystalline lattices, and these comprise all the metallic materials of restorative dentistry. In ceramics, ionic bonds form between metallic and nonmetallic elements into lattices; this arrangement is used by a wide variety of dental restorative materials. Polymers are organized into molecules via covalent bonds; molecules interact with each other to produce the diverse properties we see in common polymer restorative materials. Combinations of ceramics and polymers, called composite materials, are among the most familiar of dental restorative materials. The chapter reference to each material is shown parenthetically after the material.

Polymers

Polymers are a third major type of material found in restorative dentistry (Figure 0-5). Polymers are the most diverse class of material because their unit structure is the molecule rather than the crystal. The rich variety of molecules that form via various types of covalent bonds and many possible elements create this diversity. In many polymers, each molecule may have thousands of component atoms, typically with repeating units within them; a molecular weight of a polymer molecule may commonly exceed 100,000. Yet each molecule is discrete, and it is the interactions between polymer molecules that give polymers many of the properties we know: flexibility, moldability, and elastomeric (rubber-like) properties. The ability of the long polymer chains to slide along one another or entangle in each other on an atomic scale translates into the properties we see on a local scale.

Yet, polymer molecules may also be tied together with other small polymers and other types of covalent bonds. In these "crosslinked" polymers, the properties are quite different: more rigid, less moldable, and much harder. Still other types of polymers contain more than one type of parent molecule or more than one type of cross linker. It is thus not hard to understand why this class of materials is so diverse. In spite of the variety of materials that are possible, all stem from the basic covalent bond between atoms and its strength and directionality.

In restorative dental materials, polymers are commonplace. They find use as preventative materials (see Chapter 3), in cements (see Chapter 7), as impression materials (see Chapter 8), and as waxes (see Chapter 10). Polymers also are the basis for many removable prosthodontic restorations such as dentures (see Chapter 13).

Composite Materials

In addition to the diversity of materials possible among alloys, ceramics, and polymers, still more variety is possible when these classes of materials are combined. Composite materials result when classes of materials are mixed together. The most common examples in restorative dentistry are the direct esthetic materials (see Chapter 4) and prosthodontic polymers (see Chapter 13). We will discuss the former briefly here as an example.

In direct esthetic materials, polymers are combined with ceramics. Polymers are used for what is called the matrix of the material, providing the framework and holding the basic material form. In dentistry, these polymers are chemically formed in place ("in situ") in the tooth in a matter of seconds! The polymers also are able to bond to the enamel and dentin of the tooth. However, the polymers are not strong or hard enough to resist oral physical and chemical forces over time, and they lack appropriate esthetic properties. For this reason, ceramic particles are added to the polymer matrix, forming the composite material. Ceramics add hardness, and they define the color and optical properties of the material. Ceramic particles also limit the shrinkage of the polymer during its formation in situ. Although stronger and harder, the ceramic particles could not be used by themselves; they need the polymer to bind them together, and they cannot bond to the tooth structure by themselves. Furthermore, the ceramics could not be placed in situ because they require high temperatures to fuse them together. Thus, the composite material brings the positive attributes of each component material to the overall material. This "material synergy" is common among successful composites in restorative dentistry.

↻ QUICK REVIEW

It is truly remarkable how atoms can bond together in relatively few ways to form the diverse world of restorative dental materials. The consequences of how the electrons of each atom interact with others are far reaching. Through relatively few simple types of reactions among atoms, matter combines at an atomic level to give us a diverse palette of restorative materials that we often take for granted in the daily practice of dentistry. In this book, we will explore the nuances of that palette and the appropriate use and manipulation to achieve the best clinical outcomes. Yet, as we explore, it is always instructive to remind ourselves of what our materials are at the most fundamental level—simply a collection of bonded atoms.

💡 SELF-TEST QUESTIONS

Test your knowledge by answering the following questions. For multiple-choice questions, one or more responses may be correct.

1. If a material is formed from a specific number and ratio of atoms, it forms what type of structure?
   a. Crystal
   b. Lattice
   c. Crystalline lattice
   d. Metallic lattice
   e. Molecule
2. Ionic bonds involve a transfer of charge.
   a. True
   b. False
3. Polymers are generally formed by atoms that combine via:
   a. Ionic bonds
   b. Covalent bonds
   c. Metallic bonds
   d. All these types of bonds
4. Which structure does not have a charge?
   a. Proton
   b. Neutron
   c. Electron
5. Crystals have a molecular weight.
   a. True
   b. False

6. The number of protons and electrons in a native element are equal.
   a. True
   b. False
7. The periodic table of the elements contains all known elements in the universe.
   a. True
   b. False
8. Alloys do not have which structural attribute?
   a. Comprised of metallic elements
   b. Bonded by covalent bonds
   c. Form a crystalline lattice
   d. Are generally malleable and ductile
9. Ceramics do not have which attribute(s)?
   a. Comprised of metals and nonmetals
   b. Generally are brittle
   c. Bonded by ionic bonds
   d. Are generally opaque
   e. Form large molecules
10. Composites in restorative dentistry are comprised of:
    a. Ceramics and polymers
    b. Polymers and metals
    c. Metals and ceramics

evolve Please visit *http://evolve.elsevier.com/Powers/dentalmaterials* for additional practice and study support tools.

CONTENTS

Introduction to Restorative Dental Materials

OBJECTIVES

After reading this chapter, the student should be able to:

1. Explain why restorative materials are used in dentistry and why they are important to the patient's total health.
2. Describe the major diseases that lead to tooth damage and how materials may help restore or prevent this damage.
3. Explain the differences between intracoronal and extracoronal restorations, which oral diseases create a need for each, and which restorative materials are used for each.
4. Describe the process of endodontic treatment, when it is needed, and what materials are used for this treatment.
5. Explain which restorative materials and types of restorations are commonly used to restore the function of missing teeth and the advantages and disadvantages of each type of restoration.
6. Describe the role of restorative materials in the prevention of oral disease and trauma.

Restorative dental materials are used to prevent or repair damage to teeth caused by oral disease or trauma. The restoration of damage caused by oral disease is critical to the well-being of every individual. Tooth damage, loss, or dysfunction contribute to malnutrition, speech disorders, and deterioration of the temporomandibular joint or alveolar bone, and may inflict significant pain. Furthermore, the teeth dominate an individual's facial appearance, and missing or damaged teeth often compromise social well-being and self-esteem. Emerging data support links between oral health and systemic diseases such as heart disease, diabetes, arthritis, and abnormal pregnancy. Restorative dental materials are among the tools used by the dental team to prevent disease and alleviate pain, inflammation, and infection caused by disease, thereby improving the patient's total health. The dental auxiliary plays an important role in the delivery of care to repair damage to teeth from oral disease and trauma.

> **! ALERT**
>
> Damage to teeth may occur from infectious disease, trauma, systemic disease, or congenital disease. The dental auxiliary plays an important role in the delivery of care to repair damaged teeth with restorative dental materials.

DENTAL DISEASE AND RESTORATIVE MATERIALS

Caries

In spite of tremendous strides in its prevention, caries remains a major global problem in all countries and leads to significant destruction of teeth, pain, systemic infection, and tooth loss (Figure 1-1).

> **! ALERT**
>
> Caries remains a problem in all countries, particularly in children. The health costs of tooth damage from caries are staggering.

Caries is caused by a bacterial biofilm commonly called plaque, which accumulates on teeth in areas where patients do not remove it (see Figure 1-1). A complex community of bacteria in the biofilm adheres to teeth and secretes acids and enzymes that dissolve the enamel, dentin, and cementum. Carious lesions occur on any tooth surface but are most common in areas where plaque accumulates unchecked—in the pits and fissures, along the gingiva, and interproximally. Caries also is a significant problem on the roots of the teeth of older individuals, where it rapidly destroys the softer cementum and dentin. As caries progresses over a period of months, more and more of the coronal tooth is destroyed, and the bacteria infect the pulp of the tooth and ultimately the periapical tissues as well. If left unchecked, an infection caused by caries can be fatal, but extraction of the tooth is a far more common outcome today. Dental restorative materials are used at every stage of the caries disease process to prevent or repair damage (discussed later).

Periodontal Disease

Unlike caries, periodontal disease affects the tissues supporting the teeth, including the gingiva, periodontal ligament, cementum, and alveolar bone (Figure 1-2). Periodontal disease also is caused by a bacterial biofilm, although the strains of bacteria in the biofilm are different from those that cause caries, and the progression of the disease occurs over many years rather than months. Initially, toxins secreted by bacteria inflame the gingiva (gingivitis), but the hard tissues

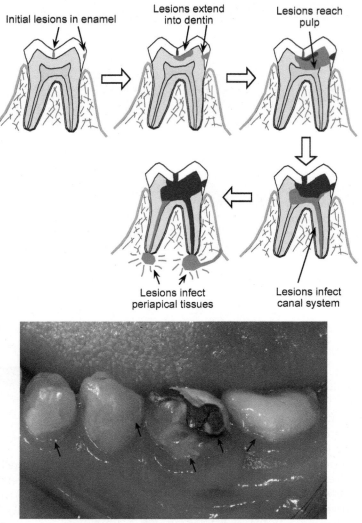

FIG 1-1 Caries is a nearly ubiquitous bacterial infection that destroys tooth structure *(arrows in photo)*. Caries occurs on any tooth surface but is common in the occlusal fissures or on proximal surfaces. Initially, the infection is restricted to the enamel, but over weeks to months, the infection spreads into the softer dentin. Once in the dentin, the infection and destruction spread laterally and deeper until the pulpal tissues are infected. At this point, the patient typically experiences some sort of sensitivity or pain. If untreated, the infection will spread through the tooth canal system and finally involve the periapical tissues. In some cases, the infection drains through the alveolar bone to the buccal or lingual. Once in the periapical tissues, the infection may spread throughout the face, usually accompanied by extreme pain, swelling, malaise, and fever. Unchecked, the infection may even cause death. Dental restorative materials are used to prevent or treat all dimensions of the damage caused by caries. (Photo courtesy Y-W Chen, University of Washington Department of Restorative Dentistry, Seattle, WA.)

(cementum or bone) are not involved. Over time, the chronic inflammation induced by the bacteria causes irreversible destruction of the alveolar bone, periodontal ligament, and cementum (periodontitis). Destruction of these tissues results in deep pockets around the teeth that harbor biofilms with even more damaging species of bacteria that grow in an anaerobic (low or no oxygen) environment. As the supporting tissues are lost, the tooth becomes mobile, and root surfaces and furcations become exposed. Exposed root dentin is often sensitive (dentin hypersensitivity) to cold, toothbrushing, or sweets, leading to even poorer cleaning. Ultimately, the support for the tooth becomes so compromised that the tooth is lost.

Periodontal disease increases the risk of caries or pulpal infection by giving cariogenic bacteria access to the tooth root or the periapical structures. Restorative dental materials are used to limit tooth mobility or replace function of lost teeth by distributing occlusal forces to healthier remaining teeth. Materials also are used to reduce sensitivity associated with exposed root surfaces.

Trauma, Systemic Disease, and Genetic Disorders

Trauma may cause diverse and significant damage to teeth and other oral structures, and restorative dental materials play

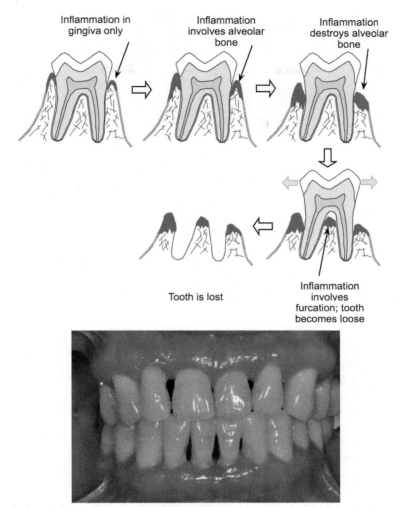

FIG 1-2 Periodontal disease is a chronic bacterial infection of the bone and soft tissues that retain the tooth (the periodontium). Bacterial biofilms adhere to teeth near the gingival tissues. Bacterial toxins cause inflammation of the periodontal tissues, initially involving only the gingiva (gingivitis). With time, the infection and associated inflammation involve the crestal alveolar bone (periodontitis). Without treatment, the infection causes loss of alveolar bone that eventually involves the furcae and increases tooth mobility *(orange block arrows)*. At this point, the risk of tooth loss is high. Unlike caries, periodontal disease is nearly always painless, although some patients experience dentin sensitivity from exposure of the root surfaces *(photo)*. These exposed surfaces sometimes require restorative procedures to mitigate pain. Advanced periodontal disease increases the risk of root caries and pulpal infection, and it is thought to contribute to systemic inflammation, for example, in the endothelial lining of arteries. Other systemic diseases such as diabetes increase the risks of periodontal disease through high glucose levels in local tissues that trigger oxidative stress. A variety of restorative materials and strategies are used to replace teeth lost to periodontal disease. (Photo courtesy Kanako Nagatomo, private practice, Seattle, WA.)

a major role in repairing trauma-induced damage. Trauma may fracture only the enamel or dentin or may cause a fracture of the tooth that involves the pulp or alveolar bone. Teeth may be completely lost (avulsion) or displaced in any direction. Restorative materials are used to repair teeth, stabilize them until the supporting tissues heal, or replace them.

Systemic disease sometimes destroys teeth and oral tissues, and restorative materials are used to repair this damage. Cancer of the head and neck region may require that a large segment of the maxilla or mandible or associated oral structures be removed for the patient to survive. Dental prostheses restore function or esthetics for these unfortunate patients.

Osteoporosis compromises the bony support for teeth, leading to edentulism and the need for major oral restoration. Diabetes accelerates and exacerbates periodontal disease. In older individuals, systemic disease often amplifies oral disease. For example, many older individuals experience decreased salivary production, which limits the body's oral immune response and promotes both caries and periodontal disease. Fluorosis, resulting from natural or iatrogenic excess ingestion of fluoride when the teeth are forming, disfigures and discolors tooth enamel and requires esthetic treatments or restoration. Gastric reflux of acids may lead to destruction of teeth by dissolving enamel.

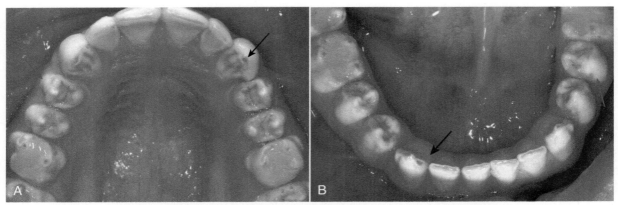

FIG 1-3 A patient with the genetic condition of amelogenesis imperfecta. In this condition, teeth in both upper **(A)** and lower **(B)** arches are affected by a genetic mutation in the genes that synthesize tooth enamel. The enamel in affected teeth is relatively soft and has numerous malformations, including a mottled, chalky appearance *(blue arrows)* on some surfaces. Premature wear *(black arrows)* occurs, exposing the dentin below. Restorative materials play a substantial role in short-term and long-term treatments of patients like this as nearly every tooth will need reconstruction. (Courtesy Y-W Chen, University of Washington Department of Restorative Dentistry, Seattle, WA.)

Genetic disorders are another significant cause of oral disease that requires the use of restorative dental materials. In several genetic diseases, teeth may be congenitally missing. Other diseases, such as amelogenesis imperfecta (Figure 1-3) or dentinogenesis imperfecta, cause major loss of tooth structure from defective enamel, dentin, or the bonds between enamel and dentin. In these patients, nearly every tooth will require restoration.

RESTORATION OF DAMAGED TEETH

Regardless of the source of damage, teeth are repaired using two basic types of restorations: intracoronal and extracoronal (Figure 1-4). If the damage to the tooth involves the pulpal or periapical tissues, then endodontic restorative treatments are used in addition to these restorations.

Intracoronal Restorations

Intracoronal restorations are used to repair damage that is restricted to the internal parts of the tooth (see Figure 1-4). Damage of this nature is nearly always caused by caries but is occasionally caused by trauma. For intracoronal restorations, the tooth is first surgically prepared to receive the restoration, a process commonly referred to as cavity preparation (Figure 1-5). Cavity preparation removes diseased or damaged tissue and creates a space that is accessible for restoration and able to stably retain the restoration. Many complex factors govern the surgical cavity preparation, although a thorough discussion of the "principles of cavity preparation" is beyond the scope of this text. Cavity preparations may be restored (Figure 1-6) with materials such as resin composites (Chapter 4), amalgam (Chapter 5), cast alloys (Chapters 11 and 12), ceramics (Chapter 14), or less often by gold foil (Chapter 11).

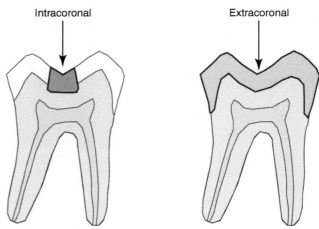

FIG 1-4 Restorations to repair tooth damage are classified into two broad categories, each requiring different types of materials and different surgical strategies. Intracoronal restorations *(left)* are retained within the body of the tooth primarily by the remaining tooth structure. Extracoronal restorations *(right)* are retained by friction with at least part of the restoration made to fit around the exterior of the tooth. Extracoronal restorations are used when the destruction or loss of tooth structure is extensive. These two categories are not entirely mutually exclusive.

Extracoronal Restorations

> **! ALERT**
>
> Extracoronal restorations are used to restore teeth with more extensive damage that cannot be managed with intracoronal restorations.

If damage to a tooth is extensive, then intracoronal restorations are not feasible and extracoronal restorations will be necessary to restore the teeth (see Figure 1-4). Extracoronal surgical tooth preparations are much more aggressive (less conservative) than intracoronal preparations (see Figure 1-5) and nearly always must be restored using restorations that are fabricated indirectly (away from the patient). Crowns, onlays, and veneers (Figure 1-7) are examples of extracoronal restorations.

Extracoronal restorations typically require that a model or die of the surgically prepared tooth be made; the die must be extremely accurate in its size, reproduction of detail, and relationship to adjacent and opposing teeth. Fabrication of dies involves making impressions (Chapter 8) and pouring the impressions with a model or die material (Chapter 9). More recently, models of the tooth can be digitally acquired. Fabricating the restoration on the die may involve waxes (Chapter 10), casting alloys (Chapters 11 and 12), polymers (Chapters 4 and 13), ceramics (Chapter 14), or some combination of these materials. Computer-aided machining (CAM) techniques may be used to fabricate indirect or direct restorations. In all cases, the design of the preparation and restoration will depend on the ability of the restorative material to withstand oral forces in service (Chapter 2).

Endodontic Treatment

> **! ALERT**
>
> Endodontic treatment is necessary if oral disease or trauma involves the pulp of the tooth. The pulpal tissues are removed, and the resulting space is cleaned and sealed with restorative materials.

When the pulpal tissue is infected and destroyed by caries, periodontal disease, or trauma, then endodontic therapy must be initiated, and the restoration of the tooth becomes more complex (Figure 1-8). The first step is to remove the infected pulpal tissue and associated root dentin. The space created when the pulpal tissues are removed must be replaced with sealers that prevent ingress of bacteria. Restoration of the coronal portion of the tooth often requires extracoronal restorations but may use intracoronal restorations in anterior teeth. Depending on the amount of tooth structure lost to the disease or trauma, a post and buildup may be placed in the root canal to strengthen the tooth and aid in fabrication of the final restoration. The physical properties of these materials, their interactions with each other, and their interactions with tooth structure are critically important to the longevity of the restoration.

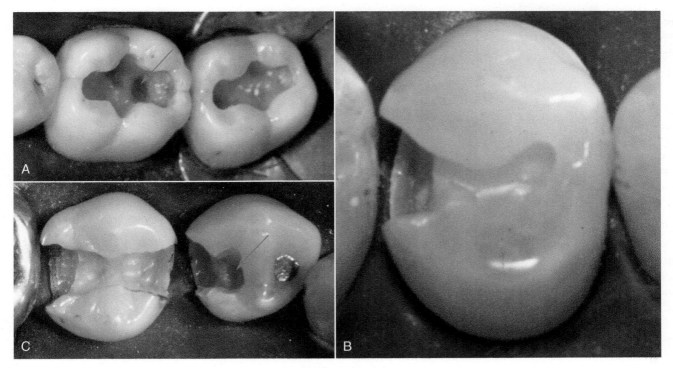

Intracoronal preparations

FIG 1-5 When the tooth is surgically modified to eliminate the destruction inflicted by caries *(red arrows)*, systemic disease, or trauma, the extent of the damage determines the type of restorative strategy and the material used. If the damage is restricted to the internal parts of the tooth **(A–C)**, surgical preparation modifies the tooth for an intracoronal restoration, and the remaining external tooth structure retains the restoration.

(Continued)

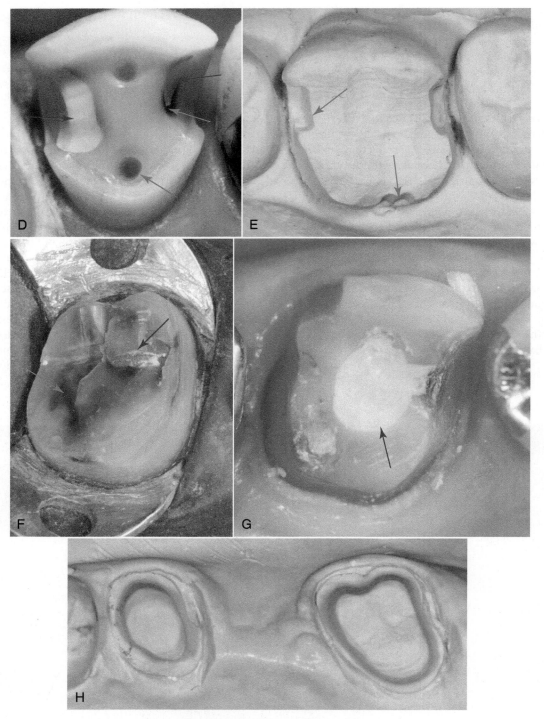

Extracoronal preparations

FIG 1-5, CONT'D With more extensive damage, the external surfaces of the tooth must be included in the surgical preparation **(D–H).** Materials to protect or restore the deepest areas (bases and liners, *blue arrows*) are often used with these more extensive preparations. Pinholes or slots are sometimes used *(green arrows)* to retain extracoronal restorations. If the restoration replaces a missing tooth **(H),** the extracoronal preparations must be designed so that the restoration can fit the retaining teeth (abutments) simultaneously. (**A, C–G,** Courtesy Richard D. Tucker, University of Washington Department of Restorative Dentistry, Seattle, WA. **B,** Courtesy J. Martin Anderson, University of Washington Department of Restorative Dentistry, Seattle, WA. **H,** Courtesy E. R. Schwedhelm, University of Washington Department of Restorative Dentistry, Seattle, WA.)

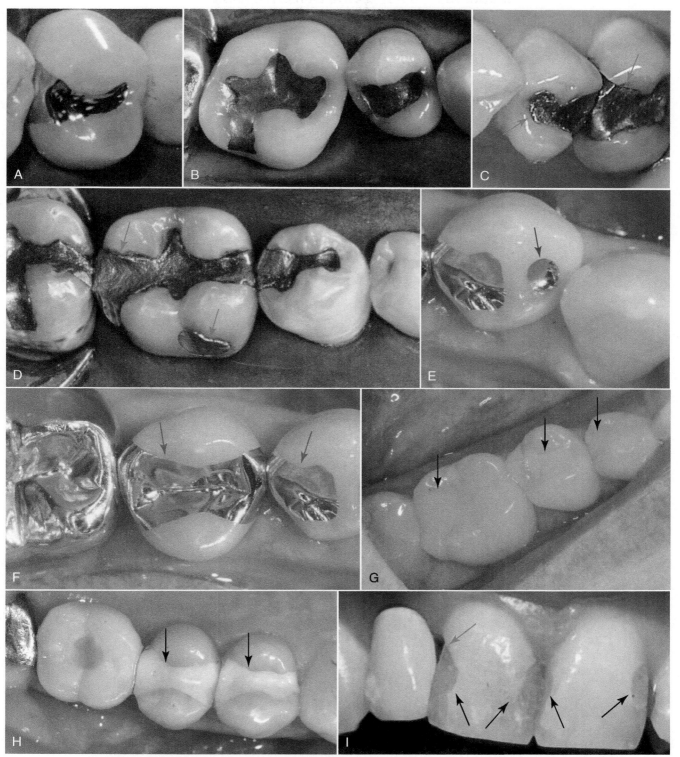

FIG 1-6 Intracoronal restorations are generally used to repair the internal structure of teeth but may involve some of the external surfaces as well **(A–I).** Today, intracoronal restorations are generally (but not always) fabricated directly, customized to fit the patient's teeth *in situ.* Several types of restorative materials are used for intracoronal restorations including amalgam **(A–D),** gold foil **(E,** *blue arrow*), cast gold **(F,** *green arrows*), and composite **(G–I,** *black arrows*). Each type of material has a different service life. For example, amalgam margins (where the restoration meets the tooth structure) are initially very good **(A, B)** but deteriorate over time, usually many years **(C, D,** *red arrows*). Gold foil and ceramics are the longest lasting of restorative materials, whereas composites and glass ionomers have shorter service lives **(I,** *red arrow*). (**A,** Courtesy J. Martin Anderson, University of Washington Department of Restorative Dentistry, Seattle, WA. **B–F,** Courtesy Richard D. Tucker, University of Washington Department of Restorative Dentistry, Seattle, WA. **G–I,** Courtesy of E. R. Schwedhelm, University of Washington Department of Restorative Dentistry, Seattle, WA.)

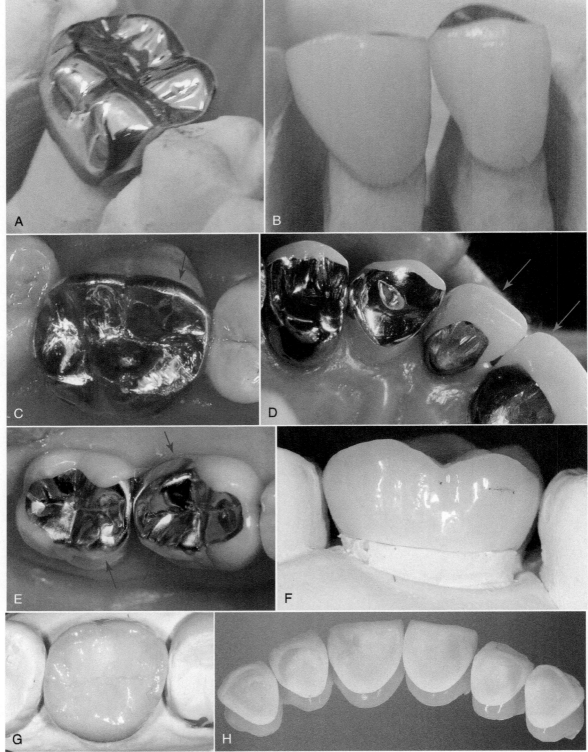

FIG 1-7 Extracoronal restorations involve at least some of the axial structure of the tooth; most extracoronal restorations are fabricated indirectly, away from the patient. A common form of extracoronal restoration in dentistry today is the crown **(A–D)**. The crown may be fabricated entirely from alloy **(A)** or may have an alloy substructure supporting a ceramic veneer **(B, D,** *ceramic shown by red arrows*). Other types of extracoronal restorations include three-quarter crowns **(C)** and onlays **(E)** in which one or more tooth cusps are restored *(blue arrows)*. Ceramics may also be used for crowns **(F, G)** or veneers **(H)**. (**C,** Courtesy Kevin Frazier, Georgia Regents University, Augusta, GA. **D, E,** Courtesy Richard D. Tucker, University of Washington Department of Restorative Dentistry, Seattle, WA. **F, G,** Courtesy E. R. Schwedhelm, University of Washington Department of Restorative Dentistry, Seattle, WA. **H,** Courtesy Kavita Shor, University of Washington Department of Restorative Dentistry, Seattle, WA.)

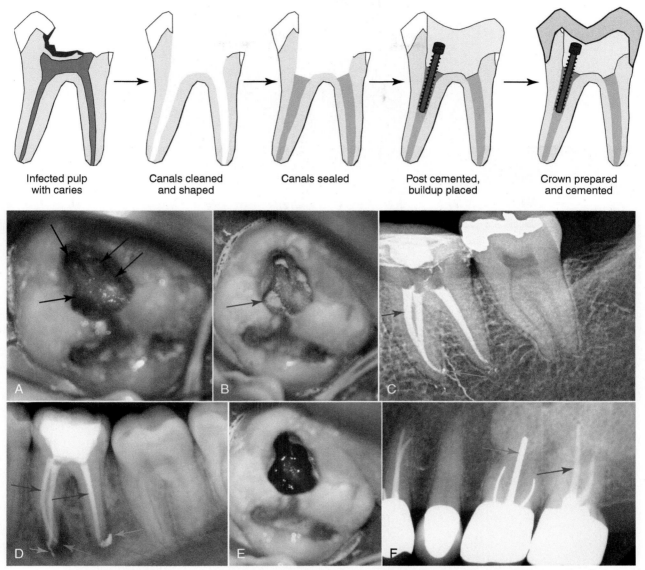

Infected pulp with caries → Canals cleaned and shaped → Canals sealed → Post cemented, buildup placed → Crown prepared and cemented

FIG 1-8 Restoration of a tooth with an infected pulp is complex and involves many restorative materials. Pulpal disease often involves the periapical tissues *(green arrows)*. The canals are identified *(black arrows)*, shaped, and cleaned using nickel–titanium files **(A)**. The shaped canals are then sealed with a natural or synthetic polymer **(B–D, F,** *blue arrows)*; on occasion, the sealing material is extruded beyond the root apex **(C, D,** *orange arrows)*. Once sealed, the canal openings are sealed using a resin composite **(E)**. A steel post may be cemented in place with a resin polymer *(red arrow)*, and the tooth is built back to full contour with amalgam or a resin composite. Finally, the tooth is surgically prepared for a crown, an impression is taken, a model made, and a crown fabricated of alloy or ceramic **(F)**. The crown is cemented with a glass ionomer or resin-based cement. (**A–F,** Courtesy Brandon Seto and James Johnson, University of Washington Department of Endodontics, Seattle, WA.)

REPLACEMENT OF LOST OR MISSING TEETH

In the event that trauma or disease has led to the loss of one or more teeth, restorative materials play a major role in replacing the function and esthetics of the missing teeth. The type of restoration depends on whether all the teeth are missing (called edentulism) or some teeth remain (partial edentulism).

Partial Tooth Loss (Partial Edentulism)

The function and esthetics of missing teeth may be restored using a fixed partial denture (also commonly known as a bridge, Figure 1-9). Classically, a bridge is prepared by placing extracoronal restorations (usually crowns) on the teeth adjacent to the edentulous space. These teeth are called abutment teeth, and the artificial replacement teeth are called pontics. Bridges

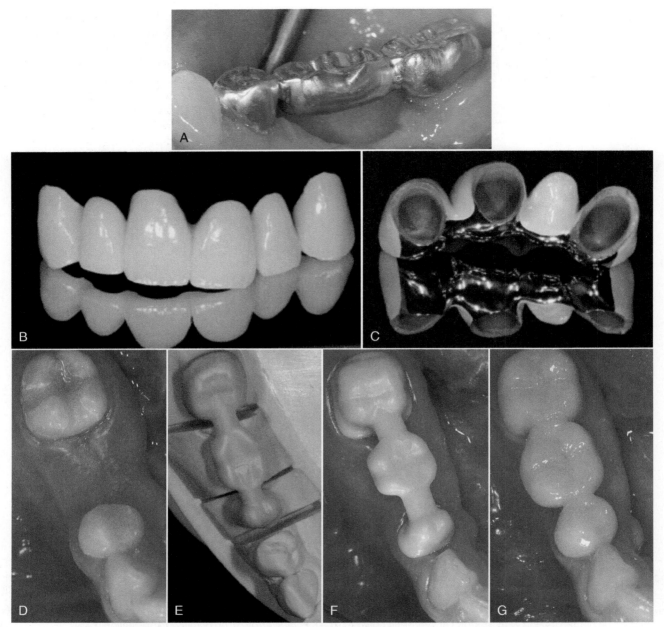

FIG 1-9 Bridges are used to replace missing teeth. A variety of materials may be used. Traditionally, bridges (more formally referred to as fixed partial dentures) were fabricated from casting alloys **(A)** or a combination of an alloy and ceramic **(B, C)**, in which the alloy serves as a substructure for strength. More recently, ceramics such as zirconia have been used to restore missing teeth **(D–G)**. In these all-ceramic bridges, a high-strength ceramic is used to form the substructure **(E, F)**, followed by a veneer of more esthetic ceramic to full contour and function **(G)**. The most contemporary of all-ceramic bridges are all zirconia (often referred to as "monolithic" zirconia restorations). (**A,** Courtesy E. R. Schwedhelm, University of Washington Department of Restorative Dentistry, Seattle, WA. **B, C,** Courtesy Y-W Chen, University of Washington Department of Restorative Dentistry, Seattle, WA. **D–G,** Courtesy Ariel Raigrodski, University of Washington Department of Restorative Dentistry, Seattle, WA. Laboratory work by Andreas Saltzer, MDT, Weinheim, Germany.)

are always made using indirect techniques and are fabricated from alloys, alloy–ceramic combinations, or ceramics alone (Chapters 11, 12, and 14). The placement of crowns on the abutment teeth requires substantial sacrifice of tooth structure regardless of the condition of the abutment tooth. Because of this, an alternative technique called a resin-bonded fixed partial denture (or Maryland bridge) is sometimes used if the abutment teeth are healthy and free of major restorations. The Maryland bridge does not require extracoronal crowns on the abutment teeth. "Arms" from the pontic are bonded to the enamel of the abutment teeth via a resin-based cement (Chapter 7). Retention of Maryland bridges is poorer than for traditional bridges, and these restorations cannot always be used because of inappropriate occlusion or positions of abutment teeth. Bridges may also be placed using implants as abutment teeth; in this case both abutments must be implants and the bridge is screwed or cemented to the abutments (Chapter 15).

> **! ALERT**
>
> Endosseous implants are increasingly used to manage the restoration of missing teeth and have reduced the need for bridges and partial dentures.

Endosseous dental implants are increasingly used to replace missing teeth (Chapter 15; Figure 1-10). Dental implants are fabricated from special titanium-based alloys or ceramics. Endosseous implants are placed into bone with special techniques to ensure integration with bone, and then indirect restorations are placed on the implants. Implants leave the adjacent teeth unrestored and are easier for the patient to clean than bridges or removable partial dentures. However, implants are expensive and involve significant surgery and treatment time. Furthermore, the bone quality may or may not be appropriate to support an implant.

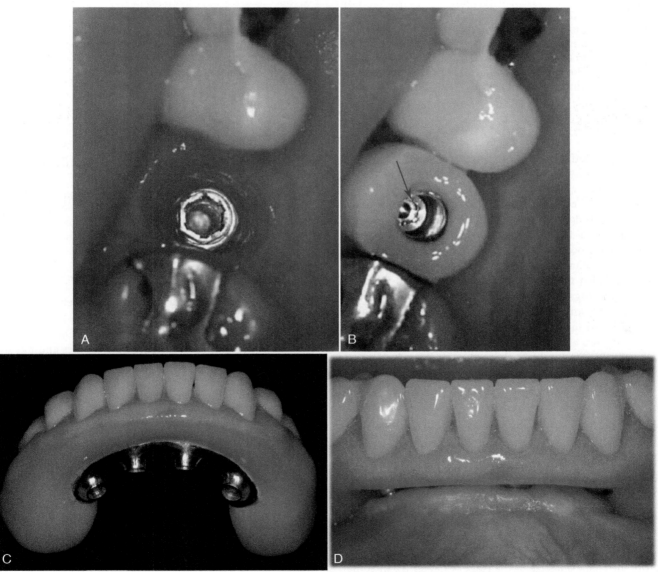

FIG 1-10 Endosseous implants are increasingly used to replace single or multiple missing teeth. In some cases, the implant is placed to the level of the bone **(A)** and an alloy–ceramic restoration shapes the gingiva and restores the missing space; a screw may be used to retain the restoration **(B,** *blue arrow)*. In other cases, multiple implants are used to restore an entire arch of missing teeth **(C).** The implants are placed to a level just above the tissue **(D),** and multiple screws retain the denture. (**A, B,** Courtesy Mats Kronström, University of Washington Department of Restorative Dentistry, Seattle, WA; **C, D,** Courtesy Y-W Chen, University of Washington Restorative Dentistry, Seattle, WA.)

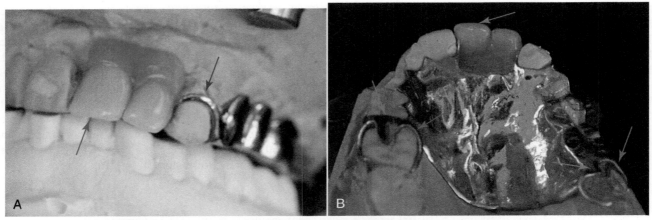

FIG 1-11 Removable partial dentures are prostheses designed to replace multiple missing teeth in the anterior or posterior areas of the mouth **(A, B)**. Teeth are made of acrylic *(green arrows)* or may be cast into the alloy framework. The appliance has rests *(red arrows)* that use the remaining teeth to absorb the forces placed on the missing teeth and clasps *(blue arrows)* to retain the appliance. The appliance should be removed for cleaning and to clean the remaining teeth. (Courtesy Richard Lee Sr., University of Washington Department of Restorative Dentistry, Seattle, WA.)

If multiple teeth are missing in multiple locations, then a removable partial denture may be indicated (Figure 1-11). Partial dentures are also common in situations in which there is no distal abutment tooth available to anchor a fixed bridge. Partial dentures use a framework of stiff alloy (Chapters 2 and 11) that rests on specific abutment teeth and distributes occlusal biting forces evenly and appropriately to the remaining teeth. Acrylic teeth (Chapter 13) are then bonded to the framework, which is held in place by clasps that engage the abutment teeth. Removable partial dentures are advantageous to the patient from the standpoint of cleaning and inspection of the remaining teeth, but they are generally less esthetic and less comfortable for the patient to wear than permanently fixed prostheses such as bridges or implants.

Loss of All Teeth (Edentulism)

Patients who have lost all teeth in an arch are described as edentulous for that arch. The edentulous patient will require a complete denture to restore function and fulfill esthetic needs. The complete denture is composed of an acrylic polymer base with acrylic denture teeth bonded into positions that are compatible with the patient's opposing arch or the denture of the opposing arch (Chapter 13; Figure 1-12). The base of the denture is constructed to provide maximum support from the edentulous ridge, and accurate impressions are critical to capture the shape and size of the ridge (Chapter 8). In some cases, the complete denture is supported (via screws and special abutments) by multiple dental implants (see Figure 1-10). This strategy is often very successful, particularly in the lower arch, but it requires meticulous cleaning by the patient and dental team and is much more expensive than a traditional complete denture.

PREVENTION OF DISEASE AND TRAUMA

> **! ALERT**
>
> Restorative materials play a role in both the repair of damage from disease and prevention of disease. Dental auxiliaries play increasingly important roles in delivery and management of preventative materials.

Fluoride gels, rinses, and varnishes are highly effective at preventing caries (Chapter 3). Fluorides also have been incorporated into direct esthetic filling materials (Chapter 4) and cements (Chapter 7). If teeth have deep fissures and pits that are at high risk for decay, sealants are highly effective at reducing the development of caries (Chapter 3; Figure 1-13). Sealants are tenaciously bonded to the tooth enamel via acid-etching procedures (Chapter 3). The dental team plays an active role in disease prevention by cleaning the teeth with various abrasives to remove calculus, stain, and plaque at regular intervals (Chapter 6). Restorations also may be polished to minimize plaque retention and corrosion, and other abrasives may be used to finish the edges (margins) of the restorations to help prevent the recurrence of caries. To prevent trauma, mouth protectors or night guards are often used (Chapters 2 and 3). Mouth protectors are made of polymers that absorb the energy of facial blows and prevent this energy from affecting the teeth and facial structures. Night guards (Figure 1-14) prevent premature wear from occlusal trauma, technically referred to as parafunction.

> **! ALERT**
>
> No branch of medicine has been as successful as dentistry in preventing disease.

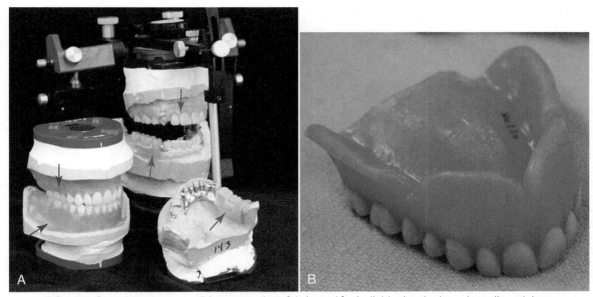

FIG 1-12 Complete dentures *(blue arrows)* are fabricated for individuals who have lost all teeth in an arch. Complete dentures are sometimes fabricated for both arches **(A,** *left*) or in combination with partial dentures **(A,** *green arrows*). A complete denture **(B)** is composed of an acrylic polymer that is used to support acrylic teeth. The tissue side of the denture often has the patient's name embedded for permanent identification. (Courtesy Richard Lee Sr., University of Washington Department of Restorative Dentistry, Seattle, WA.)

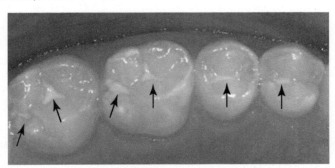

FIG 1-13 Sealants *(black arrows)* are polymers that are bonded to fissures and pits in teeth with the goals of sealing out bacterial infection and preventing caries. The sealants in this photograph are many years old and show some wear and loss of contour, yet still are protecting the major pits and grooves. (Courtesy E. R. Schwedhelm, University of Washington Department of Restorative Dentistry, Seattle, WA.)

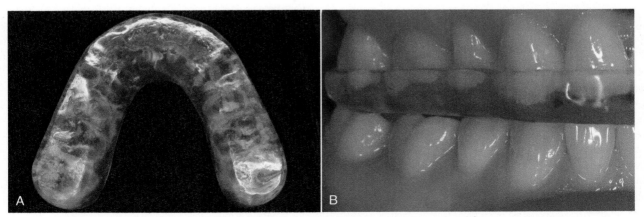

FIG 1-14 Night guard appliance to protect teeth from inappropriate occlusal forces or to prevent inappropriate occlusal contacts. Here the night guard, which is composed of an acrylic material **(A),** has been fabricated for the upper teeth. When in place **(B),** the material controls the forces that a patient can apply to any one tooth. The acrylic material can be constructed to distribute forces a number of ways and is soft enough that it wears rather than the teeth. (Courtesy Y-W Chen, University of Washington Department of Restorative Dentistry, Seattle, WA.)

❓ SELF-TEST QUESTIONS

Test your knowledge by answering the following questions. For multiple-choice questions, one or more responses may be correct.

1. A small lesion in an anterior tooth would most likely be restored with which of the following material(s)?
   a. Amalgam
   b. Resin composite
   c. Gold-based alloy
   d. Ceramic

2. A direct restorative material used to restore a small portion of an anterior tooth should have which of the following properties?
   a. Esthetics
   b. High strength
   c. Stiffness
   d. Ease of casting

3. An intracoronal restoration may be fabricated from which of the following material(s)?
   a. Amalgam
   b. Resin composite
   c. Gold-based alloy
   d. Ceramic

4. A direct restorative material used frequently to restore a portion of a posterior tooth that is subject to large biting forces would possess which of the following properties?
   a. Esthetics
   b. High strength
   c. Ease of casting
   d. Thermal insulation

5. A full crown on a maxillary anterior tooth may be restored with which of the following restorative materials?
   a. Ceramic
   b. Gold-based alloy
   c. Resin composite
   d. Ceramic–alloy combination

6. Which of the following sentences describes the construction of removable partial dentures?
   a. They are attached to natural teeth with cements.
   b. They are removable and attached to teeth with clasps.
   c. They have a framework that is composed of a stiff alloy.
   d. They have acrylic teeth bonded to an alloy framework.

7. Which of the following materials are most important for prevention of oral disease/trauma?
   a. Ceramics
   b. Resin-based sealants
   c. Fluoride-containing cements
   d. Energy-absorbing polymers

8. Complete denture bases are usually made from which of the following materials?
   a. Resin composites
   b. Gold-based alloys
   c. Acrylic resins
   d. Ceramic

9. Acrylic resins are used in which of the following types of restorations?
   a. Posterior intracoronal restorations
   b. Complete denture bases
   c. Pontics for fixed partial dentures
   d. Ceramic–alloy restorations

10. Which of the following materials are most commonly used for dental implants?
    a. Resin composite
    b. Ceramic
    c. Titanium-based alloys
    d. Acrylic

Use short answers to fill in the following blanks.

11. A posterior restoration that involves the occlusal surfaces, two proximal surfaces, and all cusps is called a(n) _____.

12. A restoration that covers the entire coronal portion of the tooth is called a(n) _____.

13. After a root canal procedure, the canal is frequently filled using _____.

14. A restoration that replaces a missing tooth that is supported by and cemented to two adjacent fully restored teeth is called _____.

15. A restoration in which artificial teeth are mounted on a metal framework containing clasps that attach it to remaining abutment teeth is called a(n) _____.

16. A restoration that replaces all the teeth in the upper or lower arch with artificial teeth that are attached to a plastic base is called a(n) _____.

17. A restoration that replaces the root of an extracted tooth and is stabilized by bone growth around it is called a(n) _____.

18. _____ materials are used to prevent damage to the teeth and oral bone from trauma.

evolve Please visit *http://evolve.elsevier.com/Powers/dentalmaterials* for additional practice and study support tools.

Properties of Materials

After reading this chapter, the student should be able to:

1. Define dimensional change and linear coefficient of thermal expansion, and give examples of their importance to clinical dentistry.
2. Give examples of where thermal and electrical properties of restorative materials are important in clinical dentistry.
3. List examples of where solubility and water sorption are important in the success of dental restorative materials.
4. Describe when wettability of tooth structure or dental materials is important clinically.
5. Define stress and strain, and illustrate how they differ.
6. Describe how elastic modulus, proportional limit and yield strength, ultimate strength, and elongation and compression are important in the selection of dental materials, as well as compare the elastic moduli of dentin, enamel, composites, bonding agents, and the hybrid layer of the tooth–composite interface.
7. Describe how resilience and toughness differ from strength properties.
8. Rank the hardness of dentin and enamel with respect to common dental restorative materials, and explain why caution is warranted in the comparison of Knoop and nano-hardness values.
9. Describe why for certain materials a strain–time curve is more informative than a stress–strain curve.

An understanding of the physical, electrical, and mechanical properties of materials used in dentistry is of tremendous importance. First, materials used to replace missing portions of teeth are exposed to attack by the oral environment and subjected to biting forces. Second, the restorative materials are cleansed and polished by various prophylactic procedures. As a result, their properties are the basis for the selection of materials to be used in particular dental procedures and restorations. Clinical experience and research have related clinical success to certain properties of materials, which have been used as guides in the improvement of dental materials. Third, the establishment of critical physical properties for various types of dental materials has led to the development of minimum standards or specifications. The American National Standards Institute (ANSI) and the American Dental Association (ADA), in conjunction with the International Organization for Standardization (ISO) and federal organizations, have established more than 100 standards or specifications for dental materials and maintain lists of materials that satisfy the minimum standards of quality. This information is available from the ADA office in Chicago or on its website (www.ada.org) and is helpful for selecting materials for dental practice and ensuring the quality control of materials.

This chapter emphasizes the dimensional change, electrical properties, solubility and sorption, and mechanical properties of dental materials. Selection of materials should be influenced by their effect on the oral tissues and by possible toxic effects if ingested. The color and optical qualities of materials also are important in the selection of restorative materials.

DIMENSIONAL CHANGE

> **! ALERT**
>
> *Dimensional change* is the percentage of shrinkage or expansion of a material.

Maintaining dimensions during dental procedures such as preparing impressions and models is important in the accuracy of dental restorations. Dimensional changes may occur during setting as a result of a chemical reaction, such as with elastomeric impression materials or resin composite restorative materials or from the cooling of wax patterns or gold restorations during fabrication. To compare materials easily, the dimensional change usually is expressed as a percentage of an original length or volume (see an example calculation in Appendix 2-1). Values for other elastomeric impression materials can be used to compare their accuracy.

Volumetric dimensional change is more difficult to measure and is not described here. The volumetric dimensional change is equal to three times the linear dimensional change for a specific material.

Thermal Dimensional Change

Restorative dental materials are subjected to temperature changes in the mouth. These changes result in dimensional changes in the materials and to the neighboring tooth structure. Because the thermal expansion of the restorative material usually does not match that of the tooth structure, a differential expansion occurs that may result in leakage of oral fluids between the restoration and the tooth.

The linear thermal expansion of materials can be measured by determination of the difference in length of a specimen at two temperatures (see an example calculation in Appendix 2-1). To make a comparison between materials easier, the linear thermal expansion is expressed as a coefficient of thermal expansion. Typical values for selected restorative dental materials and human teeth are listed in Table 2-1.

> **! ALERT**
>
> The linear thermal coefficient of expansion of a material is a measure of how much it expands per unit length if heated 1 degree higher.

The thermal coefficient of expansion is not uniform throughout the entire temperature range and is usually higher for liquids than for solids. The thermal coefficient of expansion for a solid, such as a dental wax, generally increases at some point as the temperature is increased. The linear rather than the volumetric coefficient of thermal expansion usually is reported.

The relationship between the coefficients of thermal expansion of human teeth and restorative materials is important, and Table 2-1 shows that the values for amalgam and composites are about three to five times those of human teeth. The values for unfilled polymers, however, are five to seven times those of teeth, with ceramic being ½ to ⅓ and gold alloys being approximately the same as for human teeth.

A clinical effect of this difference is as follows. If a tooth contained a poorly bonded composite restoration that was cooled by the drinking of a cold liquid, the restoration would contract more than the tooth, and small gaps would result at the junction between the two materials. Oral fluids can penetrate this space. When the temperature returns to normal, this fluid is forced out of the space. This phenomenon is called percolation and occurs with some restorative materials, depending on the relationship of the thermal coefficient of expansion of the material and human teeth and the extent of bonding. Percolation is thought to be undesirable because of the possible irritation to the dental pulp and recurrent decay. Dental amalgam is unusual in that percolation decreases with time after insertion, presumably as a result of the space being filled with corrosion products from the amalgam. If the aforementioned composite were bonded adequately to the tooth, the difference in thermal coefficient of expansion could result in stress at the interface, which could lead to failure of the bond over time.

THERMAL CONDUCTIVITY

> **! ALERT**
>
> Materials with high thermal conductivity values are good conductors of heat and cold.

Qualitatively, materials have different rates of conducting heat; metals have higher values than polymers and ceramics. When a portion of a tooth is replaced by a metal restoration such as amalgam or gold alloy, the tooth may be temporarily sensitive to temperature changes in the mouth. Individuals who wear orthodontic appliances or complete acrylic dentures also notice temperature effects different from those experienced without these appliances.

Thermal conductivity has been used as a measure of the heat transferred and is related to the rate of heat flow (see more details in Appendix 2-1). The thermal conductivity of a variety of materials is reported in Table 2-2.

Human enamel and dentin are poor thermal conductors compared with gold alloys and dental amalgam; although amalgam is substantially lower than gold. Glass ionomer cement bases closely replace lost tooth structure with respect to thermal conductivity. The reason for using cements as thermal insulating bases in deep cavity preparations is that, although dentin is a poor thermal conductor, a thin layer of it does not provide enough thermal insulation for the pulp unless a cement base is used under the metal restoration. Composite restorations have thermal conductivities comparable to tooth structure and do not present a problem with this property. Cavity varnishes and liners have low thermal conductivities but are used in layers so thin that they are ineffective as thermal insulators.

TABLE 2-1 Range of Linear Thermal Coefficient of Expansion of Dental Materials in the Temperature Range of 20° to 50°C	
Material	**Coefficient ($\times 10^6/°C$)**
Human teeth	8–15
Ceramics	8–14
Glass ionomer base	10–11
Gold alloys	12–15
Dental amalgam	22–28
Composites	25–68
Unfilled acrylics and sealants	70–100
Inlay wax	300–1000

TABLE 2-2 Thermal Conductivity of Dental Materials	
Material	**Thermal conductivity (cal/sec/cm²[°C/cm])**
Unfilled acrylics	0.0005
Zinc oxide–eugenol cement	0.0011
Human dentin	0.0015
Human enamel	0.0022
Composites	0.0025
Ceramic	0.0025
Zinc phosphate cement	0.0028
Dental amalgam	0.055
Gold alloys	0.710

ELECTRICAL PROPERTIES

> **! ALERT**
>
> *Galvanism* is the generation of electrical currents that the patient can feel.

Two electrical properties of interest are galvanism and corrosion. Galvanism results from the presence of dissimilar metals in the mouth. Metals placed in an electrolyte (a liquid that contains ions) have various tendencies to go into solution. Aluminum, alloys of which are sometimes used as temporary crowns, has a strong tendency to go into solution and has an electrode potential of +1.33 volts. Gold, on the other hand, has little tendency to go into solution, as indicated by an electrode potential of −1.36 volts. A schematic sketch of two opposing teeth, one with a temporary aluminum alloy crown and the other with a gold crown, is shown in Figure 2-1. The oral fluids function as the electrolyte, and the system is similar to that of an electrical cell. When the two restorations touch, current flows because the potential difference is 2.69 volts, and the patient experiences pain and frequently complains of a metallic taste. The same effect can be experienced if some aluminum foil from a baked potato becomes wedged between two teeth and contacts a gold restoration. Temporary polymer crowns are used to prevent this problem because they are poor electrical conductors.

> **! ALERT**
>
> *Corrosion* is the dissolution of metals in the mouth.

> **! ALERT**
>
> *Tarnish* is a surface reaction of metals in the mouth from components in saliva or foods.

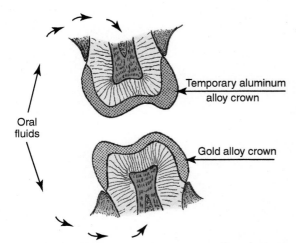

FIG 2-1 Diagrammatic sketch of opposing teeth with a gold crown and a temporary aluminum alloy crown indicating how galvanism can occur.

Oral fluids

Temporary aluminum alloy crown

Gold alloy crown

Corrosion also can result from this same condition when adjacent restorations are of dissimilar metals. As a result of the galvanic action, material goes into solution, and roughness and pitting occur. This effect also may occur if a gold alloy is contaminated with a metal such as iron during handling in the dental laboratory or because of variations in concentration of elements from one part of the restoration to another. Corrosion also may result from chemical attack of metals by components in food or saliva. Dental amalgam, for example, reacts with sulfides and chlorides in the mouth, as shown by polished amalgams becoming dull and discolored with time. This effect sometimes is referred to as tarnish.

SOLUBILITY AND SORPTION

The solubility of materials in the mouth and the sorption (adsorption plus absorption) of oral fluids by the material are important criteria in their selection. Frequently, laboratory studies have evaluated materials in distilled water. At times, these studies gave results that were inconsistent with clinical observations, because materials in the mouth are covered with plaque and therefore are exposed to various acids and organic materials. An example of the inconsistency is that zinc phosphate cements are considerably more soluble in the mouth than in laboratory tests in water indicate. Also, the loss of zinc phosphate cement retaining a gold crown is a result of dissolution followed by and accompanied by disintegration. Nevertheless, laboratory tests usually rank materials correctly, so only the actual magnitude of the numbers should be taken with a grain of salt.

Solubility and sorption are reported in two ways: (1) in weight percentage of soluble or sorbed material and (2) as the weight of dissolved or sorbed material per unit of surface area (e.g., milligrams per cm^2).

Absorption refers to the uptake of liquid by the bulk solid; for example, the equilibrium absorption of water by acrylic polymers is in the range of 2%. *Adsorption* indicates the concentration of molecules at the surface of a solid or liquid, an example of which is the adsorption of components of saliva at the surface of tooth structure or of a detergent adsorbed on the surface of a wax pattern.

WETTABILITY

> **! ALERT**
>
> *Wettability* is a measure of the affinity of a liquid for a solid as indicated by spreading of a drop.

The wettability of solids by liquids is important in dentistry; for example, the wetting of denture base acrylics by saliva, the wetting of tooth enamel by pit and fissure sealants, the wetting of elastomeric impressions by water mixes of gypsum materials, and the wetting of wax patterns by dental investments.

The wettability of a solid by a liquid can be observed by the shape of a drop of the liquid on the solid surface. Profiles of

Contact Angle (ø)

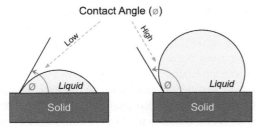

FIG 2-2 Good wetting of a solid by a liquid with a low contact angle *(left)*; poor wetting by a liquid on a solid forming a high contact angle *(right).*

drops of liquids on solids are shown in Figure 2-2. The shape of the drops is identified by the contact angle θ, by the angles through the drops bounded by the solid surface, and by a line through the periphery of the drop and tangent to the surface of the liquid.

If a low contact angle occurs, as in the left of Figure 2-2, the solid is wetted readily by the liquid (hydrophilic if the liquid is water). If a contact angle is greater than 90°, as in the right of Figure 2-2, poor wetting occurs (hydrophobic if the liquid is water).

The degree of wetting depends on the relative surface energies of the solids and the liquids and on their intermolecular attraction. High-energy solids and low-energy liquids encourage good wetting; thus, liquids generally wet higher energy solids well (e.g., water on metals and oxides). On the other hand, liquids bead up on lower-energy solids such as wax, Teflon, and many polymers. The high contact angle of water on these solids can be decreased by adding a wetting agent such as a detergent to the water, thus lowering the surface tension or energy.

MECHANICAL PROPERTIES

Knowledge of the magnitude of biting forces is essential in understanding the importance of the mechanical properties of dental materials. Maximum biting forces decrease from the molar to the incisor region, and the average biting forces on the first and second molars are about 580 Newtons (N), whereas the average forces on bicuspids, cuspids, and incisors are about 310, 220, and 180 N, respectively. To convert Newtons to pounds, Newtons are divided by 4.45.

Patients exert lower biting forces on bridges and dentures than on their normal dentition. For example, when a first molar is replaced by a fixed bridge, the biting force on the restored side is approximately 220 N compared with 580 N when the patient has natural dentition. The average biting force on partial and complete dentures has been measured to be about 111 N; therefore, patients with dentures can apply only approximately 19% of the force of those with normal dentition.

Stress

> **! ALERT**
>
> *Stress* is the force per unit area.

When a force is applied to a material, the material inherently resists the external force. The force is distributed over an area, and the ratio of the force to the area is called the stress (see more details in Appendix 2-1).

Thus, for a given force, the smaller the area over which it is applied, the larger the value of the stress. Figure 2-3 illustrates this effect. A distributed force has been applied in Figure 2-3, *A*, and the same force has been applied in a concentrated manner in Figure 2-3, *B*. The number of lines (fringes) in the plastic model of a tooth when examined in polarized light is directly proportional to the stress, and the stress is shown to be inversely proportional to the area of application. This effect can be demonstrated as follows: an unsharpened pencil is placed against the palm of the hand, a force is applied by placing a book on the end with the eraser, and any pain is noted. Then the pencil is sharpened, the procedure is repeated, and the increase in pain is noted as a result of the increase in stress.

The relationship of force, area, and stress is shown also in Table 2-3. A force of 111 N, which can readily be applied in the mouth, can produce a large stress, such as 172 megapascals (or MPa), when the area of application of the force is

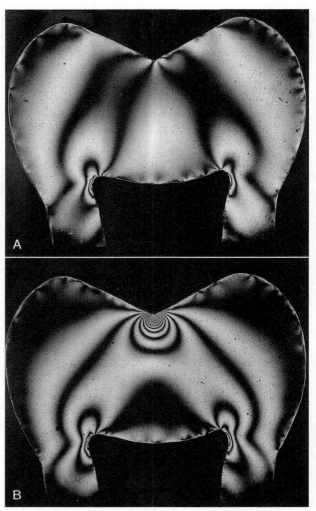

FIG 2-3 Cross-sectional model of a tooth under distributed force **(A)** and concentrated force **(B)**.

TABLE 2-3	Relationship of Force, Area, and Stress	
Force (N)	Area (mm²)	Stress (MPa)
111	645	0.1724
111	64.5	1.724
111	6.45	17.24
111	0.645	172.4
111	0.0645	1724.0

small. One megapascal equals approximately 145 lbs/in². Such conditions readily exist in the mouth, where contact areas of 0.6 mm² frequently occur.

Several types of stress may result when a force is applied to a material. These forces are referred to as compressive, tensile, shear, twisting moment, and bending moment (flexure) and are shown diagrammatically in Figure 2-4. A material is subjected to compressive stress when the material is squeezed together, or compressed, and to tensile stress when pulled apart. Shear stress occurs when one portion (plane) of the material is forced to slide by another portion. These types of stresses are considered to evaluate the properties of various materials.

Strain

> **! ALERT**
>
> *Strain* is the change in length per unit length of a material produced by stress.

The change in length or deformation per unit length when a material is subjected to a force is defined as strain. Strain is easier to visualize than stress because it can be observed directly (see an example calculation in Appendix 2-1). The units of strain are dimensionless. Some dental substances, such as elastomeric impression materials, exhibit considerable strain when a stress is applied; others, such as gold alloys or human enamel, show low strain under stress.

Stress–Strain Curves

A convenient means of comparing the mechanical properties of materials is to apply various forces to a material and to determine the corresponding values of stress and strain. A

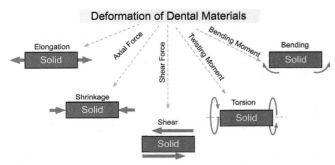

FIG 2-4 Schematic representation of tensile, compressive, shear, twisting, and bending forces and their corresponding deformations.

plot of the corresponding values of stress and strain is referred to as a stress–strain curve. Such a curve may be obtained in compression, tension, or shear. An example of a stress–strain curve in tension for a dental gold alloy is shown in Figure 2-5. The shape and magnitude of the stress–strain curve are important in the selection of dental materials. Figure 2-5 clearly shows that the curve is a straight line, or linear, up to a stress of about 276 MPa, after which it is concave toward the strain axis. The curve ends at a stress of 590 MPa and a strain of 0.2 because the sample ruptured.

Elastic Modulus

The elastic modulus is equal to the ratio of the stress to the strain in the linear or elastic portion of the stress–strain curve (see an example calculation in Appendix 2-1). The elastic modulus is a measure of the stiffness of a material, and high numbers are not unusual for this property. Values for selected materials are listed in Table 2-4, which shows that gold alloys

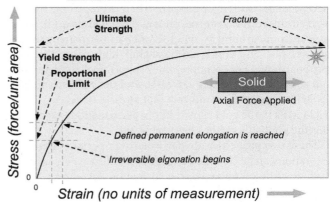

FIG 2-5 Stress–strain curve in tension for dental gold alloy with fracture point at asterisk (*).

TABLE 2-4	Elastic Moduli of Selected Dental Materials
Material	Elastic modulus (GPa)*
Silicone impression material	0.00015–0.001
Unfilled acrylic	2.8
Zinc oxide–eugenol cement	2.8
Adhesive resin layer	3.5–4.8
Zinc polyacrylate cement	3.9
Glass ionomer cement	5.5
Low-viscosity resin	5.8
Hybrid layer (composite/tooth)	8.0–9.0
Human dentin partially demineralized	13.0
Zinc phosphate cement	13.8
Composite	16.6
Human dentin	19.3
Dental amalgam	27.6
Human enamel	90.0
Gold alloy	96.6

*1 GPa = 1000 MPa.

have approximately the same stiffness as human enamel and that composites and zinc phosphate cement are in the same range as human dentin. Unfilled acrylics are much more flexible, with silicone impression material being the most flexible. Stiffness is important in the selection of restorative materials. Because large deflections under stress are not desired, low values are needed for elastic impression materials so that they can be readily removed from the mouth.

Proportional Limit and Yield Strength

> **! ALERT**
>
> Proportional limit and yield strength are measures of the stress allowed before permanent deformation.

Proportional limit and yield strength indicate the stress at which the material no longer functions as an elastic solid. The strain recovers below these values if the stress is removed, and permanent deformation of the material occurs above these values. The proportional limit is the stress on the stress–strain curve when it ceases to be linear or when the ratio of the stress to the strain is no longer proportional. The yield strength is the stress at some arbitrarily selected value of permanent strain, such as 0.001, and thus is always slightly higher than the proportional limit. For example, the proportional limit for the gold alloy in Figure 2-5 is 276 MPa, and the yield strength is 324 MPa. These values indicate that stresses in excess of 276 to 324 MPa in the gold alloy result in permanent deformation after the applied force has been removed.

These two properties are particularly important because a restoration can be classified as a clinical failure when a significant amount of permanent deformation takes place even though the material does not fracture. Materials are said to be elastic in their function below the proportional limit or yield strength and to function in a plastic manner above these stresses.

Typical yield strength values for a variety of materials are listed in Table 2-5, which shows that unfilled acrylic polymers deform permanently at a considerably lower stress than composites, but that both have much lower values than human enamel. It might seem that none of these materials would deform permanently with such high numbers for the yield strength, except that, as shown in the section on stress, biting forces can produce stresses readily that could exceed the yield strength.

TABLE 2-5 Yield Strength of Selected Dental Materials

Material	Yield strength (MPa)
Unfilled acrylics	43–55*
Composites	138–172*
Human dentin	165*
Gold alloys	207–620†
Human enamel	344*

*Yield strength in compression.
†Yield strength in tension.

Ultimate Strength

> **! ALERT**
>
> The stress at which fracture occurs is called the *ultimate strength*.

If higher and higher forces are applied to a material, a stress eventually will be reached when the material fractures or ruptures. This point on the stress–strain curve, the ultimate strength, is denoted with an asterisk in Figure 2-5. If the fracture occurs from tensile stress, the property is called the tensile strength; if in compression, the compressive strength; and if in shear, the shear strength. As Figure 2-5 shows, the tensile strength of the gold alloy was 590 MPa.

The tensile and compressive strength of a material may be significantly different, as illustrated in Table 2-6. Brittle materials, such as human enamel, amalgam, and composites, have large differences and are stronger in compression than in tension.

Limited data are available on the shear strength of dental materials. The shear strength of composites is from 55 to 69 MPa and is about 41 MPa for unfilled acrylics; these values are only slightly higher than and are comparable to the corresponding tensile strengths.

The bond between two materials is usually measured in tension or in shear and is expressed as the stress necessary to cause rupture of the bond. Depending on the system, the bond may be chemical, mechanical, or a combination of the two types. The bond between acrylic denture teeth and acrylic denture bases is essentially chemical and is frequently greater than 34 MPa measured in tension. On the other hand, the bond between composites and acid-etched tooth enamel is essentially mechanical and has a value of approximately 20 to 30 MPa in tension. Adhesives are also available for bonding composites to dentin with reported bond strengths of 15 to 35 MPa. These bonds have been shown to result from the diffusion of the bonding agent into the surface layer of etched dentin.

TABLE 2-6 Ultimate Strength of Selected Dental Materials

Material	Tensile strength (MPa)	Compressive strength (MPa)
Human enamel	10	400
Unfilled acrylics	28	97
Composites	34–62	200–345
Ceramic (feldspathic)	40	150
Dental amalgam	48–69	310–483
Human dentin	98	297
Gold alloys	414–828	–

Elongation and Compression

> **! ALERT**
>
> The amount of deformation that a material can withstand before rupture is reported as the percent elongation when the material is under tensile stress or the percent compression when it is under compressive stress.

The percent elongation at rupture of the gold alloy shown in Figure 2-5 can be determined readily from the strain at rupture simply by multiplying the strain (deformation per unit length) by 100 to convert it to percent elongation. In the example in Figure 2-5, the percent elongation is 20% (see an example calculation in Appendix 2-1). Similar calculations can be made for materials in compression and would represent the percent of plastic strain at rupture.

The percents of elongation and compression are important properties in that they are measures of ductility and malleability, respectively. These two properties indicate the amount of plastic strain, or deformation, that can occur before the material fractures, and, as such, they indicate the brittleness of the material. For example, the gold alloy with 19% elongation can be deformed considerably before fracture, and it would be classed as a ductile alloy. Considerable burnishing and adaptation of the margins of castings from this alloy could be done without fear of fracturing the margin. In general, gold alloys with elongations of less than 5% are considered brittle, and those with values higher than 5% are classed as ductile materials.

Composites are considered brittle materials because the percentage of compression at failure is in the range of 2% to 3%. Clinical observation has been that these materials fail under excessive stress as a result of brittle fracture.

Resilience and Toughness

Up to this point, properties related only to stress or strain have been discussed. Two properties involve the area under the stress–strain curve and thus involve the energy required to reach specified points on the curve.

> **! ALERT**
>
> *Resilience* and *toughness* indicate the energy absorbed up to the proportional limit and the ultimate strength, respectively, and relate to the resistance to deformation and fracture under impact.

The energy required to deform a material permanently is a criterion of its resilience, whereas the energy necessary to fracture a material is a measure of its toughness. These areas are shown as shaded portions of the stress–strain curves in Figure 2-6.

These two properties are more complex than strength or deformation, because their magnitude is a product of stress and strain. Two materials may have the same resilience, with one having high yield strength and low corresponding strain and the other having lower yield strength and higher

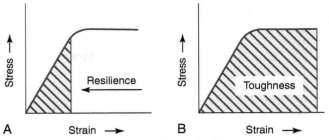

FIG 2-6 Stress–strain curves illustrating the areas that give a measure of the resilience **(A)** and toughness **(B)**.

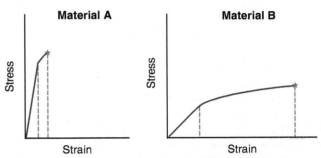

FIG 2-7 Stress–strain curves for composite (material A) and unfilled acrylic (material B). The two materials have approximately the same resilience, but material B is considerably tougher.

corresponding strain. Two such materials are composites and unfilled acrylics, both of which have a resilience of approximately 7 cm-kg/cm^3, despite considerable differences in yield strength. Toughness also is not a simple quantity; for example, although composites have considerably higher yield strengths than unfilled acrylics, the latter may be deformed so much more before rupture that they are tougher than composites (Figure 2-7).

Hardness

> **! ALERT**
>
> *Hardness* is the resistance of a material to indentation.

A material is considered hard if it strongly resists indentation by a hard material such as diamond. One would expect that hardness would be related to yield strength and wear resistance; however, the property is complex. In general, no direct relationship exists between hardness and these two properties. The only exception is in the comparison of materials of the same type, such as a series of similar gold alloys.

The hardness of dental materials generally is reported in Knoop hardness. The Knoop hardness is obtained by measurement of the length of the long diagonal of an indentation from a diamond indenter and calculating the number of kilograms required to give an indentation of 1 mm^2; thus, the larger the indentation, the smaller the hardness value. An example of indentations in dentin and cementum is shown in Figure 2-8; the larger indentations are in cementum,

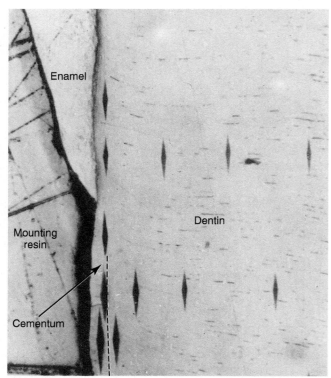

FIG 2-8 Knoop hardness indentations in dentin and cementum. Longer indentations are in cementum, indicating lower hardness than for dentin.

Material	Knoop hardness (kg/mm²)	Knoop hardness (GPa)	Nano-indentation hardness (GPa)
Unfilled acrylic resin	20	0.20	
Zinc phosphate cement	40	0.39	
Human cementum	43	0.42	
Human dentin	68	0.67	0.49*
22-Karat gold alloy	85	0.83	
Dental amalgam	110	1.08	
Human enamel	343	3.36	3.39*
Ceramic	460	4.51	
Adhesive resin			0.10*
Hybrid layer (composite/ tooth)			0.15–0.19*
Microfilled low-viscosity resin			0.19*
Fillers in composites			2.9–8.8*

*Values determined by nano-indentation are not directly comparable to Knoop hardness values.

and the smaller are in dentin. Examples of Knoop hardness values of various materials are listed in Table 2-7. Enamel and ceramic are two of the hardest materials, and unfilled acrylic is the softest of the materials listed.

The Knoop hardness is a satisfactory method for evaluating many restorative materials. Although the indentations are small, they are not small enough to evaluate the hardness of the resin–dentin bonding region of dental composites. Studies of the hardness of this region have used a nano-indentation method. The nano-indentation technique measures much smaller indentations under small loads and allows the hardness of extremely small areas to be determined. However, the nano-indentation values cannot be directly compared with Knoop values, because the Knoop hardness is calculated from the permanent surface deformation after removal of the load and the nano-indentation hardness values are calculated from the penetration while under load. This difference can be seen in the values for enamel and dentin listed in Table 2-7. In spite of this difference, the two methods rank materials in the same order. An additional advantage of the nano-indentation method is that it allows the calculation of the elastic modulus.

Strain–Time Curves

For materials in which the strain is independent of the length of time that a load is applied, stress–strain curves are important. However, for materials in which the strain is dependent on the time the load is maintained, strain–time curves are more useful than stress–strain curves in explaining their properties. Examples of materials that have strain–time-dependent behavior are alginate and elastomeric impression materials, dental amalgam, and human dentin.

A strain–time curve for an elastomeric impression material is shown in Figure 2-9. A compressive load was applied at t_0, and an initial rapid increase in strain occurred from O to A. The load was maintained until t_1, with the strain gradually increasing from A to B; this increase resulted from a combination of viscoelastic strain (time dependent but recoverable) and viscous flow (time dependent and not recoverable). The load was removed at t_1, which resulted in a rapid decrease in strain from B to C. This recovery took place because of the release of elastic strain. A continued gradual decrease in strain occurred from C to D as a result of the recovery of the viscoelastic strain. At t_2, no further decrease in strain took place, and a permanent strain remained, the magnitude of which is represented by DE.

If the load had been applied for a longer time than t_1 or the magnitude of the load had been greater, the amount of permanent strain would have been more. Clinically, this means the shorter the time and the less force applied to the

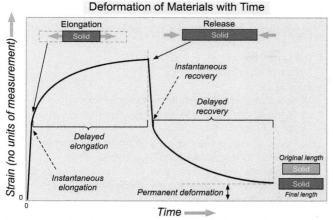

Deformation of Materials with Time

Strain (no units of measurement)

Elongation — Solid

Release — Solid

Instantaneous recovery

Delayed recovery

Delayed elongation

Instantaneous elongation

Permanent deformation

Original length — Solid

Final length — Solid

Time ⟶

FIG 2-9 Strain–time curve for elastomeric impression material.

impression material, the lower the permanent strain and the more accurate the impression.

The strengths of such materials are also dependent on the rate of application of the load. Higher tensile strengths result at more rapid rates of applying the load. As a result, it is recommended that alginate impressions be removed from the mouth in a rapid motion.

Dental amalgam is stronger the more rapidly the force is applied. However, values for the compressive strength obtained at low rates of load application have been shown to correlate better with rankings of clinical service than higher rates of loading. As a result, the testing of amalgam usually is conducted at low rates of application of force.

Dynamic Properties

The properties described so far are classified as static properties because of the relatively slow rate of application of the load. The properties at extremely high rates of loading, such as from an impact, are also important in dentistry. They are classified as dynamic properties and are important in the evaluation of materials such as athletic mouth protectors.

Properties of particular importance are the dynamic modulus and dynamic resilience. The dynamic modulus is a measure of the stiffness of the material at a high rate of strain and is important for mouth protector materials for which the mechanical properties are strain–rate dependent. The dynamic resilience measures the energy absorbed at high rates of strain such as from a blow to an athletic mouth protector.

QUICK REVIEW

The properties of materials are major criteria for the performance of dental materials in service. Dimensional stability is an important property requirement of impression and restorative materials. Thermal conductivity is important as a measure of how much heat and cold are transmitted to pulpal and soft tissues under restorations. Electrical properties are important in terms of galvanic currents generated by dissimilar metals and the discomfort they cause patients. Solubility is especially important in regard to cements that hold restorations in place. Wetting of dental materials by liquids is important in the processing of dental materials and in their relation to saliva in the mouth. Hardness is a measure of the resistance of a material to indentation and scratching. Elastic modulus indicates the stiffness of a material, yield strength the stress it can withstand before permanent deformation, ultimate strength the stress required to fracture a material, and elongation its ductility. Toughness measures the energy needed to fracture a material, and it is important for materials such as denture resins to withstand the shock of being accidentally dropped without breaking.

SELF-TEST QUESTIONS

In the following multiple-choice questions, one or more of the responses may be correct.

1. Which of the following statements describe(s) the purpose of the American National Standards Institute and the American Dental Association specifications?
   a. The specifications measure clinical properties of materials to establish minimum standards.
   b. The specifications measure critical physical and mechanical properties of materials to establish minimum standards.
   c. Knowledge of materials that meet minimum requirements ensures clinical success.
   d. Knowledge of materials that meet minimum requirements ensures quality control and is helpful in the selection of materials for dental practice.

2. An impression of the vertical dimension of a cavity preparation 8 mm in length shows a linear contraction of 0.5%. Compute the actual dimensional change in micrometers (μm).
   a. −4 μm
   b. −40 μm
   c. +40 μm
   d. +0.04 μm

3. A pattern 8 mm in length made from a wax with a linear coefficient of thermal expansion of 380×10^{-6}/°C cools from 37° to 22° C. Compute the actual dimensional change in micrometers (μm).
   a. −45.6 μm
   b. −0.0456 μm
   c. −4.56 μm
   d. +4.56 μm

4. Rank the following dental materials in order of increasing values of their coefficient of thermal expansion: dental amalgam, human teeth, ceramic, and unfilled acrylics.
   a. Human teeth, ceramic, dental amalgam, and unfilled acrylic
   b. Ceramic, human teeth, unfilled acrylic, and dental amalgam
   c. Ceramic, human teeth, dental amalgam, and unfilled acrylic
   d. Human teeth, ceramic, unfilled acrylic, and dental amalgam

5. Which of the following statements describe(s) percolation?
   a. Percolation usually decreases with time after insertion of dental amalgam.
   b. Percolation is caused by differences in the coefficient of thermal expansion between the tooth and the restorative material when heated or cooled.

c. Percolation is thought to be undesirable because of possible irritation to the dental pulp and recurrent decay.

d. Percolation is not likely to occur with unfilled acrylic restorations.

6. Which of the following restorative materials has/have values of thermal conductivity similar to human enamel and dentin?
   a. Dental amalgam
   b. Composites
   c. Zinc phosphate cements
   d. Gold alloys

7. Which of the following is/are examples of galvanism in restorative dentistry?
   a. Aluminum foil from a baked potato becomes wedged between two teeth and contacts a gold restoration.
   b. A temporary acrylic crown contacts a gold restoration.
   c. A temporary aluminum crown contacts a gold restoration.
   d. Patient complains of a metallic taste.

8. Which of the following conditions could lead to corrosion in restorative dentistry?
   a. A gold alloy contaminated with iron during handling in the dental laboratory
   b. A chemical attack of a metal by components in food or saliva
   c. Polished amalgams that have become dull and discolored with time
   d. Adjacent restorations constructed of dissimilar metals

9. The contact angle of water on a dental wax is 105°. Which of the following terms describe(s) the wettability of the wax?
   a. Hydrophobic
   b. Hydrophilic
   c. Hydroscopic
   d. Hygroscopic

10. Which of the following factors increase(s) the wetting of a solid by a liquid?
    a. High surface energy of the solid
    b. Low surface energy of the liquid

11. Which of the following statements is/are true?
    a. The average biting force on an incisor is about 180 N.
    b. The average biting force on a first molar is about 1110 N.
    c. The average biting force on complete dentures is about 111 N.
    d. When a first molar is replaced by a fixed bridge, the biting force on the restored side is about 220 N.

12. An amalgam has a force of 111 N applied over a contact area of 0.645 mm². Which of the following is the stress applied to the amalgam? Would you expect the amalgam to fracture?
    a. 17.2 MPa
    b. 1720 MPa
    c. 172 MPa
    d. 1.72 MPa

13. An alginate impression can withstand a strain of 10% without significant permanent deformation. If the impression must be deformed 0.5 mm to pass over an undercut, how thick should the material be between the tray and the tooth?
    a. 10 mm
    b. 5 mm
    c. 0.5 mm
    d. 0.05 mm

14. Which of the following dental materials has/have an elastic modulus value that is similar to human enamel?
    a. Zinc phosphate cement
    b. Human dentin
    c. Dental amalgam
    d. Gold alloy

15. Which of the following statements is/are true?
    a. The yield strength is always slightly higher than the proportional limit.
    b. Above the stress associated with the yield strength, a material no longer functions as an elastic solid.
    c. Above the stress associated with the yield strength, a material will be permanently deformed, even after the applied force is removed.
    d. Most restorations are not classified as clinical failures until fracture has occurred.

16. Rank the following dental materials in order of increasing tensile strength: dental amalgam, gold alloy, human dentin, and human enamel.
    a. Dental amalgam, human dentin, human enamel, and gold alloy
    b. Human enamel, dental amalgam, human dentin, and gold alloy
    c. Human dentin, human enamel, dental amalgam, and gold alloy
    d. Human dentin, human enamel, gold alloy, and dental amalgam

17. Rank the following dental materials in order of increasing compressive strength: unfilled acrylic, dental amalgam, human dentin, and human enamel.
    a. Human enamel, human dentin, dental amalgam, and unfilled acrylic
    b. Unfilled acrylic, human enamel, human dentin, and dental amalgam
    c. Unfilled acrylic, human dentin, human enamel, and dental amalgam
    d. Dental amalgam, unfilled acrylic, human dentin, and human enamel

18. Which of the following is/are test(s) for measuring hardness?
    a. Knoop
    b. Toughness
    c. Yield strength
    d. Resilience

19. Which of the following dental materials has/have mechanical properties that are time dependent?
    a. Human dentin
    b. Gold alloy
    c. Dental amalgam
    d. Alginate hydrocolloid
    e. Elastomeric impression materials

20. What happens if a load is applied to an elastomeric impression for a long rather than a short time?
    a. The permanent strain will be greater.
    b. The permanent strain will be less.
    c. The elastic strain will be greater.
    d. The viscoelastic strain will be less.

Use short answers to fill in the following blanks.

21. The property that measures the expansion of a material per unit length for every degree of temperature change is called the _____.

22. If the contact angle of a water droplet on the surface of a dental material is greater than 90 degrees, the material is classified as _____.
23. When the deformation of a material is divided by the length of the material, the quotient is called the_____.
24. When the force applied to a material at fracture is divided by the area over which the force was applied, the quotient is called the _____.

For the following statement, answer true or false.

25. An alginate impression material gave two different stress–strain curves (shown in the following figure) when tested rapidly and slowly. As a result, the properties (i.e., plastic and elastic) are better evaluated using a strain–time test than a stress–strain test.
   a. True
   b. False

Provide an answer for each section (a–e).

26. A dental material gave the following stress–strain curve when tested in tension. Which portions of the curve (e.g., points O, A, or B, sections OA, OAB, AB, or ab) represent the following properties?
   a. Elastic
   b. Plastic
   c. Initial permanent deformation
   d. Ultimate tensile strength
   e. Stiffness

Calculate the correct answers for each section (a–c).

27. A dental material yielded the following stress–strain curve in tension. What are the values of the following properties?
   a. Elastic modulus
   b. Proportional limit
   c. Tensile strength

SUGGESTED SUPPLEMENTARY READINGS

Craig RG, Farah JW: Stress analysis and design of single restorations and fixed bridges, *Oral Sci Rev* 10:45, 1977.

Craig RG, Peyton FA: The microhardness of enamel and dentin, *J Dent Res* 37:661, 1958.

Craig RG, Peyton FA: Elastic and mechanical properties of human dentin, *J Dent Res* 37:710, 1958.

Craig RG, Peyton FA: Thermal conductivity of tooth structure, dental cements and amalgam, *J Dent Res* 40:411, 1961.

Craig RG, Peyton FA, Johnson D: Compressive properties of enamel, dental cements, and gold, *J Dent Res* 40:936, 1961.

Craig RG, Powers JM: Wear of dental tissues and materials, *Int Dent J* 26:121, 1976.

Farah JW, Powers JW, Dennison JB, et al: Effects of cement bases on the stresses and deflections in composite restorations, *J Dent Res* 55:115, 1976.

Ferracane JL: Is the wear of dental composites still a clinical concern? Is there still a need for in vitro wear simulating devices? *Dent Mater* 22:689, 2006.

Penn RW, Craig RG, Tesk JA: Diametral tensile strength and dental composites, *Dent Mater* 3:46, 1987.

Powers JM, Farah JW, Craig RG: Modulus of elasticity and strength properties of dental inlay cements and bases, *Am Dent Assoc J* 92:588, 1976.

Van Meerbeek B, Willems G, Celis JP, et al: Assessment by nano-indentation of the hardness and elasticity of the resin–dentin bonding areas, *J Dent Res* 72:1434, 1993.

Willems G, Celis JP, Lambrechts P, et al: Hardness and Young's modulus determined by nanoindentation technique of filler particles of dental restorative materials compared with human enamel, *J Biomed Mater Res* 27:747, 1993.

evolve Please visit *http://evolve.elsevier.com/Powers/dentalmaterials* for additional practice and study support tools.

APPENDIX 2-1 EQUATIONS

Dimensional Change During Setting

A typical example is the linear dimensional change of an addition silicone impression material from a time just after setting until 24 hours after setting. An impression is taken of two marks on a metal plate approximately 51 mm apart; then the distance between the two marks transferred to the impression is measured with a measuring microscope just after the impression sets, l_0, and, again, 24 hours later, l_1. The percentage is calculated as indicated by the following formula:

$$| \; l_0 \; |$$
$$\longleftrightarrow$$
$$| \; l_1 \; |$$

$$\frac{l_1 - l_0}{l_0} \times 100 = \%$$

$$\frac{50.876 - 50.985}{50.985} \times 100 = -0.21\%$$

The result of -0.21% indicates that a linear shrinkage took place within 24 hours after setting.

Thermal Dimensional Change

To make a comparison between materials easier, the linear thermal expansion is expressed as a coefficient of thermal expansion, which is calculated according to the following formula:

$$\frac{l_{t2} - l_{t1}}{l_{t1}} \div (t_2 - t_1) = \text{Linear coefficient of thermal expansion}$$

The first term converts the change to unit length and the second to unit temperature. The value represents the change in length per unit length for each degree of temperature change. Following is a typical calculation for an unfilled dental polymer:

$$\frac{50.500-50.405}{50.405} \div (40-20) = 90.3 \times 10^{-6}/°C$$

The dimensions are per degree because the first term in the equation is dimensionless (it is a length per unit length).

Thermal Conductivity

Thermal conductivity is defined as the number of calories per second flowing through an area of 1 cm^2 in which the temperature drop along the length of the specimen is 1° C/cm.

Stress

The ratio of the force to the area is called the stress:

$$Stress = \frac{Force}{Area}$$

Strain

The change in length or deformation per unit length when a material is subjected to a force is defined as strain:

$$Strain = \frac{Deformation}{Length}$$

For example, if a rubber band 2.54 cm long is stretched 1.27 cm, the strain is as follows:

$$\frac{1.27\,cm}{2.54\,cm} = 0.5$$

Elastic Modulus

The elastic modulus is the slope of the stress–strain curve in the initial straight-line portion; thus, the value for the gold alloy (see Figure 2-5) is the following:

$$Elastic\,modulus = \frac{Stress}{Strain} = \frac{276\,MPa}{0.003} = 92,000\,MPa$$

Elongation and Compression

In practical tests, the plastic strain (the strain between the proportional limit and the ultimate tensile strength) is used in the calculations; thus, for the example in Figure 2-5, the percentage of elongation is as follows:

$$(0.20-0.01) \times 100\% = 19\%$$

Preventive Dental Materials

OBJECTIVES

After reading this chapter, the student should be able to:

Fluoride, Gels, Rinses, and Varnishes

1. Indicate the components in fluoride gels, rinses, and varnishes.
2. Compare the characteristics of different types of fluoride treatments.
3. Describe the clinical effectiveness of fluoride gels.
4. Give the pH range of many commercial fluoride gels.
5. List five steps involved in the application of a fluoride gel.

Pit and Fissure Sealants

6. Describe the uniqueness of pit and fissure caries compared with smooth-surface caries.
7. List the components in light-activated and amine-accelerated resin sealants, and indicate their function.
8. Describe factors that affect the penetration of a sealant into a fissure.
9. Discuss the retention and efficacy of sealants.
10. Describe the clinical success of sealants.
11. List four situations in which sealant should not be used.
12. List six steps involved in the application of sealants.
13. Discuss visible light-activated sealants and amine-accelerated sealants.

Mouth Protectors

14. Give the percentage of oral injuries sustained in unorganized sports.

15. List common reactions of teeth to trauma.
16. List three types of mouth protectors, and describe the material commonly used in custom-made mouth protectors.
17. Compare the characteristics of different types of mouth protectors.
18. List eight physical and mechanical properties that characterize a mouth-protector material.
19. List eight properties of a mouth protector that can be evaluated clinically.
20. Discuss the clinical implications of the properties of hardness and tearing.
21. Describe three causes of breakdown of a mouth protector.
22. List two causes of permanent deformation of a mouth protector during storage, and indicate two proper methods of storage.
23. Describe the four basic steps to prepare a custom-made mouth protector from a thermoplastic material.
24. Indicate two goals in the forming of a mouth protector.
25. Give two mistakes common in the fabrication of a mouth protector.
26. List five instructions to give to a patient for the proper care of a mouth protector.

Preventive dental materials are designed to prevent disease or injury to the teeth and supporting tissues. Three preventive materials are fluoride gels or varnishes, pit and fissure sealants, and mouth protectors. Fluoride gels are applied in a tray to the teeth after a dental prophylaxis or at home to prevent smooth-surface caries. Fluoride rinses and varnishes are also available. Pit and fissure sealants are polymers applied to the occlusal surfaces of posterior teeth to prevent pit and fissure caries. Mouth protectors are made from polymers formed by heat to fit over the teeth of the maxillary arch to protect the mouth from sudden blows that could fracture or dislodge the teeth. Mouth protectors also may be used as trays, or carriers, to provide topical fluoride or bleaching applications, or as shields to prevent damage from bruxism.

> **! ALERT**
>
> Polymers are organic molecules of high molecular weight made up of many repeating units.

FLUORIDE GELS, FOAMS, RINSES, AND VARNISHES

Numerous clinical studies have established the effectiveness of the fluoride ion in lowering the incidence of dental caries. Methods to accomplish topical application of fluoride are the use of gels in trays, rinses, and varnishes.

Composition

Typical commercial acidulated phosphate-fluoride (APF, 12,300 ppm fluoride) gels contain 2% sodium fluoride, 0.34% hydrogen fluoride, and 0.98% phosphoric acid with thickening, flavoring, and coloring agents in an aqueous gel. Some commercial gels, however, contain more sodium fluoride (2.6%) but less hydrogen fluoride (0.16%). The fluoride-ion concentration of most gels ranges from 1.22% to 1.32%. Examples of office and prescription fluoride treatments are listed in Table 3-1. APF products are contraindicated for patients with tooth hypersensitivity—they can cause erosion and worsen the hypersensitivity.

TABLE 3-1	Examples of Office and Prescription Fluoride Treatments			
Fluoride Delivery System	**Type**	**Concentration**	**Product**	**Manufacturer**
Acidulated phosphate-fluoride	Office-use foam	1.23%	ALLSolutions Fluoride Foam	DENTSPLY Professional (York, PA)
Sodium fluoride	Office-use foam	2.0%	Oral-B Neutra-Foam	Oral-B (South Boston, MA)
	Home-use rinse	0.2%	PreviDent Rinse	Colgate Professional (Canton, MA)
Stannous fluoride	Home-use gel	0.4%	Perfect Choice	Challenge Products (Louisville, CO)

> **! ALERT**
>
> A thixotropic material has low flow under no load but flows readily when placed under load.

Neutral sodium fluoride foams, gels, and rinses are available. One product is thixotropic, which contains sodium fluoride and thickening agents (polyacrylic acid and a gum). The pH is adjusted to between 6 and 8. Values of pH in this range should minimize acid etching of restorative materials, such as composites, compomers, resin-modified glass ionomers (hybrid ionomer), glass ionomers, and ceramics, caused by more acidic APF gels.

Varnishes containing 5% sodium fluoride (22,600 ppm fluoride) are available (Duraflor Halo 5% Sodium Fluoride White Varnish, Medicom, Tonawanda, NY; Kolorz Clear-Shield Fluoride Varnish, DMG America, Englewood, NJ). Some products (Enamel Pro Varnish, Premier Dental Products, Plymouth Meeting, PA) also contain amorphous calcium phosphate (ACP), which contributes to remineralization of enamel.

Stannous fluoride products are effective in providing fluoride but can cause staining of tooth surfaces and restorations.

Properties

Characteristics of different types of fluoride treatments are compared in Table 3-2. The clinical effectiveness of acidulated phosphate-fluoride gels varies, which depends in part on the method and frequency of application. Reductions in dental caries of 37% and 41% were observed in two studies of 2 years' duration in which the gel was applied annually. A reduction of

TABLE 3-2	Characteristics of Different Types of Fluoride Treatments		
Characteristic	**Acidulated phosphate-fluoride**	**Sodium fluoride**	**Stannous fluoride**
Form acidity (pH)	Gel, rinse, foam Acidic	Gel, rinse, foam Neutral	Gel, rinse Acidic
Can etch restorations	Yes	No	Yes
Can stain restorations	No	No	Yes

26% was observed at the end of 3 years in another study. A reduction of 80% after 2 years was observed in a study in which a gel with lower fluoride content (0.5% versus 1.23%) and higher pH (pH 4.5 versus pH 3) than that used in the aforementioned studies was self-applied each school day. One clinical study showed no significant reduction in the incidence of dental caries after 2 years. The typical 4-minute application appears to be more effective than a 1-minute application.

Varnish containing 5% sodium fluoride has been found to be effective in reducing caries in primary and permanent dentition. Caries reduction (Decayed, Missing, Filled Surfaces—DMFS) ranged from 19% to 48% in primary dentition and from 30% to 63% in permanent dentition. Five percent sodium fluoride varnish is also effective in reducing orthodontic decalcification.

Manipulation

Fluoride foams and gels can be applied in soft, spongy trays after a dental prophylaxis. The teeth are kept as free from saliva as possible before application of the tray. A ribbon of gel is placed in the troughs of the maxillary and mandibular trays. Then the trays are placed in position, and pressure is applied by squeezing the buccal and lingual surfaces to mold the tray tightly around the teeth so that the gel penetrates between the teeth. The patient is instructed to bite lightly for 4 minutes. After application of a gel, the patient is instructed not to eat for 30 minutes. Rinses are not recommended for children younger than 6 years.

PIT AND FISSURE SEALANTS

Smooth-surface caries has been reduced by the use of established preventive measures such as fluoridation of communal water supplies, topical application of fluoride during enamel development, and individual plaque-control programs. These measures, however, have not been completely effective in reducing the incidence of dental caries in pits and fissures, which are sites susceptible to dental caries because of their anatomic construction.

The uniqueness of pit and fissure caries is a result of the special anatomy of the occlusal surfaces of posterior teeth. A smooth-based depression on the occlusal surface of a tooth is termed a groove, an example of which is shown in a histologic section in Figure 3-1, *A*. The tip of an explorer in the upper left corner of this figure indicates the relative size of

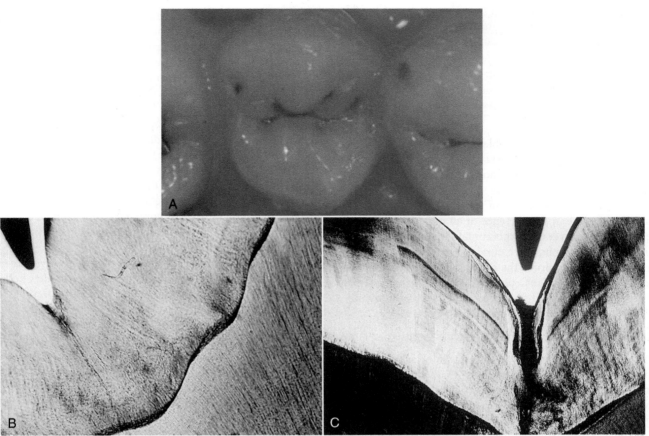

FIG 3-1 Grooves and fissures in the occlusal surface of a tooth. Clinically, **(A)** grooves and fissures in the occlusal surface of a tooth are often discolored, but the coloration belies the extent of the problem. In cross section **(B, C)** the groove may be deeper than it appears clinically, and caries may extend far beyond what the clinician can see with normal vision or detect with an explorer **(C).** Detection of caries in deep fissures requires magnification and drying of the tooth. (**A,** Courtesy Y-W Chen, University of Washington Department of Restorative Dentistry, Seattle, WA.)

such a groove. A groove is cleansed by the excursion of food or of a toothbrush bristle. The pit and fissure, however, is an enamel fault that is the result of noncoalescence of enamel during tooth formation. This lack of enamel coalescence may extend to the dentoenamel junction, or it may be incomplete, with the fissure extending some lesser depth into the enamel. The debris and microbial masses that collect in a fissure are readily apparent in Figure 3-1, *B*. Under appropriate conditions, pit and fissure caries is initiated. The unusual anatomy of the pit and fissure causes such sites to exhibit a high incidence of dental caries. In fact, 84% of dental caries in children 5 to 17 years of age involve pits.

One approach to the prevention of pit and fissure caries has been a restorative procedure in which occlusal fissures are cut away and filled with dental amalgam. Another approach is the use of pit and fissure sealants. The purpose of a pit and fissure sealant is to penetrate all cracks, pits, and fissures on the occlusal surfaces of both deciduous and permanent teeth in an attempt to seal off these susceptible areas and to provide effective protection against caries. If incipient caries are suspected in pit and fissures of a tooth, the fissures are commonly prepared with small traditional carbide burs, specialized burs called fissurotomy burs, or by air abrasion (blasting with alumina [aluminum oxide] particles). The prepared fissures are then filled with a combination of flowable composite, traditional composites, or sealants, depending on the depth of the fissure preparation. This technique is called a "preventive resin restoration."

Composition and Reaction

> **! ALERT**
>
> A monomer is a single organic molecule used to prepare a high molecular weight polymer.

Most commercial pit and fissure sealants, examples of which are listed in Table 3-3, are resins in which polymerization is activated by light. The chemistry of sealants is similar to that of the composite restorative materials that are discussed in Chapter 4. The principal difference is that sealants are more fluid to penetrate the pits and fissures in addition to the etched areas produced on the enamel, which provide for retention of the sealant.

TABLE 3-3 Examples of Light-Cured Pit and Fissure Sealants

Product	Manufacturer
Clinpro Sealant	3M ESPE (St. Paul, MN)
Helioseal Clear Chroma	Ivoclar Vivadent (Amherst, NY)
Teethmate F-1	Kuraray America (New York, NY)

Sealants polymerized by visible light (490-nm wavelength) are one-component systems that require no mixing. The resin is a diluted dimethacrylate monomer (bisphenol A-glycidyl methacrylate [Bis-GMA] or urethane dimethacrylate [UDMA]), the polymerization of which is initiated by activation of a diketone in the presence of an organic amine with the visible light. Several sealants contain up to 50% by weight of inorganic filler to improve durability, and many contain a white pigment to improve the contrast between the sealants and enamel. The sealants polymerize in the mouth when exposed to a curing light to become a cross-linked polymer, as indicated in the following simplified reaction:

Dimethacrylate + Diluent + Activator + Light = Sealant

The sealants polymerized by an organic amine accelerator are supplied as two-component systems. One component contains a monomer and a benzoyl peroxide initiator, and the second component contains a diluted monomer with 5% organic amine accelerator. The two components are mixed thoroughly before being applied to the prepared teeth.

Properties

Physical and mechanical properties of commercial pit and fissure sealants are listed in Table 3-4. Additional properties of clinical importance include retention and efficacy.

Retention of a sealant in a fissure is the result of mechanical bonding caused by penetration of the sealant into the fissure and the etched areas of enamel to form tags. Filling the fissure completely is difficult because air frequently is trapped in the bottom of the fissure (Figure 3-2, A), or the accumulation of debris at the base of the fissure prevents it from being sealed completely (Figure 3-2, B). Acid etching of the enamel surface

TABLE 3-4 Properties of Resin Pit and Fissure Sealants

Property	Typical light-cured sealant
Setting time (seconds)	Activated by light
Compressive strength (MPa)	92–150
Tensile strength (MPa)	20–31
Elastic modulus (GPa)*	2.1–5.2
Knoop hardness (kg/mm^2)	20–25
Water sorption, 7 days (mg/cm^2)	1.3–2.0
Water solubility, 7 days (mg/cm^2)	0.2
Penetration coefficient, 22°C (cm/sec)	4.5–8.8
Wear (×10^{-4} mm^3/mm)	22–23

*1 GPa = 1000 MPa.

improves the retention of the sealant by cleaning the area to be sealed, improving the wettability of the enamel, increasing the surface area, and forming spaces into which the sealant can penetrate to form tags (Figure 3-3).

Penetration of a sealant into the fissure must occur before the sealant has polymerized. The rate of penetration is determined by the configuration (length and radius) of the pit or fissure and by the penetration coefficient (PC) of the sealant (see more details in Appendix 3-1). The penetration coefficient is related to the surface tension and viscosity of the sealant and the contact angle of the sealant on the enamel.

The containers in which the sealant components are supplied must be kept closed tightly during storage to minimize the evaporation of volatile monomers, which would cause the sealant to become more viscous and limit its penetration into the pit or fissure.

Many clinical studies have been reported. However, caution is warranted when comparing some of these studies because materials, techniques, teeth studied, and clinical criteria for judging success or failure vary from study to study. Three parameters important in the evaluation of a clinical study of a sealant are (1) a statistical test of the significance; (2) the net gain as a result of treatment; and (3) the percentage of effectiveness. When pairs of teeth are studied, the net gain is the number of pairs in which the treated tooth is sound and the untreated tooth is decayed minus the number of pairs in which the treated tooth is decayed and the untreated tooth is sound. The percentage of effectiveness is the net gain divided by the total number of carious controls expressed as a percentage. A summary of a 5-year clinical study on schoolchildren is listed in Table 3-5. The effectiveness of a single application of a sealant clearly decreases with time.

In another clinical study, the teeth of schoolchildren were maintained free of caries for 5 years by reapplication of sealant as indicated by clinical reexamination at 6-month intervals. The highest retreatment rate (18%) occurred 6 months after initial treatment but was as low as 4% at subsequent 6-month recalls. The pit and fissure sealants are effective in preventing caries in sealed tooth surfaces when the sealant is retained. Periodic clinical observation is recommended to determine the success or potential failure of the sealant treatment.

One concern is what happens to dental caries that are purposely or inadvertently left beneath sealed pits and fissures. Several studies have reported that the number of cultivable microorganisms from carious dentin left *in situ* in sealed pits and fissures for up to 5 years was considerably less than before sealant was applied. Sealing a suspected carious pit and fissure appears to be a reasonable clinical service if appropriate clinical observation is maintained.

The use of sealants requires clinical judgment and continued observation. Modes of failure that have been observed include direct loss of sealant, absence of bonding of an area within an otherwise intact sealant, and wear that uncovers the ends of the fissures. Current evidence indicates that sealants should not be used on the teeth of a patient who does not cooperate in maintaining good oral hygiene, on occlusal

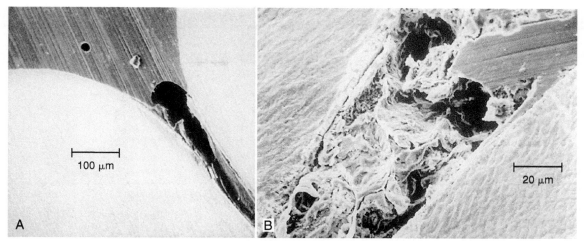

FIG 3-2 Section showing a fissure incompletely filled with sealant as a result of air **(A)** and debris **(B)**. (From Gwinnett AJ: The bonding of sealants to enamel, *J Am Soc Prev Dent* 3:21, 1973.)

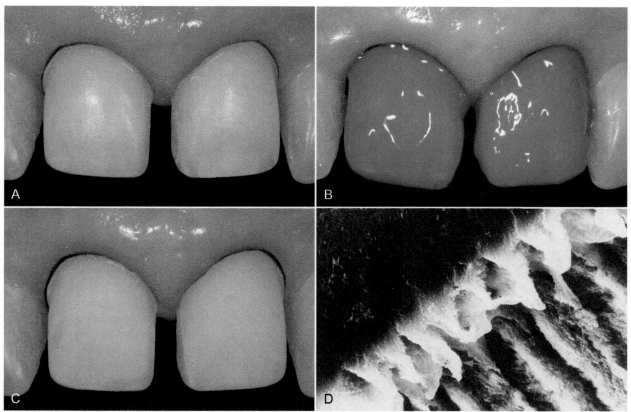

FIG 3-3 Penetration of etched enamel by sealants and resins. Normal tooth enamel **(A)** is not very porous and is shiny, reflecting light. However, etching enamel for several seconds with a phosphoric acid gel **(B)** greatly increases porosity of the enamel, which becomes apparent when the acid is rinsed away and the etched enamel dried **(C)**. Etched enamel has a dull, opaque appearance. On a microscopic level **(D)**, the enamel has thousands of small pores from the differential etch into which sealant or other types of resin bonding agents can penetrate. The many tags (*arrow*, **D**) retain the sealant in the tooth. (**A–C,** Courtesy Y-W Chen, University of Washington Department of Restorative Dentistry, Seattle, WA; **D,** from Dennison JB: Restorative materials for direct application. In Craig RG, editor: *Dental Materials: A Problem-Oriented Approach,* St Louis, 1978, Mosby.)

TABLE 3-5 Summary of a Clinical Study after Single Application of a Pit and Fissure Sealant

Type of teeth and patients	Duration of study (years)	Total retention (%)	Net gain (number of teeth)	Effectiveness (%)
First permanent molars in children 5 to 9 years of age	1	79	77	83
	2	71	96	74
	3	60	91	64
	4	52	78	54
	5	31	58	40
Second primary molars in children 5 to 9 years of age	1	72	—	—
	2	60	2	29
	3	45	7	54

Modified from Charbeneau GT, Dennison JB: Clinical success and potential failure after single application of a pit and fissure sealant: a four-year report, *J Am Dent Assoc* 98:559, 1979.

surfaces where pits and fissures do not exist, on teeth that have been free of caries for several years, or on teeth with many proximal lesions.

Manipulation of Sealants

The technique for handling the pit and fissure sealants involves six basic steps that must be followed sequentially, including cleansing and etching the occlusal surfaces, washing these areas, drying them, applying the sealant to the pit and fissure, polymerizing, and finishing.

Visible Light-Activated Sealants

The advantages of acid etching the enamel before applying a sealant were discussed earlier. Etchants are generally 37% solutions of phosphoric acid in water. Some etching agents are phosphoric acid gels. Typically, the enamel surface is cleansed with pumice before etching.

Phosphoric acid is applied liberally to the central fissure area of the occlusal surface with a small cotton pellet held by tweezers or with a fine brush. The solution is left on the tooth for 60 seconds before the surface is washed with a liberal amount of water for at least 15 seconds. Rinsing is important because residual phosphoric acid can interfere with the bonding of the sealant. The etchant should not be applied to other surfaces of the tooth, and the acid should not be allowed to overetch the enamel. If an etched tooth should become contaminated by saliva, the etching and rinsing steps are repeated.

The washed surface of the tooth is dried for 15 seconds with an air syringe. This step is critical to the success of the sealant because moisture interferes with the retention of the sealant by the fissure. At this point, the occlusal surface has an appearance similar to that shown in Figure 3-4. During application of the sealant, the isolation of the area is maintained from moisture by use of cotton rolls and high-volume evacuation or by rubber dam.

The pit and fissure sealant is applied to the occlusal surface of the tooth carefully. The application of an excessive amount of sealant is wasteful. In particular, application of the sealant to unetched areas of enamel should be avoided. Application of a light-cured bonding agent to the freshly etched surface improves retention, especially if minor contamination results from moisture or saliva.

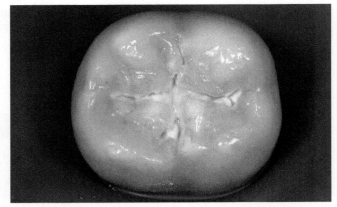

FIG 3-4 Dark areas of a preconditioned occlusal surface indicate location of pits and fissures. (From Dean JA, Avery DR, McDonald RE: *McDonald and Avery's Dentistry for the Child and Adolescent,* ed 9, St Louis, 2011, Mosby.)

Once the sealant has been applied to the etched enamel, polymerization is activated by the use of a light-curing unit (see Figure 4-10). The protective plastic tip of the light source is positioned on the occlusal surface and held there for at least 20 seconds.

Once the sealant has set, finishing can be accomplished with the use of a small cotton pellet held by tweezers. The pellet is used on the surface to remove sealant that has failed to polymerize because of exposure to air. When successfully polymerized, the sealant should offer considerable resistance to attempts to penetrate it with the tip of an explorer. The coating is inspected for areas of incomplete coverage and voids. Defects are corrected by repetition of the entire procedure and reapplication of sealant to the defective areas. A completed sealant treatment is shown in Figure 3-5. If a fluoride treatment is used in conjunction with the pit and fissure sealant, the treatment is applied after the sealant has polymerized.

Amine-Accelerated Sealants

The procedure for manipulating these sealants is similar to that just described for sealants polymerized by visible light. These sealants require mixing of the base and initiator

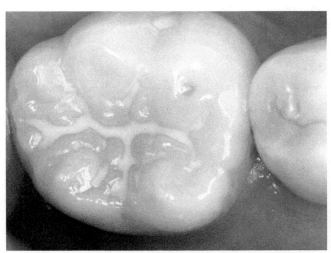

FIG 3-5 Tooth with completed sealant treatment. (From Bird DL, Robinson DS: *Modern Dental Assisting,* ed 10, St Louis, 2012, Saunders.)

components. These components are mixed thoroughly to ensure that polymerization is homogeneous but are mixed gently to minimize incorporation of air. Typically, the mixing time is 10 to 15 seconds. The sealant is applied promptly because its ability to penetrate the fissure and etched enamel decreases rapidly as it begins to polymerize. Setting will occur within several minutes after application of the liquid sealant. Once polymerized, the sealant is finished as already described.

MOUTH PROTECTORS

The Centers for Disease Control and Prevention recommends that all players of contact sports use mouth protectors. It found that football players do not sustain as many orofacial injuries as other athletes do because of required faceguards and mouth protectors. In a survey of students, 62% of injuries occurred in unorganized sports. Fifty-nine percent of injuries were suffered by children 7 to 13 years of age. Another survey found that 38% of sports participants had sustained an orofacial injury. Only 15% of the injured players stated that they were wearing a mouth protector at the time of their injury. The National Youth Sports Safety Foundation has reported that in all sporting activities the ratio of male to female injuries is 3:1. In organized sports, the ratio drops to about 2:1.

Surveys report that injuries most commonly occur in basketball, baseball, and soccer. Most injuries occurred when the athlete was not wearing a mouth protector. Common reactions of teeth to trauma include pulpitis, pulpal necrosis, resorption phenomena, replacement resorption, internal hemorrhage, pulp canal obliteration, and inflammatory resorption. Even with high rates of orofacial injuries, parents often do not perceive the need for mouth protectors.

The mouth protector program has been particularly effective in the area of preventive dentistry. The original mandate by the National Football Alliance Rules Committee that all high school athletes be equipped with internal mouth protectors has influenced other athletic programs. Most junior

colleges and many amateur hockey and football leagues have now adopted this rule, and the National Collegiate Athletic Association adopted a mouth-protector rule in 1973. Furthermore, professional hockey and football players who have worn mouth protectors in college or elsewhere usually continue to wear them in professional sports. Estimates report 1.5 million athletes have been equipped with mouth protectors, and that this number increases by 70,000 each year. In fact, each year the use of the intraoral mouth protector is estimated to prevent 25,000 to 50,000 injuries.

Types and Composition

The three types of mouth protectors, all of which offer some protection to the athlete, are stock, mouth formed (Figure 3-6), and custom made (Figure 3-7). Study results show that use of any of the mouth protectors reduces oral injuries. Players prefer the custom-made protectors because of cleanliness, lack of taste or odor, durability, low speech impairment, and comfort. Advantages and disadvantages of stock, mouth-formed, and custom-made mouth protectors are listed in Table 3-6.

> **! ALERT**
>
> A thermoplastic material becomes softer on heating and harder on cooling. The process is reversible.

Custom-made mouth protectors are generally formed from thermoplastic polymers supplied in the form of clear or colored sheets about 14 cm square. The thickness of these sheets varies from 1.6 to 3 mm, depending on the product. The most common material used in custom-made protectors is a poly (vinyl acetate)-polyethylene polymer, also called ethylene vinyl acetate (EVA). Commercial sheets for the fabrication of custom-made mouth protectors are available from companies such as Buffalo Dental, Dental Resources, and Dentsply Raintree Essix. Other products have used polyurethane, latex rubber, and a vinyl plastisol.

Properties

Laboratory studies have compared the physical and mechanical properties of numerous materials used for custom-made mouth protectors. These properties include tensile strength, percentage of elongation, tear strength, hardness, water sorption, solubility, dynamic modulus, and dynamic resilience. American National Standards Institute (ANSI)/ American Dental Association (ADA) Specification No. 99 for Athletic Mouth Protectors and Materials includes requirements for biocompatibility, Shore A hardness, tear strength, impact absorption, impact rebound, and water sorption (Table 3-7).

The properties of a poly(vinyl acetate)-polyethylene mouth protector after processing and after being worn are compared in Table 3-8. After exposure to the oral environment, the mouth protector becomes more flexible and better able to absorb an impact (energy) but has less strength in tension than previously.

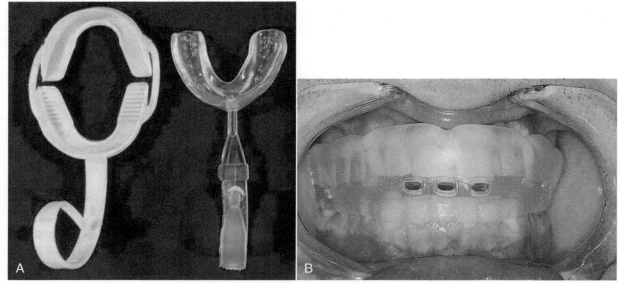

FIG 3-6 A, Stock *(left)* and mouth-formed *(right)* mouth protectors. **B,** Mouth-formed protector in use. (**A,** From Pinkham JR, Cassamassimo PS, Fields HW, et al: *Pediatric Dentistry,* ed 4, St Louis, 2005, Mosby; **B,** From Daniel SR, Harfst SA, Wilder RS: *Mosby's Dental Hygiene: Concepts, Cases, and Competencies,* ed 2, St Louis, 2008, Mosby.)

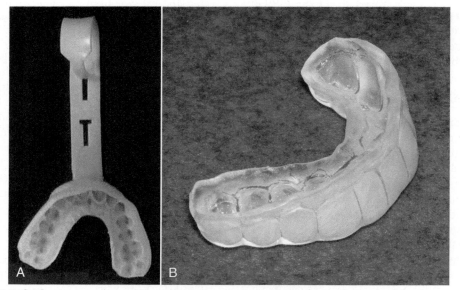

FIG 3-7 A, Custom-made mouth protector made from clear plastic. **B,** Custom-made protector properly fitted and in use. (**A,** From Pinkham JR, Cassamassimo PS, Fields HW, et al: *Pediatric Dentistry,* ed 4, St Louis, 2005, Mosby. **B,** From Dean JA, Avery DR, McDonald RE: *McDonald and Avery's Dentistry for the Child and Adolescent,* ed 9, St Louis, 2011, Mosby.)

Compared with the poly(vinyl acetate)-polyethylene material, the polyurethanes possess higher strength, hardness, and energy absorption but also have higher values of water sorption and require higher processing temperatures. The vinyl plastisols and latexes possess only slightly lower values of strength, hardness, and energy absorption than the poly(vinyl acetate)-polyethylene materials, but their greatest disadvantage is the difficulty of processing. In general, poly(vinyl acetate)-polyethylene materials are the easiest to fabricate.

Clinical studies of custom-made mouth protectors made of poly(vinyl acetate)-polyethylene have been concerned with the following clinical variables: gagging, taste, irritation, impairment of speech, feel, durability, staining, and deformation.

Gagging, presence of a taste, irritation, and impairment of speech are problems not common to properly fabricated custom-made protectors. The elimination of these four variables as potential excuses for an athlete not to wear the protector is one reason that custom-made protectors are more

TABLE 3-6 Advantages and Disadvantages of Stock, Mouth-Formed, and Custom-Made Mouth Protectors

Property	Custom-made	Mouth-formed	Stock
Fit	Excellent	Poor–good*	Poor
Thickness	Can be customized	May be too thin	
Durability	Excellent	Poor–good*	Poor
Comfort	Excellent	Poor–good*	Poor
Ease of speaking	Excellent	Poor–good*	Poor
Cost	More expensive	Inexpensive	Inexpensive

*Dependent on patient's ability to achieve a good fit.

TABLE 3-7 Requirements for Properties of Mouth Protector Materials

Property	Requirement
Shore A hardness (durometer)	55–85
Vacuum formed, stock Mouth formed	40–60
Tear strength (N/cm)	>200
Impact absorption (%)	>65
Rebound (N-cm)	<30
Water sorption (wt %)	<0.5

Modified from ANSI-ADA Specification No. 99.

TABLE 3-8 Properties of Poly(Vinyl Acetate)-Polyethylene Mouth Protector after Processing and after Being Worn

Property	Processed	Worn
Tensile strength (MPa)	3.13	2.14
Tear strength (N/cm)	240	250
Elongation (%)	975	—
Hardness (Shore A durometer)	71	60
Water sorption, 24 hours (mg/cm^2)	0.05	—
Water solubility, 24 hours (mg/cm^2)	0.001	—
Dynamic modulus, 37° C (MPa)	9.4	7.2
Dynamic resilience, 37° C (%)	23.4	20.2

desirable than the stock variety. Staining is a problem that can be expected regardless of the protector material.

Apparently, an optimal hardness exists at which an athlete will accept the protector. Complaints may be received from athletes who dislike the feel of the harder materials. If this dislike is sufficient motivation for an athlete not to wear the protector, a softer material should be selected.

As the thickness of a mouth protector material is increased from 2 to 6 mm, the energy absorption is increased, and the transmitted forces on impact are decreased. Thicker materials, however, are more uncomfortable to wear. A thickness of 4 mm of material over incisal edges and cusps of teeth is

recommended for best protection and acceptable comfort. Mouth protectors made from single sheets may be thinner than desired because of up to 30% shrinkage caused by processing. Laminated protectors formed from two 3-mm sheets provide a final thickness of 4 mm in critical occlusal areas.

The breakdown of a mouth protector usually results from one of three causes: "bitethrough," tearing, or a general deterioration that results from chewing the protector. Both bitethrough and chewing problems are compounded by the emotional involvement of the athlete. If the mouth protector is used to counteract high emotional stress during periods such as player assignments or an important game, breakdown of the mouth protector can be expected regardless of the material of construction. In addition, some athletes may react to the harder mouth-protector materials by chewing them, in which case a softer material should be selected. An example of a deteriorated mouth protector is shown in Figure 3-8.

An excessive force applied to the protector generally causes tearing of a protector. If this force were the result of a blow to the jaw, for example, tearing of the protector would be a dissipation of part of the energy of the blow. The energy absorbed by the mouth protector is not available to do damage to the mouth, and thus, from this point of view, tearing of a mouth protector from a blow is probably desirable.

As a result of the aforementioned three causes of breakdown of a mouth protector, its durability is highly dependent on both the athlete's acceptance of the protector and his or her reaction to emotional stress. A protector may last 1 week in a highly emotional high school athlete or a whole season (4 months) in a more experienced college player. As a general rule, mouth protectors should be evaluated for breakdown on a game-to-game basis and replaced when necessary.

Observations have shown that mouth protectors become permanently deformed. A primary cause is the mode of storage. Permanent deformation can occur as the result of

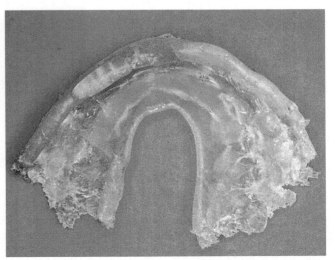

FIG 3-8 Example of a deteriorated mouth protector. (From Pinkham JR, Cassamassimo PS, Fields HW, et al: *Pediatric Dentistry*, ed 4, St Louis, 2005, Mosby.)

pressure (such as that occurring when the mouth protector is squeezed together in a locker) or heat (such as that resulting when the mouth protector is stored in a helmet left in the hot sunlight). When not in use between games and practice, the mouth protector is stored in a rigid plastic container or on the model on which it was fabricated.

An attempt to provide additional protection has resulted in the development of a laminated protector that contains a hard sheet bonded to the softer poly(vinyl acetate)-polyethylene material.

The use of extraoral instead of intraoral mouth protection on young athletes has been advocated because of the continued eruption of teeth. However, in view of the fact that many injuries result from a blow that drives the mandible into the maxillary arch, the protection afforded by the extraoral protector is not considered adequate. Therefore, starting the athlete with the intraoral protector is ideal.

Fabrication of Mouth Protectors

The fabrication of a custom-made mouth protector from a thermoplastic material such as poly(vinyl acetate)-polyethylene requires four basic steps: taking an impression of the arch, pouring a model, forming the thermoplastic material over the model, and finishing the mouth protector. The goal is to attain an optimal fit so that the mouth protector will distribute a blow over the entire dental arch. In addition, the protector should provide as little distortion of normal occlusion as is necessary for maximum protection.

An alginate impression is made of the maxillary arch. If many protectors are being made in a short time, as in a clinic, it is convenient to use disposable impression trays. Trays are modified as necessary with utility wax (Figure 3-9) to provide adequate extension of the labial portion of the tray and to prevent the patient from gagging. Further information on manipulation of alginate and impression making can be found in Chapter 8.

Athletes should not wear any removable appliances when participating in contact sports. Thus, impressions for mouth protectors should be made with such appliances removed. Orthodontic appliances that are fixed to the teeth need not be removed because an impression can be made with them in place. The areas occupied by the appliances then can be blocked out on the model with dental stone or wax (Figure 3-10) so that the mouth protector will fit over them.

After disinfection, the impression is poured immediately in stone. Because the model may be reused to form many mouth protectors, high-strength stone provides the most durable model. It is not necessary to pour the palate in the model

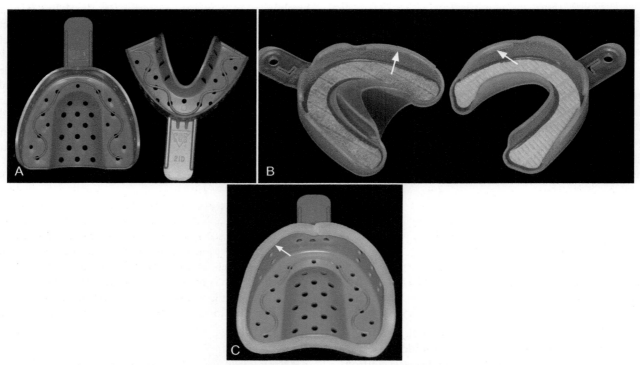

FIG 3-9 Disposable impression trays. Disposable impression trays are used to make impressions, usually with alginate impression materials. They come in several styles **(A, B)**. In **A,** the tray has holes and ridges to retain and support the alginate material in the tray. The maxillary tray is on the left and mandibular tray on the right. In **B,** there are ridges on the periphery of the trays *(arrows)* to retain the impression material. The maxillary tray is on the left and mandibular tray on the right. To prevent the hard plastic from irritating the soft oral tissues, utility wax (**C,** *arrow*) is often applied to the periphery of the disposable tray. When constructing a night-guard or mouth protector, it is often not necessary to pour the full palate in the maxillary impression. (Courtesy Y-W Chen, University of Washington Department of Restorative Dentistry, Seattle, WA.)

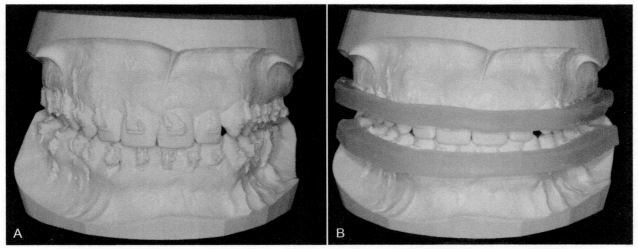

FIG 3-10 On occasion, a patient will have a clinical situation that requires block out prior to the fabrication of a mouth protector. Patients with orthodontic brackets **(A)** can have the alginate taken with the brackets in place. Then prior to mouthguard fabrication, utility wax can be used to block out the brackets **(B).** The block out prevents the mouthguard material from bonding to the impression of the brackets, and it also provides space in the final mouthguard to protect the brackets. (Courtesy Y-W Chen, University of Washington Department of Restorative Dentistry, Seattle, WA.)

(see Figure 3-9) because only areas to be included in the mouth protector are poured. The model is identified with the athlete's name written in pencil. Further information on the manipulation of gypsum products can be found in Chapter 9.

Forming the mouth protector can be accomplished by a vacuum machine, by a pressure-lamination machine, or by hand. The vacuum and pressure methods of forming the protector are desirable because they reproduce the occlusal anatomy more accurately than forming by hand does. Vacuum-forming and pressure-lamination machines are available. An illustration of a vacuum-forming machine is shown in Figure 3-11. An example of a pressure-laminate machine is Dreve Drufomat (Westone Laboratories, Colorado Springs, Colorado).

To form the protector, a square sheet of mouth-protector material is clamped in the frame with the attached handles (see Figure 3-11), and the frame is raised to the top position just below the heating element. The model is centered on the vacuum former platform. By elimination of the palatal area of the model, a higher vacuum can be attained more readily, and thus adaptation of the material will be better. The heating element is turned on, and the center of the sheet of mouth-protector material must sag approximately 3 cm. The vacuum is turned on, and the frame holding the material is lowered over the model. The vacuum pulls the material over the model and adapts it. The heating element is turned off, and it is swung away to the right. The vacuum is maintained for a minute, and the material is allowed to cool for an additional minute. The model and mouth protector are removed from the vacuum platform and chilled thoroughly in cold water or allowed to air cool before the mouth protector is removed from the model.

If the athlete has rapidly emerging deciduous teeth, space in the mouth protector is allowed to accommodate this growth by placing portions of a damp towel over these teeth on the model. The damp towel serves as a spacer during fabrication but can be removed easily once the material has cooled.

The mouth protector is removed from the model and trimmed 3 mm short of the labial fold (Figure 3-12) with a curved pair of surgical scissors. Clearance must be provided for the buccal and particularly the labial frenum by notching the mouth protector in these areas. The mouth protector on the model is replaced and its edges flamed with an alcohol torch. These edges are smoothed with moist fingers. A simpler method of smoothing the edges of a mouth protector is to use a Moore's Satin Buff Wheel available for use at chairside (2.5-cm wheel) or with a laboratory lathe (10-cm wheel).

Only a small percentage of mouth protectors need adjustment to equalize the occlusion. Should equalization be necessary, this procedure is followed. The contacting surfaces of the mouth protector are heated gently with an alcohol torch. Only enough heat is used to barely soften the material. The appliance is dipped in warm water and is placed in the athlete's mouth; the athlete is asked to close the mouth gently until all the teeth contact the mouth protector. The athlete is asked to open his or her jaws, and the mouth protector is removed to cool. The protector is replaced in the mouth to examine the occlusion. All the teeth must contact the appliance. If it is desirable to open the athlete's vertical dimension, a strip of the thermoplastic material is heated and adapted to the occlusal surface of the stone model. A second layer is vacuum-processed over the entire model, which encloses the strip. The increased occlusal thickness of the appliance allows the vertical dimension and the occlusion to be adjusted.

When a mouth protector is formed by hand, the thermoplastic mouth-protector sheet is warmed in boiling water for about 20 seconds. Because the material has a tendency to lose its shape, it is heated by holding first one corner and then

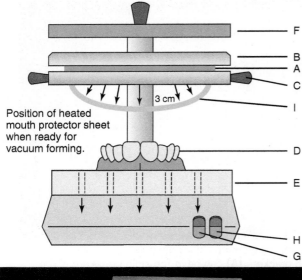

Position of heated mouth protector sheet when ready for vacuum forming.

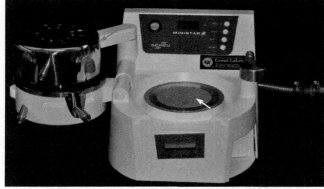

FIG 3-11 Illustration of typical vacuum-forming machine. The sheet of mouth protector material **(A)** is held between the upper clamp **(B)** and lower clamp **(C)**. The model **(D)** is centered on the perforated support plate **(E),** and the heater **(F)** is turned on by a switch **(H)**. Heating continues until the sheet sags about 3 cm (shown as **I,**) and then the vacuum switch **(G)** is turned on. The heated sheet is lowered quickly over the model using the plastic handles attached to the lower clamp **(C)**. The sheet is vacuum sealed to the support plate via the perforations and is then vacuum formed over the model. The heater is turned off and swung away 90 degrees using the attached handles; the vacuum is turned off after 30 to 60 seconds. The vacuum-formed mouth protector remains on the model until cool, and then trimming and finishing can begin. In the lower figure, an alternative newer device is shown that is used for mouthguard fabrication. This device uses positive pressure rather than a vacuum to adapt the softened mouthguard material to the model. The model is placed on the platform *(white arrow)*, then the upper member of the device *(red arrow)* is then swung over the platform, after which the mouthguard material is added, heated, and pressure applied. The positive pressure technique generally provides superior adaptation. (Lower figure: Courtesy Y-W Chen, University of Washington Department of Restorative Dentistry, Seattle, WA.)

another. Fingers are protected from the sticky material by wetting them with cold water or by using tongs. The material is draped over the model, and it is adapted to the model with the use of finger pressure. A wet towel helps in the adaptation. The mouth protector is trimmed and finished in the same manner described for the vacuum technique.

A strap can be attached to a custom-made mouth protector. Heat-seal a wide strap into a slit made in the mouth protector at the incisal edge of the maxillary central incisors. A tubular strap can be fabricated from three sizes of Tygon tubing. Both straps break away at low forces of 5 to 25 N (0.5 to 5 kg).

Two mistakes that are common to the fabrication of mouth protectors are (1) the use of a sooty flame during smoothing and (2) the reproduction of flaws in the model that do not exist in the arch. The use of a sooty flame during smoothing operations should be avoided because this type of flame blackens the mouth protector. When a model is handled and trimmed, the anatomy should not be changed because the protector will reproduce any changes in the model and thus not fit properly or comfortably on the arch.

The athlete is instructed in the proper hygiene of a mouth protector. The following instructions are enclosed in the plastic storage case given to the athlete.

After each use, the following steps should be performed:
1. Rinse your mouth protector under cold tap water.
2. Occasionally clean your mouth protector in a solution of soap and cool water.
3. Do not scrub your mouth protector with an abrasive dentifrice.
4. Do not use alcohol solutions or denture cleansers to clean your mouth protector.
5. Store your mouth protector in the container provided.

If necessary, identification may be placed on the buccal flange of the mouth protector with a laundry-marking pencil. Technique tips for mouth protectors are summarized in Box 3-1.

◉ QUICK REVIEW

Fluoride gels, rinses, and varnishes, pit and fissure sealants, and mouth protectors are dental materials designed to prevent disease or injury to the teeth and supporting tissues. Fluoride treatments are effective in lowering the incidence of dental caries depending on the method and frequency of application. Pits and fissures are responsible for the majority of dental caries in children. Sealants are effective in preventing caries when properly applied and completely retained. Intraoral mouth protectors prevent numerous athletic injuries each year. Players prefer custom-made protectors. Mouth protectors should be evaluated for breakdown frequently and replaced when necessary.

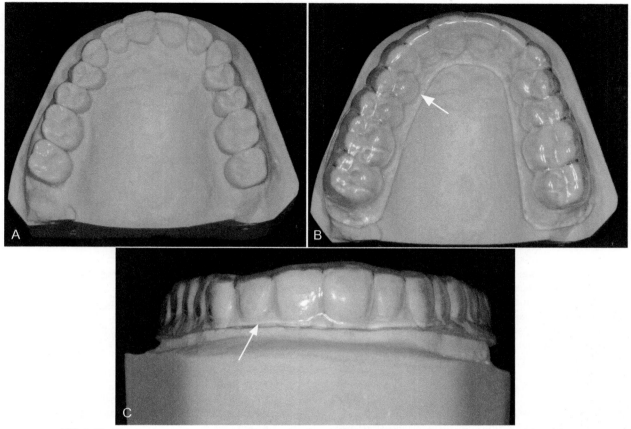

FIG 3-12 Finished mouth protector. The patient's original maxillary teeth are shown in **A**. After fabrication the mouth protector (**B,C,** *arrows*) is adapted closely to the teeth. The periphery is trimmed to just cover the teeth, and the edges are rounded to prevent intraoral soft tissue irritation. (Courtesy Y-W Chen, University of Washington Department of Restorative Dentistry, Seattle, WA.)

BOX 3-1   Technique Tips for Mouth Protectors

1. Ask the athlete to remove any removable appliances when taking the impression.
2. Block out fixed orthodontic appliances on the model.
3. Do not pour the palatal portion of the model.
4. Trim the mouth protector to avoid impinging on soft tissues.

5. Polish (round) the edges of the mouth protector with lab wheels and finish with an alcohol or butane flame.
6. Attach a strap at the incisal edge of the maxillary central incisors of the mouth protector by heat sealing it.

SELF-TEST QUESTIONS

In the following multiple-choice questions, one or more of the responses may be correct.

1. Which of the following statements best describe(s) the clinical effectiveness of fluoride gels?
   a. The clinical effectiveness of fluoride gels varies, depending in part on the method and frequency of application.
   b. The incidence of dental caries is not reduced significantly.
   c. Reductions in dental caries vary between 37% and 41% when a gel is applied monthly.
   d. A 1-minute application of APF gel is equally effective as a 4-minute application.

2. Which of the following statements is/are true?
   a. The reduction of pit and fissure caries has been accomplished by fluoridation of communal water supplies, topical application of fluoride during the development of enamel, and individual plaque-control programs.
   b. A smooth-based depression on the occlusal surface of a posterior tooth is termed a fissure.
   c. The uniqueness of pit and fissure caries is the result of the special anatomy of the occlusal surfaces of posterior teeth.
   d. The anatomy of the pit and fissure causes difficulty in diagnosing the early stages of dental caries.

3. A light-cured sealant contains which of the following?
   a. A dimethacrylate monomer diluted with a low molecular weight monomer
   b. An organic amine
   c. An organic peroxide initiator
   d. An absorber of visible light, such as a diketone

4. Which of the following statements is/are true?
   a. The compressive strength of pit and fissure sealants is less than that of enamel but more than that of dentin.
   b. The hardness of pit and fissure sealants is less than that of enamel and dentin.
   c. Retention of sealants is the result of chemical bonding to enamel.
   d. The penetration of a sealant could be reduced if evaporation of the diluent caused the viscosity of the sealant to increase.

5. Which of the following statements is/are true?
   a. The evaluation of any clinical study on sealants requires a statistical test of significance, the net gain as a result of treatment, and the percentage of effectiveness.
   b. A patient with sealant treatment should be recalled at 6-month intervals and have sealant reapplied after 2 years.
   c. After 2 years, values of retention and effectiveness of sealants on first permanent molars in children 5 to 9 years of age are both about 70%.
   d. Sealants appear to be retained better on permanent than on primary teeth.

6. Which of the following statements is/are true of the etching solution?
   a. It is usually a 37% phosphoric acid solution or gel.
   b. It is allowed to overetch the immediate vicinity of the fissure.
   c. It is applied liberally to the central fissure area but not allowed to contact other surfaces of the tooth.
   d. It is left on the tooth for 60 seconds and then rinsed away with water for 15 seconds.

7. Which of the following is/are true of application of the sealant?
   a. Can be done with a small tube (cannula)
   b. Should be done carefully to avoid overextending the sealant to unetched areas of enamel
   c. Should be done with isolation to prevent contamination of the etched surface with saliva
   d. Should be preceded by re-etching, rinsing, and drying if contamination of the enamel occurs

8. Which of the following statements is/are true?
   a. The setting time of an amine-accelerated sealant is about 60 seconds.
   b. A visible light-activated sealant will polymerize within 15 to 20 seconds after the light source is applied.
   c. A cotton pellet is used to remove sealant that fails to polymerize because of exposure to air.
   d. When successfully polymerized, the sealant should offer considerable resistance to attempts to penetrate it with the tip of an explorer.

9. Which of the following is/are used as athletic mouth protectors?
   a. Stock protector
   b. Mouth-formed protector
   c. Custom-made poly(methyl methacrylate) protector
   d. Custom-made poly(vinyl acetate)-polyethylene protector

10. Which of the following statements concerning the properties of a mouth protector is/are true?
    a. Select a harder material if the athlete complains about the feel of the protector and will not wear it.
    b. Pressure and heat can cause a mouth protector to become deformed permanently.
    c. Staining is generally not a problem with a mouth protector.
    d. Tearing of a mouth protector may be desirable if the tearing dissipates the energy of a blow.

11. When not in use, a mouth protector is stored in which of the following places?
    a. In distilled water
    b. In an immersion denture cleanser
    c. In a rigid plastic container
    d. On the model on which it was fabricated

12. The fabrication of a custom-made mouth protector requires which of the following?
    a. A silicone impression of the mandibular arch
    b. An alginate impression of the maxillary arch
    c. An alginate impression of the mandibular arch
    d. Alginate impressions of both arches
    e. Removable appliances to remain in the mouth when the impression is made

13. Which of the following statements concerning the fabrication of a mouth protector is/are true?
    a. High-strength stone provides the most durable model.
    b. Pour the model within 24 hours.
    c. It is not necessary to pour the palate in the model.
    d. Block out orthodontic appliances in the model with dental stone or wax.

14. Steps involved in finishing a mouth protector include which of the following?
    a. Trimming 3 mm short of the labial fold
    b. Notching the protector in the areas of the buccal and labial frenum
    c. Flaming the edges of the protector to smooth them
    d. Polishing the labial surfaces with extra-fine pumice

15. To form the protector from a poly(vinyl acetate)-polyethylene material using a vacuum-forming machine, which of the following steps is/are performed?
    a. Center the stone model on the vacuum former.
    b. Heat the thermoplastic sheet until it sags 3 cm.
    c. Lower the heated sheet in the frame over the model before turning on the vacuum.
    d. Cool the material for 1 minute before chilling it thoroughly in cold water.

Use short answers to fill in the following blanks.

16. The range of pH of neutral sodium fluoride gel is _____.

17. The penetration of a sealant into a fissure is affected by the configuration (_____ and_____) of the pit or fissure.

For the following statements, select true or false.

18. The recommended thickness of a mouth protector on occlusal surfaces is 2 mm.
    a. True
    b. False

19. The recommended Shore A hardness of a mouth protector is 55 to 85.
    a. True
    b. False

20. Laminating two sheets of mouth protector material will produce a desirable thickness by offsetting the shrinkage that results from forming the protector.
    a. True
    b. False

SUGGESTED SUPPLEMENTARY READINGS

Fluoride Gels and Varnishes

Academy of Dental Therapeutics and Stomatology: *Fluoride guide,* 2010, PennWell www.ineedce.com.

Farah JW, Powers JM, editors: Products for the dental hygienist, *Dent Advis* 23(6):1, 2006.

Farah JW, Powers JM, editors: Innovations in prevention: fluoride varnish and calcium phosphates, *Dent Advis* 27(2):1, 2010.

Pit and Fissure Sealants

Berry EA III: Air abrasion in clinical dental practice. In Hardin JF, editor: *Clark's clinical dentistry,* St Louis, 1996, Mosby.

Farah JW, Powers JM, editors: Pediatric dentistry, *Dent Advis* 23 (9):1, 2006.

Fiegel RJ: The use of pit and fissure sealants, *Pediatr Dent* 24:415, 2002.

Gilpin JL: Pit and fissure sealants: a review of the literature, *J Dent Hyg* 71:150, 1997.

Manton DJ, Messer LB: Pit and fissure sealants: another major cornerstone in preventive dentistry, *Aust Dent J* 40:22, 1995.

Seppä L, Leppänen T, Hausen H: Fluoride varnish versus acidulated phosphate fluoride gel: a 3-year clinical trial, *Caries Res* 29:327, 1995.

Simonsen RJ: Retention and effectiveness of dental sealant after 15 years, *J Am Dent Assoc* 122:34, 1991.

Simonsen RJ: Pit and fissure sealant [review of the literature], *Pediatr Dent* 24:393, 2002.

Waggoner WF, Siegal M: Pit and fissure application: updating the technique, *J Am Dent Assoc* 127:351, 1996.

Mouth Protectors

Craig RG, Godwin WC: Properties of athletic mouth protectors and materials, *J Oral Rehabil* 29:146, 2002.

DeYoung AK, Robinson E, Godwin WC: Comparing comfort and wearability: custom-made vs. self-adapted mouthguards, *J Am Dent Assoc* 125:1112, 1994.

Farah JW, Powers JM, editors: Mouth protectors and laboratory handpieces, *Dent Advis* 17(6):2, 2000.

Godwin WC, Craig RG, Koran A, et al: Mouth protection in junior football players, *Phys Sportsmed* 10:41, 1982.

Padilla RR, Lee TK: Pressure-laminated athletic mouth guards: a step-by-step process, *Calif Dent Assoc J* 27:200, 1999.

Soporowski NJ: Fabricating custom athletic mouthguards, *Mass Dent Soc J* 43(4):25, 1994.

Westerman B, Stringfellow PM, Eccleston JA: EVA mouthguards: how thick should they be? *Dent Traumatol* 18:24, 2002.

Wilkinson EE, Powers JM: Properties of custom-made mouth protector materials, *Phys Sportsmed* 14:77, 1986.

Wilkinson EE, Powers JM: Properties of stock and mouth-formed mouth protectors, *J Mich Dent Assoc* 68:83, 1986.

evolve Please visit *http://evolve.elsevier.com/Powers/dentalmaterials* for additional practice and study support tools.

APPENDIX 3-1 EQUATIONS

Penetration Coefficient

The rate of penetration is determined by the configuration (length, *l*, and radius, *r*) of the pit or fissure and by the penetration coefficient (PC) of the sealant:

$$\text{Rate} = \frac{r(\text{PC})}{2l}$$

The penetration coefficient is related to the surface tension (γ) and viscosity (η) of the sealant and the contact angle (θ) of the sealant on the enamel:

$$\text{PC} = \frac{\gamma(\cos\theta)}{(2\eta)}$$

4

Direct Esthetic Restorative Materials

OBJECTIVES

After reading this chapter, the student should be able to:

Composites
1. Describe the uses of universal composites.
2. Indicate components used in composites.
3. Describe properties of composites, and indicate their clinical importance.
4. Describe the manipulation of composites.

Composites for Special Applications
5. Describe the uses of composites for special applications, including flowable, bulk-fill, laboratory, core buildup, and provisional composites and repair of composites and ceramics.
6. Indicate components used in composites for special applications.
7. Describe properties of composites for special applications.
8. Describe the manipulation of composites for special applications.

Compomers
9. Describe the uses of compomers.
10. Indicate components used in compomers.
11. Describe properties of compomers.
12. Describe the manipulation of compomers.

Glass Ionomers
13. Describe the uses of glass ionomers.

14. Indicate components used in glass ionomers.
15. Describe properties of glass ionomers.
16. Describe the manipulation of glass ionomers.

Resin-Modified Glass Ionomers
17. Describe the uses of resin-modified glass ionomers.
18. Indicate components used in resin-modified glass ionomers.
19. Describe properties of resin-modified glass ionomers.
20. Describe the manipulation of resin-modified glass ionomers.

Bonding Agents
21. Indicate components used in bonding agents.
22. Describe properties of bonding agents, and indicate their clinical importance.
23. Describe the manipulation of bonding agents.
24. List dental materials that can interfere with the polymerization of bonding agents.

Light-Curing Units
25. List desirable features of light-curing units.
26. Describe precautions for protecting eyes of patients and staff.
27. Describe four factors that influence exposure times for polymerization of composites.

The need for restorative materials that have the appearance of natural tooth tissue and that can be placed directly into a cavity preparation in a paste condition is great (Figure 4-1). The patient desires esthetic restorations, particularly in the anterior portion of the mouth, and a direct filling material is advantageous in terms of the time required and the cost of the restoration. Selection of a material is made based on a need for esthetics, fluoride release, wear resistance, strength, and ease of use.

Currently, four types of materials are being used as direct esthetic dental restorations: (1) composites; (2) compomers; (3) resin-modified glass ionomers; and (4) glass ionomers (Figure 4-1). Composites were introduced about 1960 and now dominate the materials used for direct esthetic restorations. Glass ionomers were introduced in 1972 and have been used primarily for restoration of cervically eroded areas. Resin-modified glass ionomers were introduced in the early 1990s to provide better esthetics than glass ionomers. Compomers were introduced in 1995 to provide improved handling and fluoride release compared with composites.

Composites are esthetically pleasing, strong, and wear resistant but have low or no fluoride release. Compomers are less wear resistant but are esthetically pleasing and release fluoride. Resin-modified glass ionomers release more fluoride than compomers do but are not as wear resistant and are not used in posterior restorations. Glass ionomers release the most fluoride and are best for patients with a high risk of caries in low-stress applications. Uses of composites, compomers, resin-modified ionomers, and glass ionomers are listed in Table 4-1. Typical products, including composites for special applications, are listed in Table 4-2.

COMPOSITES

Composite restoratives generally are recommended for Classes III to V and for Class I when occlusal stress is not a problem and appearance is crucial. Although less durable than amalgam, composites designed for Class II posterior applications are used in about 50% of these restorations.

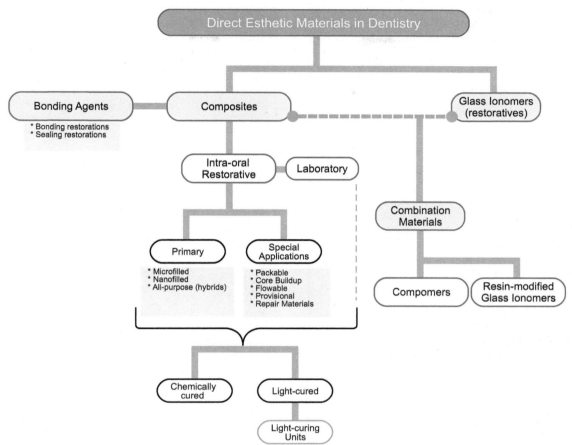

FIG 4-1 Direct esthetic materials have increased in use and in complexity over the years. Originally, composites and glass ionomers were completely separate classes of materials, but combination materials have evolved to provide more treatment options. Initially, no bonding of composites was possible to enamel or dentin, but over time, bonding agents were developed from composite components that allowed bonding to enamel and dentin. Finally, the activation ("curing") of composites also has evolved. The use of visible (mostly blue) light to activate the polymerization of composites has revolutionized composite use; original composites were chemically activated only.

Composites also can be classified as universal, flowable, laboratory, microfilled, and nanofilled composites, uses of which are listed in Table 4-1. Typical products are listed in Table 4-2. Composites are also used for provisional restorations and core buildups and in fiber-reinforced posts.

Composition and Reaction

Composites consist of three phases: resin matrix, dispersed inorganic filler particles, and silane coupling agent on the filler particles to produce a good bond between the matrix and the filler.

Filler Size

Currently, most composites have fillers with average diameters of 0.2 to 3 μm (fine particles) or 0.04 μm (microfine particles). The fraction of particles having diameters of 0.04 μm varies from a few percent to 35% by weight. The volume percentage of filler particles is lower than the weight percentage because of the higher density of the filler compared with that of the polymer matrix. Nanofilled composites have fillers ranging in size from 1 to 10 nanometers (nm), although these fillers may be present as clusters of a larger size.

Figure 4-2 illustrates the two main classes of composites. Microhybrid composites (Figure 4-2, *A*) contain blends of fine and microfine filler particles with as much as 84% filler by weight. The microfine filler particles fit in spaces between the fine filler particles, producing a total filler concentration of 70% by volume, which results in improved properties.

Microfilled composites (Figure 4-2, *B*) contain microfine fillers with high surface areas. Only 35% to 50% by volume of these particles can be used with the resin matrix and still produce a paste of acceptable viscosity. Some microfilled composites use fillers that are polymer particles reinforced with microfine particles, which are then mixed with the resin matrix; these reinforced filler particles may be as large as 10 to 20 μm. These products allow the incorporation of more microfilled fillers and yield a paste with reasonable viscosity.

Filler Composition

Quartz, lithium aluminum silicate, and barium, strontium, zinc, or ytterbium glasses have been used as fine fillers. Microfine fillers are colloidal silica particles. Fine fillers that contain barium, strontium, zinc, or ytterbium atoms are radiopaque,

TABLE 4-1 Uses of Composites, Compomers, Resin-Modified Glass Ionomers, and Glass Ionomers

Type	Uses
Universal composite	Class I, II, III, IV, V, patients with low risk of caries
Microfilled composite	Class III, V
Nanofilled composite	Class I, II, III, IV, V
Bulk-filled composite	Class I, II, VI (mesial, occlusal, distal=MOD)
Flowable composite	Cervical lesions, pediatric restorations, small, low-stress-bearing restorations
Universal flowable composite	Class I, II, III, IV, V, patients with low risk of caries
Laboratory composite	Class II, three-unit bridge (with fiber reinforcement)
Compomer	Cervical lesions, Class III primary teeth, Class I, II restorations in children, Class II (with sandwich technique), patients with medium risk of caries
Resin-modified glass ionomer	Cervical lesions, Class III, V, II (with sandwich technique), pediatric restorations primary teeth, Class I restorations in children, sandwich technique (Class II), patients with a high risk of caries
Glass ionomer	Cervical lesions, Class V restorations in adults in whom esthetics is less important than that of other types, patients with a high risk of caries

TABLE 4-2 Typical Composites, Compomers, Resin-Modified Glass Ionomers, and Glass Ionomers, Including Composites for Special Applications

Type	Product	Manufacturer
Microhybrid composites	Estelite Sigma Quick	Tokuyama Dental America (Burlingame, CA)
Microfilled composites	Durafill VS	Heraeus (South Bend, IN)
Nanofilled composites	Filtek Supreme Plus Universal Restorative	3M ESPE (St. Paul, MN)
Bulk-filled composites	Tetric EvoCeram Bulk Fill Nano-Hybrid Composite Restorative	Ivoclar Vivadent
	Surefil	DENTSPLY Caulk (Milford, DE)
Flowable composites	Filtek Supreme Plus Flowable Restorative	3M ESPE
	Surefil SDR flow	DENTSPLY Caulk
Flowable composites (self-adhesive)	Fusion Liquid Dentin	Pentron Clinical
Laboratory composites	Tescera ATL	Bisco Dental Products (Schaumburg, IL)
Laboratory composites (milled)	Lava Ultimate	3M ESPE
Compomers	Dyract eXtra	DENTSPLY Caulk
Glass ionomers	GC Fuji II	GC America
Resin-modified glass ionomers	GC Fuji II LC	GC America
	Ketac Nano Light-Curing Glass Ionomer Restorative	3M ESPE
Composites for special applications		
Core buildup	LuxaCore Z-Dual	DMG America (Englewood, NJ)
	Clearfil PhotoCore PLT	Kuraray America (New York, NY)
Provisional composites	Luxatemp Fluorescence	DMG America

with the radiopacity proportional to the volume fraction of the filler. Quartz (crystalline silica) and lithium aluminum silicate are not radiopaque. Manufacturers specify if a composite is radiopaque or not. Radiopaque composites are used to restore posterior teeth.

Coupling Agents

To provide a good bond between the inorganic fillers and the resin matrix, manufacturers treat the surface of the filler with silane, which has groups that react with the inorganic filler and other groups that react with the organic matrix.

> **! ALERT**
>
> Silanes are bifunctional, silicon-organic compounds that couple inorganic filler particles and resin matrix.

Resin Matrix

The most common resins are based on dimethacrylate (Bis-GMA, bisphenol A-glycidyl methacrylate) or urethane dimethacrylate (UDMA) oligomers. A highly simplified formula in which R represents any of a large number of organic groups (e.g., phenyl-, methyl-, carboxyl-, hydroxyl-, and amide-) follows:

$$CH_2 = C - R - C = CH_2$$
$$| \qquad |$$
$$CH_3 \quad CH_3$$

Bis — GMA or UDMA

> **! ALERT**
>
> An oligomer is a moderate molecular weight organic molecule made from two or more organic molecules.

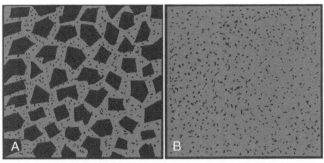

FIG 4-2 Two-dimensional diagrams of microhybrid composite **(A)** and microfilled composite **(B)**.

Bis-GMA and UDMA oligomers are viscous liquids to which low-molecular-weight monomers (dimethacrylates) are added to control the consistency of the composite paste. Oligomers and the low molecular weight monomers are characterized by carbon double bonds that react to convert them to a polymer.

Initiators and Accelerators

The principal system used to achieve polymerization (setting) is the visible light-curing system. In this system, the composite is polymerized by exposure to an intense blue light. The light is absorbed by a diketone, which, in the presence of an organic amine, starts the polymerization reaction. Exposure times of 20 to 40 seconds are needed for polymerization. Because blue light is necessary to start the reaction, the diketone and amine can be in the same composite paste, and no reaction occurs until it is exposed to blue light. Light-curing units are described later in this chapter.

In self-curing systems, polymerization is accomplished with an organic peroxide initiator and an organic amine accelerator. The initiator and accelerator must be kept separated and not mixed until just before the restoration is placed.

Regardless of the system used, the following general reaction takes place:

Dimethacrylate + Initiator + Accelerator

+ Treated inorganic filler → Dental resin composite

Pigments

Inorganic pigments are added in small amounts so that the color of the composite matches the tooth structure. Typically, composites are provided in 10 or more shades, which cover the normal range of human teeth (yellow to gray). Highly pigmented tints can be mixed with the standard shades to match the color of teeth outside the normal range. Special shades for bleached teeth are also available.

Composites have been developed with enamel, dentin, cervical, and opaque shades for special techniques in esthetic dentistry. These multipurpose composites can be placed in one layer or several layers to improve esthetics. Examples of these special composites are listed in Table 4-2.

PROPERTIES

Important properties of composites include the following:
1. Low polymerization shrinkage
2. Low water sorption
3. Coefficient of thermal expansion similar to tooth structure
4. High fracture resistance
5. High wear resistance
6. High radiopacity
7. High bond strength to enamel and dentin
8. Good color match to tooth structure
9. Ease of manipulation
10. Ease of finishing and polishing

Some of these qualities are more important for anterior or posterior applications. Values for a variety of properties are presented in Table 4-3 for microhybrid and microfilled composites. The nanofilled composites have values similar to those for the microhybrid composites.

Polymerization Shrinkage

Microhybrid composites shrink less during setting than microfilled types because the microhybrid composites have less resin. Even with acid etching of enamel and dentin and use of bonding agents, stresses from polymerization shrinkage can exceed the bond strength of a composite to tooth structure, and, as a result, marginal leakage can occur.

Low-shrinkage and low-stress composites (GC Kalore, GC America, Alsip, IL; N'Durance, Septodont, Louisville, CO)

TABLE 4-3 Properties of Microhybrid and Microfilled Composites

Property	Microhybrid composite*	Microfilled composite
Polymerization shrinkage (% linear)	1.0–1.7	2–3
Thermal conductivity (10^{-4} cal/sec/cm^2 [°C/cm])	25–30	2–15
Linear coefficient of thermal expansion ($\times 10^{-6}$/°C)	25–38	55–68
Water sorption (mg/cm^2)	0.3–0.6	1.2–2.2
Radiopacity (mm Al)[†]	2.7–5.7	—
Compressive strength (MPa)	200–340	230–290
Diametral tensile strength (MPa)	34–62	26–33
Flexural strength (MPa)	90–140	—
Elastic modulus in compression (GPa)	8–14	3–5
Flexural modulus (GPa)	5–18	—
Knoop hardness (kg/mm^2)	55–80	22–36
Bond strength to enamel and dentin with bonding agent (MPa)	14–30	14–30

*Nanofilled composites have properties similar to microhybrid composites.
[†]If advertised as radiopaque. Enamel is 4.0 mm Al (millimeters of aluminum) and dentin is 2.5 mm Al.

have been introduced. These composites have modified resin and filler systems that result in reduced polymerization shrinkage and stress.

Two techniques have been proposed to overcome or minimize the effect of polymerization shrinkage. One method is to insert and polymerize the composite in layers, which reduces the effective shrinkage. The second method is to prepare a laboratory (indirect) composite inlay on a die and then to cement the inlay to the tooth with a thin layer of low-viscosity resin cement as discussed later in this chapter.

Thermal Conductivity

The thermal conductivity of a composite is much lower than that for metallic restorations (see Table 2-2) and closely matches that of enamel and dentin. Therefore, composites provide good thermal insulation for the dental pulp.

Thermal Expansion

Typical values for microhybrid and microfilled composites are shown in Table 4-3. Because the thermal expansion of composites is greater than that of tooth structure (see Table 2-1), composite restorations have a greater change in dimensions with changes in oral temperatures than tooth structure. The more resin matrix, the higher is the linear coefficient of thermal expansion because the polymer has a higher value than the filler. As a result, microfilled composites have higher values for thermal expansion than microhybrid composites.

Water Sorption

Values of water sorption of microhybrid and microfilled composites are given in Table 4-2. The microfilled composites have a greater potential for discoloration by water-soluble stains. Water sorption is accompanied by swelling of the composite, but this has not been an effective way to counteract polymerization shrinkage. However, the effect of water sorption on degradation of properties of composites is irreversible.

Radiopacity

Most microhybrid composites are radiopaque. One microfilled composite (Heliomolar, Ivoclar Vivadent, Amherst, NY) contains ytterbium trifluoride, which makes it radiopaque. Most composites are radiopaque when compared with dentin but are radiolucent when compared with enamel. Argument exists whether radiopacity is an advantage in diagnosis; nevertheless, not all composites appear radiopaque on dental radiographs.

Compressive and Flexural Strengths

The compressive strength of microhybrid composites is higher than that of microfilled composites. Strength generally increases linearly with the volume fraction of filler. Because composite restorations most likely fail in tension or bending, their tensile and flexural strengths are of special interest (see Table 4-3).

Elastic Modulus

The elastic modulus, or stiffness, of the composites is dominated by the amount of filler and increases exponentially with the volume fraction of filler. The lower filler content of the microfilled composites results in elastic moduli of one fourth to one half of the more highly filled microhybrid composites. This stiffness is important in applications in which high biting forces are involved and wear resistance is essential. However, the rate of bond failure of Class V cervical restorations was higher for microhybrid composites when compared with microfilled composites; the lower modulus of the microfilled composites probably reduced the stress on the bond of the restoration to dentin. Values of elastic modulus in compression and bending are listed in Table 4-3.

Hardness and Wear

Knoop hardness of composites (see Table 4-3) is related exponentially to the volume fraction of filler and is less related to the hardness of the filler. The higher filler content of microhybrid composites is important to provide higher resistance to nonrecoverable penetration and abrasive wear. Abrasive wear is, however, only one aspect of the wear process and is described in the section on clinical qualities.

Bond Strength

The bond strength of composites to acid-etched enamel and dentin is about the same (14 to 30 MPa) when a universal bonding agent is used.

Etching of the enamel and dentin are recommended to remove the smear layer, which results from cavity preparation, before application of the bonding agent. Most bonding agents require polymerization before placement of the composite. Because polymerization stresses are of the same magnitude as the bond strengths to tooth structure, marginal leakage may not be prevented entirely. Bond strength of 20 MPa is an estimated requirement to prevent marginal gaps as a result of polymerization shrinkage. Bonding agents are described in detail later in this chapter.

Qualitative ranking of properties of various types of composites and other restorative materials are listed in Table 4-4.

Clinical Qualities
Wear

Clinical studies have shown that composites are superior materials for anterior restorations in which esthetics is essential and occlusal forces are low. Color changes are minimal; marginal adaptation is good; recurrent decay is low. One problem with composites is the loss of surface contour of composite restorations in the mouth, which results from a combination of abrasive wear from chewing and tooth brushing and erosive wear from degradation of the composite in the oral environment.

Wear of posterior composite restorations is observed at the contact area where stresses are the highest. Ditching at the margins within the composite also is observed for posterior composites, probably as a result of inadequate bonding and stresses. Currently accepted composites for posterior

TABLE 4-4   Ranking of Selected Properties of Microhybrid and Microfilled Composites, Compomers, Resin-Modified Glass Ionomers, and Glass Ionomers

Property	Microhybrid composite	Microfilled composite	Compomer	Glass ionomer	Resin-Modified Glass ionomer
Compressive strength	High	Med–high	Med–high	Low–med	Med
Flexural strength	High	Med–high	Med–high	Low–med	Med
Flexural modulus	High	Med–high	Med–high	Med–high	Med
Wear resistance	High	Med–high	Med–high	Low	Med
Fluoride release	Low	Low	Low–med	High	Med–high
Fluoride rechargeability	Low	Low	Low–med	High	Med–high
Esthetics	Excellent	Excellent	Excellent	Poor	Good

applications require clinical studies that demonstrate over a 5-year period a loss of surface contour less than 250 μm or an average of 50 μm per year of clinical service. Products developed as posterior or packable composites usually have better wear resistance than anterior or all-purpose composites.

Postoperative Sensitivity

Sensitivity associated with composite restorations has been reported in about 10% of cases. It most likely results from microleakage of bacteria or induced internal stress. Incremental placement of the composite, excellent isolation during placement, and use of bases to protect the pulp, as described in the next section, are recommended solutions.

Manipulation
Etching and Bonding

To achieve a bond between the composite and the tooth structure, the tooth must be etched and primed. With fourth- and fifth-generation bonding agents, the enamel and dentin of the cavity preparation are etched with acid for 30 seconds with an etchant supplied by the manufacturer, frequently 37% phosphoric acid solution or gel. The acid is flushed away with water, and the surface is dried gently with a stream of air. The etched enamel will appear dull; a magnified view of an etched enamel surface is shown in Figure 4-3. With sixth- and seventh-generation and universal bonding agents, etching and priming are accomplished at the same time, and no rinsing is required. The bonding agent penetrates the etched enamel and dentin surfaces and provides micromechanical retention of the restoration. Bonding agents and their interactions with tooth structure are discussed later in this chapter.

Single-Paste Composites

These composites are supplied in various shades in disposable syringes and compules, examples of which are shown in Figure 4-4. The syringes are made of opaque plastic to protect the material from exposure to light and thus provide adequate shelf life. The compule is placed on the end of the syringe, and the paste is extruded after removal of the protective tip. The advantages of compules are ease of placement of the composite paste, decrease in cross infection, and protection of the paste from exposure to ambient light. Single-paste composites are light activated, a process that is discussed later in this chapter.

Two-Paste Composites

Self-cured core composites are supplied in an auto-mixed cartridge (Figure 4-5, *A*) with mixing and intraoral tips or an auto-mixed syringe (Figure 4-5, *B*). The paste with the peroxide initiator, or catalyst, and the paste with the amine accelerator are mixed with the special mixing tip and placed directly on the preparation with the intraoral tip. After mixing, self-cured composites have a working time of 1 to 11/2 minutes. The mix will begin to harden, and the material should not be disturbed from this time until the setting time of about 4 to 5 minutes from the start of the mix.

Dual-cured composites are also supplied in auto-mixed cartridges and contain chemical accelerators and light activators so that polymerization can be initiated by light and then continued by the self-cured mechanism. Because some dual-cured composites set by a self-curing mechanism without activation by light, the manufacturer's instructions must be reviewed carefully before use.

Pulpal Protection

Before the composite is inserted, the pulp may be protected with a cavity liner ($Ca[OH]_2$) or glass ionomer, resin-modified glass ionomer, compomer or bioceramic base. Liners and bases are described in Chapter 7.

Insertion

The composite can be inserted into the cavity preparation by several methods. It can be placed with a plastic or an instrument with disposable elastomeric tips (Figure 4-6), which do not stick to the composite during insertion. The composite also may be placed into the plastic tip of a syringe and then injected into the cavity preparation. The syringe allows the use of small mixes, reduces the problem of incorporating voids in the composite during insertion, and facilitates placement of the material in the areas of retention.

Finishing and Polishing

For gross reduction, diamonds, carbide finishing burs, finishing disks, or strips of alumina are used. For final finishing, abrasive-impregnated rubber rotary instruments or disks or a rubber cup with various polishing pastes is used. Finishing is performed in a wet field with a water-soluble lubricant. Final finishing of light-cured composites can be started

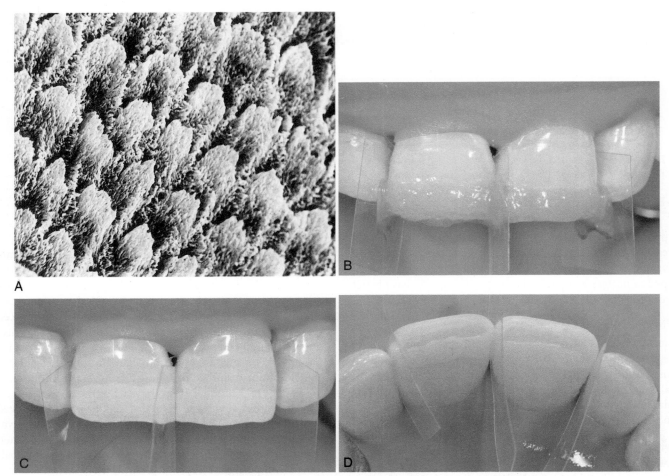

FIG 4-3 Enamel acid etching. **(A)** At a microscopic level, the enamel rods are differentially etched when subjected to a 37% phosphoric acid solution for 10–15 seconds. The rods do not all etch away at the same rate, leaving a rough post-etch surface that facilitates bonding. **(B)** The acid is generally in a blue gel; the gel sequesters the acid to the desired location. The blue color allows the operator to see where the acid is. The clear matrix strips prevent undesirable etching of the adjacent teeth. **(C, D)** After rinsing and drying, the etched area may be identified by the dull, opaque, whiter appearance. The change in surface color is a result of the roughness seen in **A** at the microscopic level. (**A,** Courtesy J. B. Dennison, University of Michigan School of Dentistry, Ann Arbor, MI; **B–D,** Courtesy Y-W Chen, University of Washington Department of Restorative Dentistry, Seattle, WA.)

immediately after light curing. Finishing of composites is important because a smooth surface is desired to prevent retention of plaque and is needed to maintain good oral hygiene. Microfilled and nanofilled composites have lower surface roughness and higher gloss than microhybrid composites after polishing. Various finishing and polishing instruments for composites are described in Chapter 6. Technique tips for resin composites are summarized in Box 4-1.

COMPOSITES FOR SPECIAL APPLICATIONS

Flowable Composites

Traditional low-viscosity composites (see Table 4-2) are light-cured and recommended for cervical lesions, pediatric restorations, and other small, low-stress-bearing restorations. They contain dimethacrylate resin and inorganic fillers with

a particle size of 0.4 to 3.0 μm and filler loading of 42% to 53% by volume. Newer universal flowable (syringeable) composites have higher filler content and can be used in load-bearing restorations.

Flowable composites have a low modulus of elasticity, which may make them useful in cervical erosion and abfraction areas. A cervically eroded tooth (Figure 4-7, *A*) can be restored with flowable composite (Figure 4-7, *B*). Because of their lower filler content, flowable composites exhibit higher polymerization shrinkage and lower wear resistance than microhybrid composites. The low viscosity of these composites allows them to be dispensed by a syringe for easy handling. Recently, a low-stress flowable composite (Surefil SDR flow, DENTSPLY Caulk, Milford, DE) with modified resin chemistry has been introduced. Universal flowable composites have properties similar to universal composites.

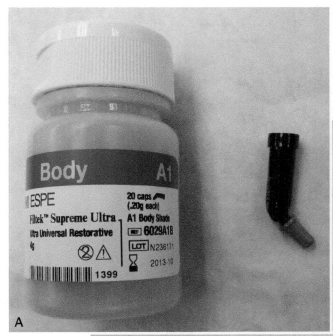

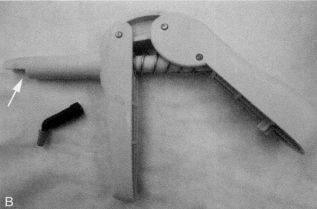

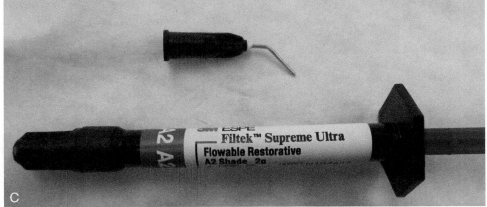

FIG 4-4 Today most composites come in syringes or compules. Compules **(A)** are disposable aliquots of single-paste composite, in a black light-proof container to prevent premature setting from exposure to visible light. The compules fit into a dispensing syringe **(B,** *at arrow)*; the compule is discarded after a single clinical use. Other single paste composites are dispensed in a syringe, which may have various types of dispensing tips. The flowable composite shown in **C** has a very small tip for precise placement and control of this low viscosity composite.

Another innovation is the self-adhesive flowable composite (Fusio Liquid Dentin, Pentron Clinical, Wallingford, CT; Vertise Flow, Kerr Corporation, Orange, CA). These composites bond to dentin without the use of a separate bonding agent.

Bulk-Fill Composites

These composites (see Table 4-2) are recommended for use in Class I, II (MOD, mesial-occlusal-distal), and VI cavity preparations. They are composed of light-activated, dimethacrylate resins with fillers that are fibers or porous or irregular particles with a filler loading of 66% to 70% by volume. The interaction of the filler particles or modifications of the resin matrix cause these composites to be packable.

Important properties include high depth of cure, low polymerization shrinkage, radiopacity, and low wear rate (3.5 μm/year), which is similar to that of amalgam. The bulk-fill technique has been demonstrated to be effective in short-term clinical studies. Light-cured bonding agents are used with these composites.

Laboratory Composites

Crowns, inlays, veneers bonded to metal substructures, and metal-free bridges are prepared indirectly on dies from composites processed in the laboratory (see Table 4-2) using various combinations of light, heat, pressure, and vacuum, which increase the polymerization and the wear resistance. Recently, precured composites for in-office and laboratory milling have become available. Restorations usually are cemented with resin cements. Cavity preparations for indirect composites must be nonretentive rather than retentive as typically prepared for direct placement.

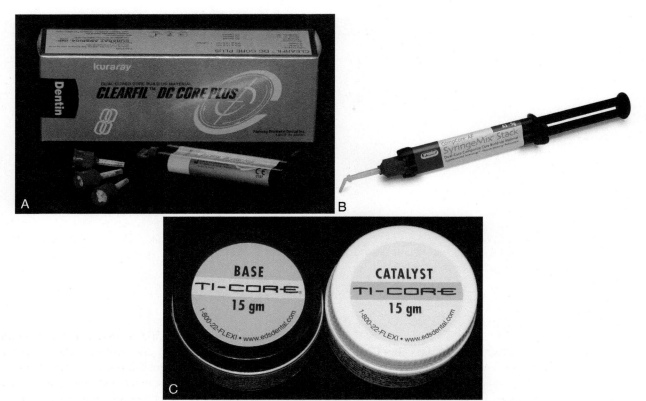

FIG 4-5 Two-paste composites. These composites have the ability to cure without exposure to light; these are needed because often it is impossible to adequately irradiate the restorative material in large or deep areas of buildup restorations or in root canals. They can be formulated in an auto-mixed cartridge **(A)** or an auto-mix syringe **(B)** or as two pastes that are mixed by hand **(C)**. In some cases (as in **A**), the core materials are dual cured, which permits faster clinical initial setting times. In any case, the manufacturer's instructions for use should be consulted and closely followed. (**A, C,** Courtesy Y-W Chen, University of Washington Department of Restorative Dentistry, Seattle, WA; **B,** Courtesy Premier Dental Products, Plymouth Meeting, PA.)

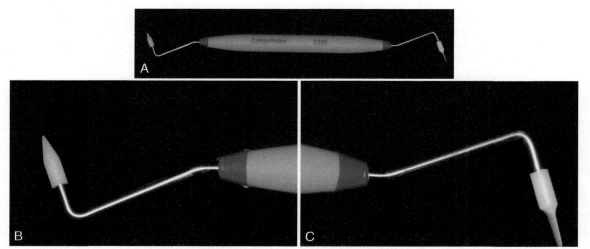

FIG 4-6 Instruments for manipulating dental composites. Composite instruments like the one in **(A)** are designed to facilitate shaping of the composite prior to photo-activation; in this manner, less time can be spent polishing and less material is needed. A variety of instrument shapes **(B, C)** are available. The instrument materials (generally plastic, specially coated alloys, or Teflon® materials) are designed to minimize sticking of the paste composite material to the instrument. (Courtesy Y-W Chen, University of Washington Department of Restorative Dentistry, Seattle, WA.)

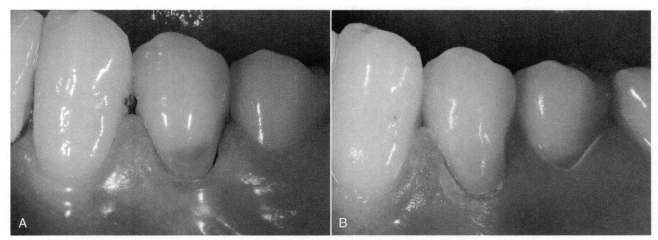

FIG 4-7 (A) Cervically eroded tooth. **(B)** Tooth (viewed immediately postoperatively) restored with a flowable composite. (Courtesy K. L. O'Keefe, Houston, TX.)

Core Buildup Composites

At times, so much tooth structure is lost from caries that the crown of the tooth must be built up to receive a crown. Amalgam is the most common core material, but composite is popular, especially as cores for all-ceramic restorations. Composite core materials are typically two-paste, self-cured composites, although light-cured and dual-cured products are available. Core composites usually are tinted (blue, white, opaque) to provide a contrasting color with the tooth structure. Some products release fluoride. Examples of composite core buildup materials are listed in Table 4-2. An example of a core composite is shown in Figure 4-5.

Composite cores have the following advantages as compared with amalgam: they can be bonded to dentin, can be finished immediately, are easy to contour, have high rigidity, and have good color under all-ceramic restorations. Bonding agents are used to bond composite cores to remaining enamel and dentin. A bonding agent recommended by the manufacturer of the core material should be used because some self-cured composite core materials are incompatible with some light-cured bonding agents.

Provisional Composites

Temporary inlays, crowns, and long-span bridges typically are fabricated from composite or acrylic resins. The purposes of provisional restorations are to maintain the position of the prepared tooth, seal and insulate the preparation and protect the margins, establish proper vertical dimension, aid in diagnosis and treatment planning, and evaluate esthetic replacements. Examples of composite provisional materials are listed in Table 4-2. The properties of acrylic and composite provisional materials are compared in Table 4-5.

Repair of Ceramic or Composite

One of the main concerns in these repairs is the bond strength between the remaining silica-based ceramic or composite and the added composite. To achieve the maximum bond strength, the remaining porcelain is cleaned and surface-treated with a silane supplied in a liquid form. The silane is supplied separately, and a chosen composite is used with it. Zirconia-based ceramics require special primers (Clearfil Ceramic Primer, Kuraray America, New York, NY; Monobond Plus, Ivoclar Vivadent, Amherst, NY).

The repair of composites is accomplished by abrading of the surface of the remaining composite with 50 µm alumina and then keeping the surface well isolated from saliva and moisture. The surface of the composite is treated with silane, and the new composite is added. Repair bond strength is about 60% to 80% of the cohesive strength of the original composite.

COMPOMERS

Compomers are composites modified with polyacid groups and are used for restorations in low-stress-bearing areas, although a recent product (Dyract AP, DENTSPLY Caulk, Milford, DE) is recommended by the manufacturer for Class I and II restorations in adults (see Table 4-1). Compomers are recommended for patients with medium caries risk.

BOX 4-1 Technique Tips for Resin Composites

1. Cover dispensed composite with an orange shield to minimize initiation of curing by operatory lights.
2. Place and cure universal composites in 2-mm increments and cure for 20 seconds. Darker shades may require a longer light activation of 40 seconds. Bulk-fill composites can be cured in 4-mm increments.
3. Perform finishing and polishing in a wet field.

TABLE 4-5   Comparison of Properties of Acrylic and Composite Provisional Materials

Characteristics of acrylic	Characteristics of composite
Advantages	
Better color stability	Lower heat release during curing
Esthetic, with many shades	Less shrinkage on curing
Doughy stage for easy handling	Higher flexural strength
Less expensive	Better wear resistance
	Excellent tissue biocompatibility
Disadvantages	
Higher heat release during curing	Harder, more brittle
Higher shrinkage on curing	Expensive
Poor smell and taste	

Composition and Reaction

Compomers contain monomers modified by polyacid groups with fluoride-releasing silicate glasses and are formulated without water. Some compomers have modified monomers that provide additional fluoride release. Among current products, the filler-volume percentage ranges from 42% to 67%, and the average filler-particle size ranges from 0.8 to 5.0 μm. Compomers are packaged as single-paste formulations in compules and syringes. Setting occurs primarily by light-cured polymerization, but an acid-base reaction also occurs as the compomer absorbs water after placement and on contact with saliva. Water uptake is also important for fluoride transfer.

Properties

Compomers release fluoride by a mechanism similar to that of glass and resin-modified glass ionomers. As a result of the lower amount of glass ionomer present in compomers, the amount of fluoride release and its duration are lower than those of glass and resin-modified glass ionomers. Also, compomers do not recharge from fluoride treatments or brushing with fluoride dentifrices as much as glass and resin-modified glass ionomers.

Manipulation

Compomers are formulated as a single paste packaged in unit-dose compules. Because of their resin content, compomers require a bonding agent to bond to tooth structure.

GLASS IONOMERS

Glass ionomers are used in cervical and Class V restorations in adults where esthetics is not critical. They are recommended for patients with a high risk of caries (see Table 4-1).

Composition and Reaction

Glass ionomers are supplied as powders of various shades and as a liquid and can be packaged as unit-dose capsules (Figure 4-8). The powder is an aluminosilicate glass, and the liquid is a water solution of polymers and copolymers of acrylic acid. The material sets as a result of the metallic salt bridges between the Al^{+3} and the Ca^{+2} ions and the acid groups on the polymers. The reaction goes to completion slowly and is protected from saliva with a varnish.

Properties

The properties of glass ionomer restoratives are compared qualitatively with other restorative materials in Table 4-4. Properties especially noteworthy are a modulus that is similar to dentin, bond strength to dentin of 2 to 3 MPa, an expansion coefficient comparable to that of tooth structure, low solubility, and fairly high opacity.

Although the bond strength of glass ionomers to dentin is lower than that of composites, clinical studies have shown that the retention of glass ionomers in areas of cervical erosion is considerably better than the retention for composites. When the dentin is etched, the glass ionomer may be used without a cavity preparation. Available enamel should be acid-etched to provide additional retention. Four-year clinical data showed a retention rate for glass ionomer cervical restorations of 75%. The surfaces of the restorations seen in the studies were noticeably rough, and some shade mismatches were present. Pulp reaction to glass ionomers was mild; if the thickness of dentin is less than 1 mm, a calcium hydroxide liner should be used. Also, cervical restorations did not contribute to inflammation of gingival tissues. The fluoride in the glass ionomer is released over a period

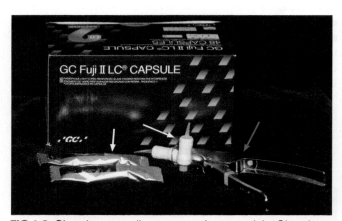

FIG 4-8 Glass ionomer direct restorative materials. Glass ionomers are available in unit dose capsules *(white arrows)* that are mixed in a triturator and then loaded into a delivery device *(red arrow)*. Setting times are much faster than for chemically activated composites; light curing is available (dual-cure) if the glass ionomer constituents have been modified with resins and photo-activators. (Courtesy Y-W Chen, University of Washington Department of Restorative Dentistry, Seattle, WA.)

of 2 years. Less *Streptococcus mutans* exists in plaque adjacent to glass ionomer restorations.

Manipulation

Glass ionomers are packaged in bottles and in capsules. The powder and liquid are dispensed in proper amounts on the paper pad, and half the powder is incorporated to produce a homogeneous milky consistency. The remainder of the powder is added, and a total mixing time of 30 to 40 seconds is used with a typical setting time of 4 minutes. After the restorative is placed and the correct contour carved, the surface should be protected from saliva by an application of varnish. Trimming and finishing are done after 24 hours.

The liquid in the capsule is forced into the powder by use of a press and is mixed by means of a mechanical mixer for amalgam (see Chapter 5). The mixture is injected through the use of the special syringe.

Clinical techniques for glass ionomers should be adhered to rigidly, with maintenance of isolation, adequate etching procedures, protection of the restoration from saliva after placement, and delay of final finishing for 1 day or longer with most products.

RESIN-MODIFIED GLASS IONOMERS

Resin-modified glass ionomers, or hybrid ionomers, are used for restorations in low-stress-bearing areas and are recommended for patients with a high risk of caries (see Table 4-1). These restorations are more esthetically pleasing than glass ionomers because of the resin content.

Composition and Reaction

The powder of resin-modified glass ionomers is similar to that of glass ionomers. The liquid contains monomers, polyacids, and water. Resin-modified glass ionomers set by acid-base and both light-cured and self-cured resin polymerization reactions. Placing a dentin-bonding agent before inserting a resin-modified glass ionomer is contraindicated because it decreases fluoride release.

Properties

Resin-modified glass ionomers bond to tooth structure without the use of a dentin-bonding agent. Typically, the tooth is conditioned (etched) with polyacrylic acid or a primer before placement of the resin-modified glass ionomer. Resin-modified glass ionomers release more fluoride than compomers and composites do but less fluoride than glass ionomers. Resin-modified glass ionomers recharge when exposed to fluoride treatments or fluoride dentifrices.

Manipulation

Resin-modified glass ionomers are packaged as powder-liquid encapsulated or paste-paste forms. Their manipulation is like that of glass ionomers. Unlike glass ionomer restorations, resin-modified glass ionomers set immediately when light cured and can be finished immediately.

BONDING AGENTS

Bonding agents are used with composites to provide an adequate bond to enamel and dentin. An adequate bond resists forces caused by polymerization of the composite and by forces of occlusion. Bonding agents are available as light-cured and dual-cured, multi-bottle systems (fourth generation); light-cured, single-bottle systems (fifth generation); and self-etching systems (sixth and seventh generation). Fourth- and fifth-generation bonding agents are called total-etch or etch-and-rinse systems. Universal bonding agents can be either total-etch or self-etch systems. Characteristics and examples of fourth, fifth, sixth, and seventh generations and universal bonding agents are listed in Tables 4-6 and 4-7.

Composition and Reaction

A bonding agent consists of three components: etchant, primer, and adhesive. The etchant for fourth- and fifth-generation bonding agents typically is 34% to 37% phosphoric acid in a gel. Many bonding agents contain a multifunctional monomer (primer/adhesive) with both hydrophilic groups to improve wetting and penetration of the treated dentin and hydrophobic groups to polymerize and form a bond with

TABLE 4-6	Characteristics of Fourth-, Fifth-, Sixth-, and Seventh-Generation Bonding Agents				
Generation	Type	Components	Application	Phosphoric acid etching and rinsing	Smear layer on dentin
Fourth	Total-etch, multiple bottle	Etchant, primer, adhesive*	Apply components separately	Yes	Removed
Fifth	Total-etch, single bottle	Etchant, primer-adhesive*	Apply components separately	Yes	Removed
Sixth (Type I)	Self-etching primer, adhesive	Acidic primer, adhesive*	Apply components separately	No	Modified
Sixth (Type II)	Self-etching adhesive	Acidic primer-adhesive	Mix components and apply	No	Modified
Seventh (Type I)	No-mix, self-etching adhesive	Acidic primer-adhesive*	No mixing, apply	No	Modified
Universal	Total-etch or self-etch	Acidic primer-adhesive*	No mixing, apply	Yes or no	Removed or modified

*Dual-cured activator available—mixing required.

TABLE 4-7	Examples of Fourth-, Fifth-, Sixth-, and Seventh-Generation Bonding Agents	
Type	**Product**	**Manufacturer**
Fourth	All-Bond 3	Bisco Dental Products (Schaumburg, IL)
	Scotchbond Multipurpose	3M ESPE (St. Paul, MN)
Fifth	Prime & Bond NT	DENTSPLY Caulk (Milford, DE)
Sixth (Type I)	Clearfil SE Protect	Kuraray America (New York, NY)
Sixth (Type II)	Adper Prompt L-Pop	3M ESPE
Seventh	Clearfil S3 Bond	Kuraray America
	Optibond All-In-One	Kerr Corporation (Orange, CA)
	Xeno IV DC	DENTSPLY Caulk
Universal	Scotchbond Universal Adhesive	3M ESPE

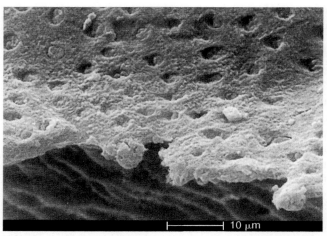

FIG 4-9 Hybrid layer formed by bonding agent penetrating collagen from demineralized dentin. (From Powers JM, Finger WJ, Xie J: Bonding of composite resin to contaminated human enamel and dentin, *J Prosthodont* 4: 28, 1995.)

the composite. The primer and adhesive components usually are carried in a solvent such as acetone, alcohol, or water. In total-etch (or etch-and-rinse), multiple-bottle systems (fourth generation), these components are packaged separately. In total-etch, single-bottle systems (fifth generation), the primer and adhesive are combined. Self-etching, sixth- and seventh-generation and universal systems contain acidic primers/adhesives, which allow them to be used without prior etching with phosphoric acid and without rinsing. Universal bonding agents may contain special primers for bonding to silica- and zirconia-based ceramics and metals.

Bonding to etched enamel is micromechanical and results from good wetting and penetration of the surface as shown in Figure 4-3. Bonding to dentin requires the removal of the smear layer, which consists of hydroxyapatite and partially denatured collagen, and decalcification of intertubular dentin to a depth of 1 to 5 μm. The bonding agent penetrates the exposed collagen and, unlike bonding to enamel, forms a hybrid layer (Figure 4-9). The formation of a hybrid layer provides micromechanical retention to the dentin. Because the morphology of dentin varies with its location, such as number and size of tubules, bonding varies, especially in areas of high tubule density (deep dentin) and sclerotic dentin.

Manipulation

Application of a bonding agent may require a drying step to evaporate the solvent. An acetone-based bonding agent dries more readily after application to the tooth than does a water-based system. Ethanol-based bonding agents require an intermediate time for evaporating the alcohol solvent on the tooth. Some bonding agents have been introduced that are solvent free and do not require drying before curing.

Frequently, the bonding agent is polymerized separately from the composite to minimize problems from shrinkage

during polymerization. As listed in Table 4-3, considerable variation exists among reported bond strengths to tooth structure. Modern bonding agents, however, bond equally well to enamel and dentin. Regardless of the system, these general directions should be followed:

1. Isolate the surface to be bonded.
2. Maintain a clean, moist surface.
3. Follow the manufacturer's directions carefully.
4. Use a protective liner for deep cavities.
5. Provide mechanical retention in the cavity design when no enamel is available for etching and retention.

Most bonding agents bond more effectively to a moist tooth surface than to one that is dry or very wet. Technique tips for total-etch and self-etch bonding agents are summarized in Box 4-2.

LIGHT-CURING UNITS

Visible light-curing units are used to activate polymerization of light-cure materials. Light-emitting diode (LED) units are cordless and rechargeable (Figure 4-10). A less common light source is a quartz-tungsten halogen (QTH) bulb. Light from a QTH bulb is transmitted to the hose tip by a fiber-optic bundle. Examples of LED light-curing units are listed in Table 4-8. Desirable features of LED light-curing units are listed in Box 4-3.

Although the light is filtered to provide only blue light, the tip or the reflected light from the teeth should not be looked at directly because of the high intensity. An eye protection device (usually an orange plastic shield) may be attached to a light curing unit such as the one shown in Figure 4-10. Some lamps produce considerable heat, which can produce pulpal irritation. Too much heat is generated if a finger cannot be held 2 to 3 mm from the tip for 20 seconds.

Exposure times for polymerization vary, depending on the type of lamp, depth of the composite, shade of the composite, and type of composite. For typical LED lights, times may vary from 10 to 60 seconds for a restoration 2 mm thick.

BOX 4-2 Technique Tips for Total-Etch and Self-etch Bonding Agents

Total-Etch Bonding Agents
1. Apply phosphoric acid etchant with a microbrush for the recommended time.
2. Rinse phosphoric acid for 15 seconds after etching.
3. Dispense the bonding agent just before use—don't dispense early.
4. Dry (evaporate) the solvent in the bonding agent for the recommended time. Water takes longer to dry than ethanol. Ethanol takes longer than acetone.
5. Recap bottles immediately to prevent evaporation of solvent.
6. Store at the temperature indicated in the manufacturer's instructions.

Self-Etch Bonding Agents
1. Self-etch bonding agents may require scrubbing with a microbrush or a waiting time before curing.
2. Select a compatible bonding agent when bonding self- and dual-cured composites and resin cements.

Microfilled composites require longer exposure than microhybrid composites because the small filler particles scatter the light more. Darker shades or more opaque composites require longer exposure times (up to 60 seconds longer) than lighter shades or more translucent composites. In deep restorations, the composite may be added and polymerized in layers, with one layer bonding to another without any loss of strength. Bulk-fill composites can be cured in layers up to 4 mm thick. Technique tips for LED light-curing units are summarized in Box 4-4.

⟳ QUICK REVIEW

Composites can be classified as microhybrid, microfilled, and nanofilled, based on the particle size and distribution of the filler. The trend has been toward the microhybrid and nanofilled composites, which contain mostly submicron filler particles with some nanofilled particles. These composites permit high concentrations of filler, which can be polished to a smooth surface. Both Bis-GMA and UDMA oligomers are used. Currently, most composites are polymerized using blue light to initiate the reaction and thus are single-paste systems supplied in syringes or compules. Universal composites are used routinely for both anterior and posterior restorations. Graded-sized fillers have allowed the volume fraction of filler to be increased, in addition to the wear resistance. Composites for special applications include flowable, bulk-fill, laboratory, provisional, and core buildup composites. When higher fluoride release is desirable in low-stress-bearing restorations, compomers and glass and resin-modified glass ionomers can be used. Compomers and resin-modified glass ionomers are more esthetically pleasing than glass ionomers. Fourth-, fifth-, sixth-, and seventh-generation and universal bonding agents used with composites bond well to both enamel and dentin. However, bonding of composites to tooth structure is micromechanical, and acid etching of enamel and dentin or the use of self-etching primers is required. Most direct restorative resins are polymerized by visible light-curing units.

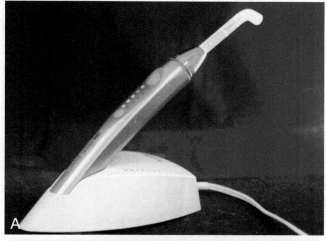

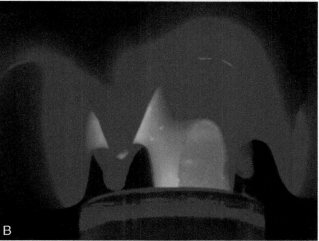

FIG 4-10 Most curing units today are light-emitting diodes (LED) designed **(A)** to emit high intensity blue light that activates photo-chemicals in the composite, triggering an addition polymerization. The units are generally cordless and have controls for time and, in some cases, intensity. LED units are intense enough to travel through translucent parts of the tooth **(B)** and bright enough to damage the retina of the eye. Thus, measures to limit visual exposure should be used at all times. (Courtesy Y-W Chen, University of Washington Department of Restorative Dentistry, Seattle, WA.)

TABLE 4-8 Typical Light-Curing Units

Type	Product	Manufacturer
LED light	Bluephase Style	Ivoclar Vivadent (Amherst, NY)
	Elipar S10 LED Curing Light	3M ESPE (St. Paul, MN)
	Demi Plus LED Light Curing System	Kerr Corporation

BOX 4-3   Desirable Features of Light-Emitting Diode (LED) Light-Curing Units

- Portable with stable docking station/stand
- Good ergonomics—lightweight
- Easily accessible controls
- Digital readout clearly displayed
- Probe is long enough (>7 mm) to reach posterior surfaces
- Sensor to indicate low battery
- Light tip 8–10 mm in diameter
- Built-in radiometer
- Battery holds a charge for several hours of use—extra battery provided
- Durable—diode lasts 5000 hours
- Compatible with variety of initiators (third-generation)
- Autoclavable light tip or protective barrier
- Easy to disinfect

Data from Farah JW, Powers JM, editors: LED light-curing units, *Dent Advis* 23(5):1, 2006.

BOX 4-4   Technique Tips for LED Light-Curing Units

1. Minimize direct exposure of eyes to intense blue light from light-curing unit—provide orange glasses or shields for dental team and patient.
2. Minimize heat by directing a stream of air or high-volume vacuum over the tooth during light curing.
3. Monitor output of curing light over time with radiometer.

⚡ SELF-TEST QUESTIONS

In the following multiple-choice questions, one or more of the responses may be correct.

1. Which of these statements applies to the filler particles of composites?
   a. Microhybrid composites contain as much as 84% filler by weight.
   b. Fine-particle fillers range in size from 0.2 to 3 μm.
   c. Microfilled composites contain more filler than all-purpose composites.
   d. All-purpose composites contain more filler than flowable composites.

2. Which of the following statements about curing of composites is/are true?
   a. Exposure times of 2 to 3 seconds are needed for polymerization with visible light.
   b. Before light activation, the base and catalyst pastes are mixed.
   c. Lights with both blue and red wavelengths are equally effective for polymerization.
   d. Light from an argon laser will activate polymerization.

3. Which of the composites with the following fillers may be radiopaque?
   a. Quartz
   b. Lithium aluminum silicate
   c. Colloidal silica
   d. Barium glass

4. Which of the following polymer systems is used for the organic matrix in composites?
   a. Bisphenol A-glycidyl methacrylate (Bis-GMA)
   b. Poly(methyl methacrylate)
   c. Urethane dimethacrylate (UDMA)
   d. Polystyrene

5. Which of the following initiator-accelerator systems is/are needed for a light-activated composite?
   a. Peroxide-amine
   b. Diketone-amine
   c. Organic acid–peroxide
   d. Organic acid–metal ion

6. Which of the following properties is/are higher for microhybrid composites than for microfilled composites?
   a. Polymerization shrinkage
   b. Thermal expansion
   c. Water sorption
   d. Modulus of elasticity

7. Which of the following is the best choice of restorative material to achieve moderate to high strength, fluoride release, and esthetics?
   a. Composite
   b. Compomer
   c. Resin-modified glass ionomer
   d. Glass ionomer

8. Which of the following statements about laboratory composites is/are true?
   a. Curing using light, heat, and pressure increases the wear resistance.
   b. Bridges prepared from laboratory composites require a metal substructure.
   c. Fiber reinforcement increases their strength but decreases their rigidity.
   d. Restorations prepared from laboratory composites typically are cemented with zinc phosphate cement.

9. Which of the following statements about adhesion of composite restorations to tooth structure is/are true?
   a. Bonding is achieved to enamel by application of an acid etchant followed by application of a bonding agent and then the composite resin.
   b. The bonding agent forms a hybrid layer with enamel.
   c. The bonding agent forms a micromechanical bond with enamel but a chemical bond with dentin.
   d. Bonding agents with water as a solvent dry more readily after application to the prepared tooth than bonding agents with an acetone solvent.
   e. Most bonding agents bond more effectively to a dry tooth surface.

10. Which of the following statements about compomers is/are true?
    a. They are two-paste systems that self-cure within 2 to 3 minutes.
    b. Because of their resin content, they require a bonding agent for adhesion to tooth structure.
    c. They typically are recommended for Class II restorations.
    d. They also are known as polyacid-modified composites.
11. Which of the following statements about provisional composites is/are true?
    a. Provisional composites are more color stable than provisional acrylics.
    b. Provisional composites have less shrinkage on curing than provisional acrylics.
    c. Provisional composites are more wear resistant than provisional acrylics.
    d. Provisional composites release more heat on curing than provisional acrylics.
12. Which of the following statements apply to the packable composites?
    a. Their depth of cure allows bulk polymerization, which has been shown to be clinically effective.
    b. Their wear rate is low (3.5 μm/year), which is similar to that of amalgam.
    c. They are radiolucent.
    d. They have similar or slightly less polymerization shrinkage than all-purpose composites.

13. Which of the following statements applies to resin-modified glass ionomer restorations?
    a. The powder is an aluminosilicate glass, and the liquid is a low-viscosity Bis-GMA polymer.
    b. Resin-modified glass ionomers set immediately when light cured and can be finished immediately.
    c. The fluoride can be recharged by fluoride treatments or brushing with fluoride-containing toothpaste.
    d. They release fluoride better than fluoride-containing composites do.

Use short answers to fill in the following blanks.
14. Bonding agents with self-etching primers (sixth- and seventh-generation) do not require _____ and _____ _____.
15. LED light-curing units are typically _____ and _____.

For the following statements, select true or false.
16. Nanofilled composites generally will have lower surface roughness and higher gloss than microhybrid composites when polished by the same technique.
    a. True
    b. False
17. PAC light-curing units allow composites to be cured in a shorter time than typical QTH lights without adversely affecting properties.
    a. True
    b. False

SUGGESTED SUPPLEMENTARY READINGS

American Dental Association Council on Scientific Affairs: Statement on posterior resin-based composites, *J Am Dent Assoc* 129:1627, 1998.

Berg JH: Glass ionomer cements, *Pediatr Dent* 24:430, 2002.

Bunek SS, editor: Composite cores and fiber posts, *Dent Advis* 29 (5):1, 2012.

Bunek SS, editor: LED curing lights—evolving at the speed of light, *Dent Advis* 29(3):1, 2012.

Bunek SS, editor: Looking back over 30 years—composites and bonding agents, *Dent Advis* 31(3):1, 2014.

Bunek SS, editor: Simplifying composite restorations, *Dent Advis* 30 (7):1, 2013.

Bunek SS, editor: Understanding the newest generation of adhesives: universal bonding agents, *Dent Advis* 30(2):1, 2013.

Bunek SS, editor: Provisionalization in restorative dentistry, *Dent Advis* 29(7):1, 2012.

Burgess JO, Walker R, Davidson JM: Posterior resin-based composite: review of the literature, *Pediatr Dent* 24:65, 2002.

Croll TP, Nicholson JW: Glass ionomer cements in pediatric dentistry: review of the literature, *Pediatr Dent* 24:423, 2002.

Donly KJ, Garcia-Godoy F: The use of resin-based composite in children, *Pediatr Dent* 24:480, 2002.

Farah JW, Powers JM, editors: Glass ionomers and resin-modified glass ionomers, *Dent Advis* 28(4):1, 2011.

Farah JW, Powers JM, editors: Powers JM, editors: Provisional composites and liquid polishes, *Dent Advis* 27(4):1, 2010.

Ferracane JL: Is the wear of dental composites still a clinical concern? Is there still a need for in vitro wear simulating devices? *Dent Mater* 22:689, 2006.

Garcia-Godoy F, Donly KJ: Dentin/enamel adhesives in pediatric dentistry, *Pediatr Dent* 24:462, 2002.

Swift EJ Jr.: Dentin/enamel adhesives: review of the literature, *Pediatr Dent* 24:456, 2002.

evolve Please visit *http://evolve.elsevier.com/Powers/dentalmaterials* for additional practice and study support tools.

5

Dental Amalgam

OBJECTIVES

After reading this chapter, the student should be able to:

1. Define amalgam and discuss its diminishing use in modern dental practice.
2. Explain the clinical advantages and disadvantages of using spherical or admixed types of amalgams.
3. Describe precapsulated amalgam, and explain why its use is mandatory today.
4. Compare the clinical advantages and disadvantages of amalgam versus more esthetic alternative restorative materials.
5. Explain why the strength, dimensional change, creep, and corrosion of amalgam are clinically important.
6. Discuss the clinical success of an amalgam based on the appropriate manipulation and explain why the proper condensation of amalgam into a cavity preparation is clinically important.
7. Understand the rationale for limiting the patient's and dental personnel's exposure to mercury.
8. Understand the sources of mercury important to human exposure, and put the exposure to mercury from amalgam into context of total exposure.
9. List steps the dental team can take to limit the exposure of the patient and dental personnel to mercury and mercury vapor.

In general terms, an amalgam is a mixture of any metallic element with the liquid element mercury. More specifically, dental amalgam is a mixture of a silver alloy with mercury. When the silver alloy—a powder composed mostly of silver, copper, and tin—is mixed with mercury, a chemical reaction ensues. For 1 to 2 minutes after mixing, dental amalgam has a putty-like consistency, but it progresses to a carvable consistency for an additional 2 to 4 minutes. During this time, the amalgam is packed into a cavity preparation in a tooth and carved to the desired shape (Figure 5-1). In the following minutes to hours, the amalgam reaction proceeds, reaching maturity and full strength in about 24 hours.

> ⚠ **ALERT**
>
> *Dental amalgam* is a mixture of an alloy of silver, copper, and tin with the liquid element mercury.

On a global scale, amalgam restorations are a rapidly shrinking proportion of all dental restorations. Today, many modern dental practices in the United States and other countries use amalgam sparingly or not at all. Prior to the development of tooth-colored restorations, amalgams were used to restore teeth throughout the mouth. However, because of their gray color, today these restorations are limited to the posterior teeth where esthetics is less of a concern (Figure 5-2). More esthetic ceramic or direct resin composite materials are now used in situations where esthetics is important. However, these alternative materials have problems such as expense and technique sensitivity in placement. Thus, amalgam remains a viable clinical choice where longevity, ease of placement, and clinical performance are paramount, especially when clinical conditions are challenging (Table 5-1). Concerns over mercury toxicity from amalgams remain despite no credible evidence that adverse health effects stem from the mercury in amalgam materials. Concerns about the effects of mercury from dental sources on the environment also remain.

SILVER ALLOYS FOR DENTAL AMALGAMS

Historically, the silver alloy used in dental amalgams had low (2 to 4 wt%) amounts of copper (Figure 5-3). These alloys were combined with mercury to form "low-copper amalgam." However, the development of silver alloys with higher (13% to 30%, generally about 20%) copper (Figure 5-3) has replaced low-copper alloys because high-copper alloys produce amalgams with higher strength, less corrosion, less creep, and better longevity at the margins (edges of the cavity preparation). Other elements such as palladium and indium are sometimes included to reduce corrosion of high-copper amalgams. Although low-copper amalgams had small amounts of zinc, today's high-copper silver alloys are essentially free of zinc (<0.01 wt% per ADA Specification No. 1) because zinc causes a significant, long-term, and clinically unacceptable expansion of the amalgam if it is contaminated with saliva or other moisture during placement.

Particles of the silver alloy powder can be either irregularly shaped, spherical, or a mixture of the two (Figure 5-4). The shape of these particles will significantly influence the setting reaction and manipulation of the

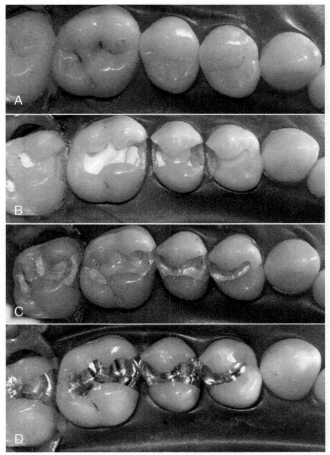

FIG 5-1 Overview of placement of amalgam restorations. Teeth that require restoration **(A)** are prepared using cavity preparations that have undercuts to retain the amalgam, which does not bond effectively to the tooth **(B).** The amalgam is mixed (triturated), then quickly placed into the preparations, and carved into appropriate anatomic and occlusal form **(C).** After 24 hours or more, the amalgams may be polished **(D)** to assure good contours, a smooth surface, and closed margins. (Courtesy J. Martin Anderson, University of Washington Department of Restorative Dentistry, Seattle, WA.)

amalgam. If a mixture of particles is used, the resulting amalgam is referred to as an admixed amalgam. Amalgams containing irregular particles with or without spherical particles added require greater packing or condensation forces during placement than amalgams with spherical particles alone. Most practitioners feel that amalgams containing irregular particles produce better proximal contacts and are easier to carve. Spherical amalgams, containing only spherical alloy particles, require less mercury and set somewhat faster. Practitioners generally select either a spherical or admixed amalgam, depending on the clinical situation. The importance of proper manipulation of each type cannot be over-emphasized. For example, if a condensation force that is appropriate for a spherical amalgam is applied to an admixed amalgam, the restoration will likely contain voids and lack adequate proximal contacts.

MERCURY

Mercury is a dense metal (density = 13.5 g/mL) and the only metallic element in the periodic table that is a liquid at room temperature. Mercury's liquid form facilitates mixing of mercury with the alloy particles to create a putty-like mass that is condensed into a cavity preparation prior to setting. Historically, excess mercury was added to the alloy particles and mixed with a mortar and pestle by hand until the proper consistency was achieved for placement. The excess mercury was removed by "wringing it out" with a cheesecloth. This practice was abandoned because of concerns about mercury toxicity and inconsistencies in the consistency of the putty state. Later, the powder was compressed into tablets of specific mass, and the proper amount of mercury was added with a dispensing device into a reusable mixing capsule. This new method of trituration resulted in consistently strong amalgams and reduced the exposure of the dental staff to mercury. However, the mercury in this dispensing device was exposed to air and dust particles that increased the risk of contamination leading to inferior clinical properties of the mixed amalgam. The risk of spilling significant amounts of mercury during filling or use of the device was another disadvantage.

Today, nearly all practitioners use silver alloy powder and mercury sealed into disposable hard plastic capsules (Figure 5-5). Both the mercury and alloy powder are apportioned by the manufacturer. The mercury is sequestered from the alloy powder by a plastic membrane inside the capsule that is easily ruptured during mixing. Sometimes, a small inert cylinder called a pestle is added to facilitate mixing. This pre-capsulated method provides the proper ratio of alloy powder to mercury, limits handling of pure mercury by the dental team, produces amalgams with consistent physical properties, and keeps the mercury clean.

REACTION OF SILVER ALLOY WITH MERCURY

The reaction of the silver alloy with mercury is called amalgamation. When high-copper alloy particles contact the mercury, the copper, silver, tin, and other elements in the alloy dissolve from the surfaces of the particles into the mercury much as sugar would dissolve in water (Figure 5-6). Dissolution rates vary for each element and occur from the surface of the alloy particles. Almost immediately, new solid products begin to crystallize as the dissolved elements react with the mercury. The crystallization of new products continues until all the liquid mercury is consumed, and the amalgam becomes stiffer and eventually hardens completely. The ratio of alloy to mercury is formulated so that the hardening of the amalgam occurs before all the original alloy particles can dissolve. Thus, the set amalgam contains many of the original alloy particles

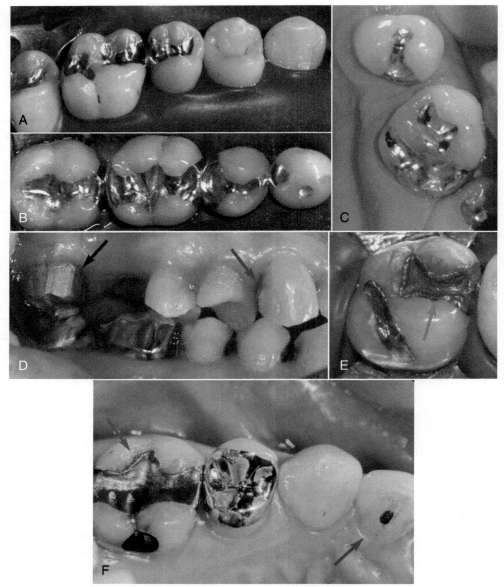

FIG 5-2 Examples of amalgam restorations. In most modern dental practices today, amalgam restorations are placed in posterior teeth where esthetic concerns are secondary. New amalgams have highly adapted margins and longevity **(A–C)**. Restorations on canines or other anterior teeth are used rarely (*blue arrows* in **D** and **F**). Amalgam also may be used to build up the tooth in preparation prior to a crown preparation (*black arrow* in **D**). The value of amalgam is that it can be placed with good clinical success under diverse and even nonideal conditions. For example, amalgam may be successfully placed when isolation of the tooth is impossible and bonding of composites would be compromised. **E,** Amalgam generally fails due to deterioration of its margins with the tooth *(red arrows)*. (**A–C, E,** Courtesy J. Martin Anderson, University of Washington Department of Restorative Dentistry, Seattle, WA. **D,** Courtesy E. R. Schwedhelm, University of Washington Department of Restorative Dentistry, Seattle, WA; **F,** Courtesy Richard D. Tucker, University of Washington Department of Restorative Dentistry, Seattle, WA.)

surrounded by several new products of mercury with tin, copper, or silver (see Figure 5-6). The reaction products are collectively called the **matrix** of the amalgam. In the set mass of most contemporary amalgams, the original particles comprise more than 50% of the volume and are important to the strength and corrosion resistance of the clinical restoration.

Once the amalgamation reaction is complete, little or no mercury remains unreacted. In its reacted state, mercury is not easily released from the amalgam. This fact is important because free mercury can pose a health risk if it occurs in sufficient concentrations. In practice, minute amounts of mercury vapor (approximately 1 to 2 µg per day) are released from dental amalgams as a result of chewing. Higher release may occur during the setting reaction, during removal of old amalgams, or if the amalgam is heated above 80° C (Figure 5-7). To further limit mercury release during the

TABLE 5-1	Dental Amalgam versus Esthetic Alternatives					
Material	Placement method	Ease of placement	Proximal contacts	Clinical versatility	Bonding to tooth?	Longevity
Amalgam	Direct	Relatively simple, even in diverse clinical situations	Reliable	High, intermediate in preservation of tooth structure	Controversial*	Proven long term
Resin composite	Direct	Somewhat complex; requires isolation, multiple steps, time	More difficult to achieve	Moderate, but most conservative of tooth structure	Yes	Very good, improving
Ceramic inlay	Indirect	More complex; requires isolation, multiple steps	Reliable	Lowest and least conservative of tooth structure	Yes, via resin bonding	Good, relatively unknown long term

*Studies of amalgam-tooth bonding have been done but are inconclusive about the clinical utility.

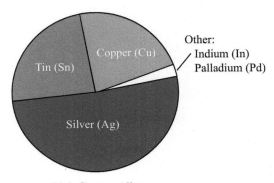

High Copper Alloy

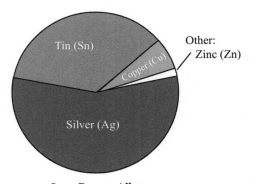

Low Copper Alloy

FIG 5-3 The composition by weight of a typical silver alloy powder used for high-copper and the older low-copper amalgams. Copper contents average about 20 wt% (vs. <13 wt% for the old low-copper amalgams). Trace elements such as indium and palladium are added by some manufacturers to reduce intra-oral corrosion or improve mechanical properties of high-copper amalgams. Low-copper amalgams contained zinc, which increased alloy corrosion and caused slow amalgam expansion.

setting reaction, newer mercury–indium liquid alloys have been substituted for pure mercury in a few products.

Early alloys for amalgams were much lower in copper (2 to 4 wt%) than–contemporary products (Figure 5-3). In low-copper amalgams, the chemical reaction of amalgamation produced a tin–mercury product in the matrix called

gamma-2 (γ_2). Gamma-2 has poor corrosion properties that significantly shorten the clinical lifetime of amalgam restorations. The current high-copper amalgams have eliminated the gamma-2 product; high-copper amalgams have greatly increased resistance to corrosion and marginal breakdown in clinical use.

> **! ALERT**
>
> The absence of the mercury-tin compound gamma-2 (γ_2) is responsible for the exceptional clinical longevity of today's high-copper amalgam restorations.

PROPERTIES OF AMALGAM

Clinically relevant properties of amalgam include strength, dimensional change, creep, tarnish, and corrosion. The clinical importance of these properties are listed for spherical and admixed high-copper amalgams in Table 5-2; the properties themselves are listed in a table in Appendix 5-1. Several examples of commercial products are listed in Table 5-3.

Strength

The strength of an amalgam must withstand oral mechanical forces. Insufficient strength may lead to bulk fracture or marginal fracture requiring replacement (Table 5-2). When amalgam restorations are subjected to occlusal forces in service, both compressive and tensile stresses result inside the amalgam restoration. If those stresses exceed the compressive or tensile strengths of amalgam, the restoration fractures. The table in Appendix 5-1 lists the compressive and tensile strengths of amalgam. Tensile strengths for amalgam are about 12.5% of compressive strengths at 1 day and are therefore an important clinical parameter to consider, because they are weaker. The tensile strength of amalgam at 1 day is approximately the same as human dentin.

Generally, amalgam restorations are subjected to occlusal loads immediately after placement. The rate at which an amalgam develops strength is therefore an important clinical characteristic; compressive strengths for 30 minutes, 1 hour, and 1 day after mixing are listed in the table in Appendix 5-1

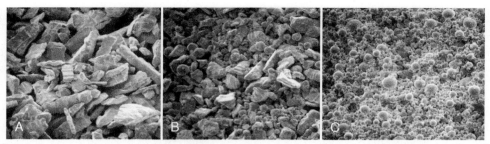

FIG 5-4 Scanning electron micrographs of silver alloy particles used in dental amalgam. Particles may have irregular **(A)** or spherical **(C)** shapes or may be mixed together to form "admixed" amalgam **(B)**. Each micrograph has a horizontal field of view of approximately 500 microns.

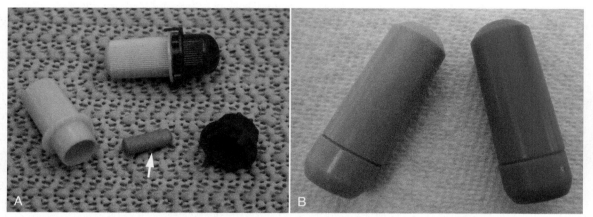

FIG 5-5 Capsules used for trituration (mixing) of amalgam. Some capsule types **(A)** have a pestle *(arrow)* inside that is required to activate or adequately triturate the alloy power and mercury. In these types, the pestle is removed before transfer of the amalgam to the amalgam well. Other types of capsules **(B)** have no pestle inside. To sequester the liquid mercury before trituration, a small plastic membrane is used in one end of either type of capsule the capsule *(not visible)*. Historically, dentists manually added silver alloy and mercury into a reusable capsule. Today, all capsules are prepackaged as in **A** and **B,** disposable, and come sealed and ready for use from the manufacturer, a strategy referred to as "precapsulated" amalgam. Precapsulated amalgam capsules is the standard of care in dentistry today, as it reduces exposure of auxiliaries, the dentist, and the patient to mercury vapor. Auxiliaries should appropriately dispose of capsules, the pestle (if present), and any unused amalgam scrap.

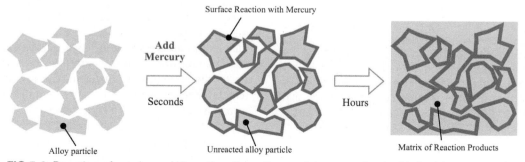

FIG 5-6 Reaction of amalgam. When the silver alloy particles are mixed with liquid mercury, elements such as copper, silver, and tin dissolve into the mercury from the surface of the particles. These elements then react with the mercury to form solid compounds, forming the amalgam matrix. As the reaction progresses, all the liquid mercury is consumed to form the solid matrix. The amount of mercury is controlled to assure that much of the original particle mass remains, thereby giving the amalgam better strength and corrosion resistance. An amalgam with too much or too little matrix will have inferior properties and a higher risk of clinical failure.

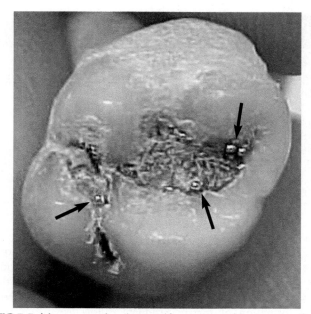

FIG 5-7 Mercury oozing *(arrows)* from an amalgam restoration that has been inadvertently autoclaved. Note that the extreme temperature of the autoclave (>130° C) has caused substantial corrosion of the amalgam. Although this treatment of amalgam is not clinically relevant, it illustrates that the mercury normally chemically bound within the matrix of the amalgam may be released if sufficient heat is applied and corrosion occurs. Exposure of amalgam to less extreme heating that occurs during polishing or cutting with a high-speed handpiece will cause local corrosion and release of small but significant amounts of mercury vapor. For this reason, heat generation should be minimized during the polishing of amalgam or replacement of amalgam restorations. (Courtesy K. Frazier, Georgia Regents University, Augusta, GA.)

and illustrated in Figure 5-8. If an amalgam restoration is subjected to chewing or other oral forces before sufficient strength develops, it is at risk for fracture and failure. As Figure 5-8 shows, spherical and admixed alloys develop compressive strength at different rates during amalgamation. In general, spherical high-copper amalgams develop strength most rapidly. Because of its clinical importance, the early (1 hour) compressive strength of amalgam is regulated by the American Dental Association/American National Standards Institute (ADA/ANSI) and must be at least 80 MPa.

The manipulation of amalgam also affects its strength. Inadequate condensation results in voids, which weaken the set mass. Mixing the amalgam for too long or too short a time also weakens the final strength by changing the ratio of unreacted particles to matrix products (see Figure 5-6). In general, the manufacturer's instructions for mixing should be followed precisely to ensure maximum strength.

Dimensional Change

Ideally, a freshly mixed amalgam would neither expand nor contract as it sets after it is condensed into a cavity preparation (Table 5-2). Expansion may result in post-placement sensitivity or even protrusion from the cavity, whereas contraction would leave gaps between the restoration and the tooth prone to leakage and recurrent decay. The net contraction or expansion of an amalgam during setting is defined as dimensional change. Dimensional change is negative if the amalgam contracts and positive if it expands during setting. The table in Appendix 5-1 lists the 24-hour dimensional change for several types of amalgams. In general, most amalgams expand or contract only slightly during setting, but the ANSI/ADA requires that the dimensional change be no more than 20 μm/cm (expansion or contraction).

TABLE 5-2 Properties of Amalgam and Clinical Use

Property (units)	Description	Clinical importance
Tensile strength (MPa)	Amount of stress required to fracture the amalgam when forces are applied in opposite directions along an axis	The weakest amalgam strength. Low tensile strength increases the risk of bulk fracture of restorations with narrow dimensions (isthmus) as well as at restoration margins.
Compressive strength (MPa)	Amount of stress required to fracture the material when forces are applied toward each other along an axis	The strongest amalgam strength, which increases rapidly after trituration. Low compressive strength increases the risk of early failure of a newly placed restoration. For this reason, the American Dental Association requires that amalgams have ≥80 MPa compressive strength 1 h after trituration.
Creep (%)	The slow deformation of the amalgam under chronic, usually cyclical loads	High creep is strongly associated with gradual failure of the amalgam at the margins of a restoration. Creep is highest in amalgams that use low-copper alloys. Today's amalgams have low creep values.
Dimensional change (μm/cm)	The expansion or contraction of an amalgam upon setting after trituration, usually 24 h	Either excessive expansion or contraction is clinically undesirable. Contraction will increase marginal leakage of the restoration, leading to pulpal sensitivity and recurrent caries at the margins. Expansion will increase the risk of tooth fracture, post-placement sensitivity, or extrusion from the cavity preparation. Most contemporary amalgams have a dimensional change near zero.
Tarnish	Discoloration of the amalgam at its surface due to chemical reactions with oral fluids or foods	Undesirable esthetically but of little clinical consequence.
Corrosion	Chemical degradation of the amalgam at the surface and throughout the bulk of the material	Corrosion leads to loss of physical strength and reduced restoration integrity, ultimately causing restoration failure. The corrosion products pose some biological risk.

APPENDIX 5-1   Amalgam Properties Clinically Important Properties of Typical High-Copper Amalgams (compared with enamel, dentin and ADA requirements where relevant)

Property (units)	Admixed amalgam	Spherical amalgam	Enamel	Dentin	ADA requirement
Tensile strength (MPa)	50	54	10	50–105	
Compressive strength (MPa)				275–300	
30 minutes	67	111			
1 hour	109	188			80
1 day	402	451			
Creep (%)	0.44	0.15	Near 0	0.3	<3
Dimensional change at 24 hours (μm/cm)	−3	−5	NA	NA	<20, >−20
Knoop hardness (kg/mm^2)	143	166	342	20–70	

TABLE 5-3   Examples of Commercial Amalgam Restorative Materials

Alloy type	Manufacturer
Spherical type	
Megalloy EZ	DENTSPLY (York, PA)
Tytin	Kerr Corp. (Orange, CA)
Valiant	Ivoclar Vivadent (Amherst, NY)
Admixed type	
Contour	Kerr Corp.
Dispersalloy	DENTSPLY (York, PA)
Valiant Ph.D.	Ivoclar Vivadent

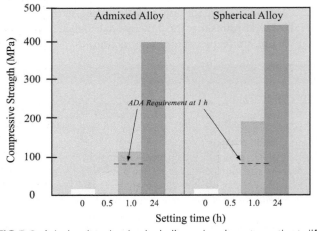

FIG 5-8 Admixed and spherical alloys develop strength at different rates after mixing with mercury. Spherical amalgams are stronger at 30 minutes and 1 hour (h) after mixing, which is important clinically. The patient is often dismissed in this time interval, and if the restoration is subjected to too much biting force, it will fail. Therefore, practitioners often use spherical amalgams in clinical situations with a high risk of early force application (for example, in children). The early strength also allows spherical amalgams to be polished at 1 hour, according to some studies. For both types of amalgams, the compressive strength reaches its final strength after about 7 days (d), but it is essentially (>95%) complete after 24 hours. Because of the importance of early strength to clinical success, the American Dental Association requires a 1-hour compressive strength of 80 MPa *(dashed lines)*.

Although it is somewhat confusing, expansion and contraction occur simultaneously during the setting reaction of amalgam. The dissolution of the alloy particles into the liquid mercury generally leads to contraction, whereas the formation of matrix products causes expansion (see Figure 5-6). The overall dimensional change is therefore the sum of these two processes. Improper manipulation such as inappropriate mixing time or mixing force that alters the ratio of original particles to matrix will affect the dimensional change. For this reason, the dental team should follow the manufacturer's recommendations closely when mixing amalgam.

Historically, amalgams that contained zinc expanded sufficiently to fracture the tooth if they were contaminated with moisture during placement. The expansion occurred slowly over months after placement; restorations sometimes appeared to bulge out of the cavity preparation. Zinc was added to the silver alloy to facilitate machining needed to create the irregularly shaped particles (Figure 5-3), but techniques were developed that did not require zinc, and all alloys today are free of zinc (<0.01%, "zinc-free").

Creep

> **! ALERT**
>
> *Creep* is a dimensional change that occurs over months to years under cyclical loads such as chewing.

The repeated chewing forces applied to amalgam restorations over time cause the amalgam to creep (Figures 5-9 and 5-10). Clinically, high creep is associated with a breakdown at the margins of the restoration as the thin margins gradually "stretch" beyond their limit, ultimately leading to clinical failure (Table 5-2). High-copper amalgams have values of creep far below the old low-copper amalgams (Appendix 5-1). Figure 5-9 shows the clinical effect of creep. Low-copper amalgams have far more breakdown at the margins than high-copper amalgams over the same period of service. More than any other property, the reduced creep of high-copper amalgams led to their predominance in dental amalgam restorations in the 1970s and the virtual disappearance of low-copper amalgams from the marketplace.

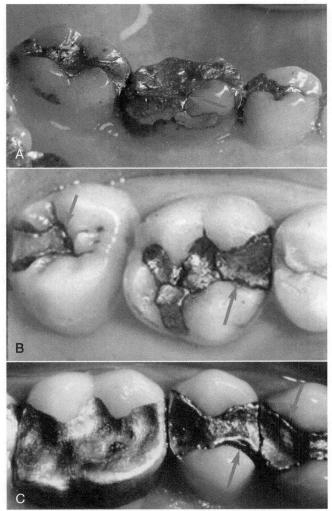

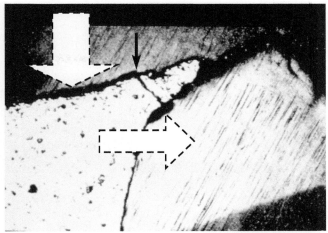

FIG 5-10 Creep in amalgam results from the cyclical application of nondestructive occlusal forces over a period of months to years *(symbolized by vertical block arrow)*. As the application of force continues over months to years, the amalgam material responds by gradually changing shape (creeping, *horizontal block arrow*), ultimately leading to fracture *(smaller solid arrow)*. Creep-mediated fracture results in loss of marginal integrity and failure of the restoration. The creep of high-copper amalgams is generally very low, ranging from 0.05% to 0.15%. However, creep and marginal fracture were a significant drawback of low-copper amalgams used in prior years because they had creep values of nearly 6%. (Courtesy D. Smith, Georgia Regents University, Augusta, GA.)

FIG 5-9 Low-copper amalgams have poor marginal integrity in restorations over time. **A–C,** Red arrows indicate areas of marginal breakdown. **C,** A 3-year postoperative placement photograph of restorations using high-copper *(left)* or low-copper *(center, right)* amalgam. The margins of the high-copper amalgam retain integrity, whereas significant corrosion, creep, and fracture at the margins of the low-copper restorations have occurred. The poor performance of low-copper amalgam is caused by the presence of the gamma-2 phase, which is not present in high-copper amalgam but leads to corrosion, creep, and fracture at the margins of low-copper restoration. These marginal defects are at high risk for caries. Low-copper amalgam is no longer used in the United States. (**A, B,** Courtesy E. R. Schwedhelm, University of Washington Department of Restorative Dentistry, Seattle, WA; **C,** Courtesy D. Smith, Georgia Regents University, Augusta, GA.)

Tarnish and Corrosion

Tarnish is a surface phenomenon that can result in a discolored restoration (Table 5-2). With tarnish, the chemical reaction between the amalgam and the oral cavity is restricted to the amalgam surface. Corrosion results from chemical reactions that penetrate into the body of the amalgam (Table 5-2). Although tarnish may be undesirable esthetically, it will not often cause a restoration to fail. Corrosion, on the other hand, eventually leads to failure of the restoration. Tarnish and corrosion occur more on amalgams with rough surfaces. Thus, a well-polished amalgam limits these problems.

MANIPULATION OF AMALGAM

The clinical success of an amalgam restoration depends on the appropriate manipulation of the amalgam during placement. In general, manipulation is divided into four steps: mixing (or trituration), condensation, carving, and finishing (which may include polishing). The practitioner must first select the appropriate type of amalgam for the clinical situation. The rate of setting, size of the restoration, proximity of adjacent teeth, occlusion, and final restorative goal for the tooth must all be considered before selecting an admixed or spherical amalgam.

Mixing the Amalgam (Trituration)

The process of mixing the silver alloy together with mercury is called trituration. Proper trituration ensures appropriate properties of the amalgam during and after setting and increases the chances of long-term success of the amalgam restoration. Trituration is accomplished mechanically with an amalgamator (Figure 5-11). Amalgamators agitate the capsule containing the silver alloy and mercury back and forth at a high speed and mix the alloy and mercury together in less than 20 seconds. Amalgamators generally have a timer and may have a speed control to regulate the trituration.

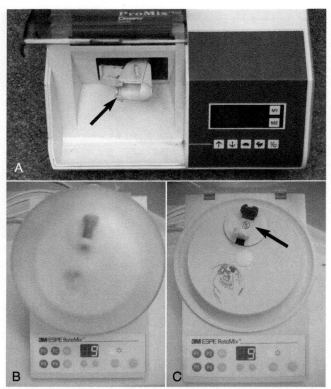

FIG 5-11 Photographs of a two common types of amalgamators: linear oscillating **(A)** and centrifugal **(B** and **C).** A precapsulated amalgam capsule is placed in holders *(arrows)*, and the covers are closed before trituration is started. These devices have controls for on and off, duration of mixing, and speed of mixing. In addition, preprogrammed settings may be stored and accessed by pushing specific buttons *("M" in top figure; "P" in bottom figures).* Settings to optimally mix different types of amalgam are always available from the manufacturer and should be followed.

In today's dental practice, the use of precapsulated amalgam is mandatory. Precapsulated amalgam (discussed previously; see Figure 5-5) is available with capsules containing different amounts of silver alloy and mercury. These different amounts are generally delineated by color-coded capsules. A "single mix" (also called "single-spill," a term used before precapsulated packaging) contains about 600 mg of silver alloy and is sufficient for a small restoration. A "double mix" contains 800 mg of silver alloy and is sufficient for most moderately sized restorations. If larger amounts of amalgam are needed for a single restoration, several capsules should be mixed in succession rather than mixing more than one capsule simultaneously.

> **⚠ ALERT**
>
> *Trituration* is the process of mixing the silver alloy and mercury together.

The speed, time, and force of trituration all affect the amalgam setting reaction. Of these factors, the clinician has control

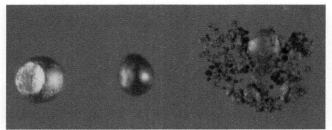

FIG 5-12 The effect of trituration time on amalgam. Undertrituration *(right)* results in a crumbly, dull mass that cannot be effectively condensed into the cavity preparation. The undertriturated amalgam also is weak because inadequate matrix forms to hold the amalgam together (see Figure 5-6). Overtriturated amalgam *(left)* has a shiny appearance and soupy texture and has low resistance to condensation. Overtriturated amalgam is weak because of overproduction of matrix, which is weaker than the original alloy particles. Properly triturated amalgam *(center)* is somewhat shiny and has a putty-like consistency yet offers firm resistance to condensation. (Courtesy D. Smith, Georgia Health Sciences University, Augusta, GA.)

only over speed and time; force is determined by the design of the amalgamator. In general, speed and time should be set as recommended by the manufacturer, considering the type of amalgam, amount mixed, and type of amalgamator. A deviation of only 2 to 3 seconds in mixing time will adversely affect the handling and properties of the amalgam and the long-term clinical success of the restoration. As an amalgamator ages, increases in speed or time may be necessary to compensate for a reduction in force to ensure a proper mix.

Under- or over-trituration generally both lead to amalgams with inferior physical properties and an increased risk of failure of the restoration. Under-triturated amalgam has a dull, crumbly appearance (Figure 5-12). Under-triturated amalgam has poor compressive and tensile strengths because an insufficient matrix (see Figure 5-6) is formed to hold the mass together and because the crumbly texture increases voids in the restoration. Over-triturated amalgam is soupy and adheres to the inside of the capsule. It will have poorer strength and creep and may have poorer corrosion properties, all caused by formation of too many matrix products. A properly triturated amalgam is shiny but offers resistance to condensation. With experience, the practitioner and auxiliaries generally develop a sense about the appearance of a properly triturated amalgam.

Transfer and Condensation

After trituration, the amalgam must be transferred and condensed into the cavity preparation in the tooth before its putty-like consistency decreases. The goals of condensation are to produce a mass without voids that adapts closely to the cavity walls and margins of the cavity preparation. In the past, condensation also was used to reduce excess mercury from the mass, thereby ensuring optimal strength and minimal creep of the restoration. However, the use of precapsulated amalgam greatly reduces the need to try to remove excess mercury from the setting mass, and this is no longer a goal of condensation.

The triturated amalgam is transferred from the mixing capsule to an amalgam well and then to the cavity preparation via an amalgam carrier (Figure 5-13). Amalgam carriers generally have two ends, one smaller than the other. The assistant selects the end of the instrument appropriate for the clinical needs as directed by the operator; generally, smaller increments are used initially, graduating to larger increments. Once delivered to the desired areas of the preparation, condensing may be accomplished by hand or mechanical condensers. Each increment is condensed before adding the next. Hand condensation is far more common and probably more desirable than mechanical condensation in most cases. Hand condensers come in a variety of shapes and sizes and are selected on the basis of the type of amalgam, the shape and size of the cavity, and the stage of condensation. In general, smaller condensers (2 to 3 mm in diameter) are more effective in achieving the goals of condensation. The amalgam must be condensed with 30 to 40 N of force using overlapping "steps" and lateral (sideways) condensing to adapt the amalgam to all cavity walls. Spherical amalgams are more plastic and require larger condensers or lower forces. Condensation must commence immediately after mixing. A delay in condensation of even 1 to 2 minutes may reduce strength or increase creep of the final restoration.

Mechanical condensers are available that use a tapping or vibrating motion. Mechanical condensation is not a substitute for good condensation pressure and selection of the proper size instrument. Ultrasonic condensers, used previously, are rare today, but they are strongly discouraged because they greatly promote the evaporation of mercury from the setting amalgam, which poses a significant health risk to dental personnel via exposure to mercury vapor.

Carving and Finishing

The cavity preparation is always overpacked with amalgam and carved back to final contours. Overpacking allows the

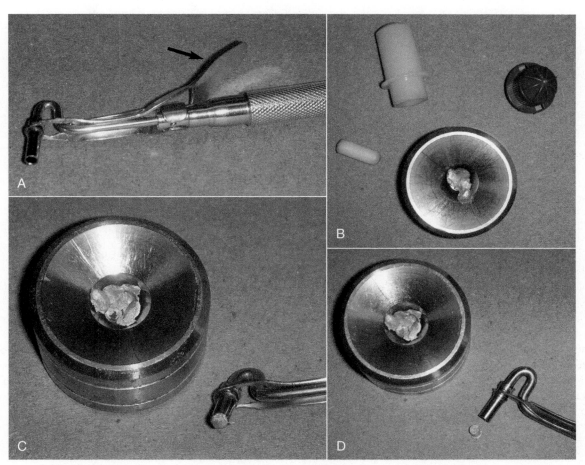

FIG 5-13 **A,** Transfer of amalgam into the cavity preparation is accomplished using an amalgam carrier. The carrier has two ends, one shown here, and a lever *(arrow)* that is used to express the setting amalgam into the cavity preparation. **B,** After trituration, the capsule is opened and its contents are placed in the amalgam well. **C,** The amalgam carrier has a small hole that is filled with the amalgam, and the unset amalgam is transferred from the well into the carrier temporarily. **D,** By pushing the lever on the carrier, the amalgam can be expelled into any specific part of the cavity preparation. The amalgam is moved incrementally from the well to the cavity preparation using the carrier in this manner. Each increment is condensed prior to addition of the next to assure a well-adapted, void-free restoration.

practitioner to control the final shape and occlusion of the restoration more closely than would be possible otherwise. Carving of an amalgam restoration is done with a variety of hand instruments (Figure 5-14). Depending on the type of amalgam, carving may start 2 to 3 minutes after mixing and should cease when the amalgam mass becomes hard (5 to 10 minutes). Carving after an amalgam is set may cause fracture of the amalgam, particularly at the restoration margins.

The finishing and polishing of the amalgam generally are performed at least 24 hours after placement. However, if a spherical high-copper amalgam is used, polishing may be done at the time of placement because these amalgams set much faster than irregular or admixed amalgams (see Figure 5-8). Clinical studies have shown that a well-finished and polished amalgam is easier to keep clean and corrodes less. Polishing is achieved through a series of steps (see Figure 5-14). Generally, the amalgam surface is contoured with use of finishing burs, or abrasive disks. The margins of the amalgam are checked and contoured until they are smooth and congruous with the tooth. The next step is to smooth the alloy surface. This step is accomplished using a polishing agent such as fine pumice or silux or rubber abrasive points. The final step is to put a luster (high shine) on the surface using a very fine abrasive paste or rubber abrasive point. Polishing always should be done wet (with water) because dry polishing may overheat the amalgam and tooth. Overheating may damage the pulp of the tooth and damages the amalgam surface by driving mercury from the amalgam.

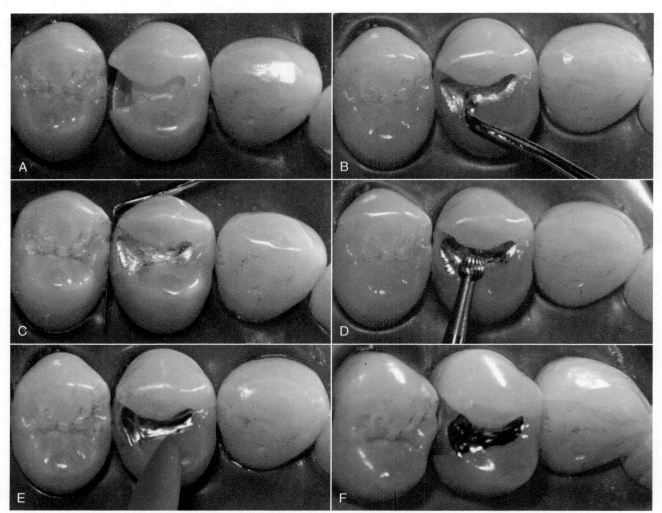

FIG 5-14 Carving and polishing the amalgam. Once the amalgam is condensed into the cavity preparation **(A)**, it is burnished and carved into its final form before it sets. Various instruments are used to burnish and carve the amalgam to appropriate contours, including a discoid cleoid **(B)** or interproximal carving instruments **(C)**. After carving is completed, the amalgam will have appropriate contours, proximal contacts, occlusal contacts, and occlusal function. After the amalgam sets completely (usually more than 24 hours after placement), it is then polished using burs **(D)** and rubber points **(E)**, producing a surface with high luster **(F)**. (Courtesy J. Martin Anderson, University of Washington Restorative Dentistry, Seattle, WA.)

LIMITING EXPOSURE TO MERCURY

The element mercury is particularly toxic, and precautions should be taken to limit exposure of the patient and dental team to its various forms. Human exposure to mercury is especially problematic because it is eliminated slowly from the body. For example, the time to eliminate elemental or organic forms of mercury is greater than 300 days. Thus, even small daily exposures may build up to toxic levels in the body. Mercury gains access to the body through skin contact, through ingestion, or through the lungs as a vapor. The most likely route of exposure for the dental patient and dental personnel is by inhalation of vapor. However, good mercury hygiene limits exposure from all of these routes. Finally, although the exposure of the patient is always a concern, the occupational exposure of dental personnel is more critical because of daily exposure to amalgam during its most mercury-labile periods: mixing, placement, polishing, and removal. Furthermore, environmental concerns have prompted government agencies to increasingly regulate mercury efflux from users, including dental offices.

> **! ALERT**
>
> *Mercury hygiene* is the practice of handling amalgam and mercury to minimize exposure of the dental staff, the patient, and the environment to mercury.

Mercury occurs in three forms: elemental (Hg^0), inorganic (Hg^{2+}), and organic. Each of these forms has different dynamics of entry into and excretion from the body. Furthermore, we are exposed to the different forms from different sources (Table 5-4). For example, the most common source of organic forms is fish. In general, the organic forms are the most toxic because they are most efficiently distributed to long-term storage sites in the nerve and fat tissues. Exposure to inorganic mercury is less critical because it is poorly absorbed.

Mercury vapor occurs in the elemental form and is most relevant to dental amalgam. In service, amalgam generates a minute amount of mercury vapor. For an average individual with amalgam restorations in posterior teeth, 1 to 2 micrograms (μg) of mercury vapor are generated every day.

TABLE 5-4   Estimates of Daily Human Exposure to Mercury (μg/day)

Source	Elemental mercury (Hg^0)	Inorganic mercury (Hg^{2+})	Organic mercury
Air	0.12	0.038	0.034
Water	—*	0.05	—
Fish	0.94	—	3.76
Food	—	20.0	—
Amalgam	1–2	—	—

*A dash (—) indicates that amounts are not significant.

If vapor reaches the lungs, it is rapidly absorbed into the blood and gains access to body tissues. The lowest known dose of mercury that has been documented to cause mild, reversible symptoms in humans is 3 micrograms (μg) per kilogram of body weight. For the average 70-kg individual, this means they would have to absorb and retain over 200 μg of mercury to experience even mild reversible symptoms. This level is 100 times what an individual is exposed to from amalgam-generated mercury vapor in a day. Because not all the vapor generated reaches the lungs, the risk is even less. More serious symptoms of mercury toxicity do not occur until exposure is 500 μg/kg or more and would require 35,000 μg of retained mercury in the average individual. Given these facts, the risk of toxicity from mercury vapor from amalgam is low.

Good mercury hygiene involves simple, commonsense strategies. Freshly mixed amalgam should never be touched, even with gloved hands. A mask should be worn during placement, polishing, or removal of amalgams to decrease inhalation of particulate (although masks offer little protection against mercury vapor). The use of precapsulated amalgam limits handling of liquid mercury and reduces the possibility of a spill of liquid mercury in the office. The use of high-volume evacuation during placement, polishing, and removal of amalgam restorations reduces the exposure of the patient and the dental team to mercury vapor. Ultrasonic amalgam condensers should not be used. The dental operatory should not be carpeted so that spills of particulate amalgam may be cleaned effectively. Amalgam scrap should be stored in containers containing x-ray fixer or other reducing agents and should be capped tightly and kept cool. The office should have a comprehensive plan for mercury hygiene, including an amalgam separator to limit mercury efflux into the water waste; there are building codes and requirements for these separators in many jurisdictions.

The dental staff is at highest risk for mercury exposure because they work in the dental environment every day. Studies indicate that the mercury vapor levels in most offices are well below the maximum of 0.05 mg/m^3 per 40-hour week set by the Occupational Safety and Health Administration (OSHA). Other studies have shown that 99% of 1555 dentists tested had blood mercury values less than 30 ng/mL, which is well below the 100 ng/mL required to cause early symptoms of toxicity and comparable to blood levels in the general population. The ADA recommends a monitoring program for the dental office for mercury vapor. Private companies provide this service.

Despite the toxicity of mercury, dental amalgams are unquestionably safe restorations. No evidence currently exists that links amalgam use with health problems in patients. However, on rare occasions, a person with allergy to mercury is encountered, and amalgam use should be avoided in these persons. Information on the safety of amalgam and the hazards of mercury is sometimes promulgated by individuals with questionable motives. Patients are especially vulnerable to this misinformation, particularly if they have chronic disease or other life problems. Patients will look to the dental team for reliable information. Thus, the dental health team should pay close attention to quality of sources of information (the ADA, Food and Drug Administration [FDA], or peer-reviewed literature) when they consider whether to use amalgam and how they respond to patients' questions about the safety of amalgam restoration and mercury exposure.

QUICK REVIEW

The use of amalgam as a restorative material continues to decline at the expense of more esthetic materials. The introduction of high-copper amalgams in the late 1970s dramatically improved the clinical longevity of amalgam restorations by eliminating a corrosion-prone gamma-2 phase from amalgam. These high-copper formulations are still excellent choices for long-term, posterior restorations in which esthetics is not a primary concern or isolation of the tooth is difficult. The use of precapsulated amalgam has significantly reduced the risk of exposure of dental personnel to liquid mercury and has improved the predictability of the mechanical properties of amalgam. A successful amalgam restoration depends on the proper trituration (mixing), condensation, carving, and finishing of the amalgam. Each of these manipulation steps significantly affects the physical properties and clinical performance of the amalgam. Amalgam does not bond to tooth by itself, although some products have been developed that promote some bonding. Amalgam–tooth bonding does not appear to significantly improve long-term retention of these restorations. Although minute amounts of mercury vapor are released from amalgam restorations in service (approximately 1 to 2 µg/day), all evidence indicates that amalgams are safe restorations. Still, dental offices are under increasing regulatory pressures to limit contributions of mercury to solid or liquid waste streams.

SELF-TEST QUESTIONS

Test your knowledge by answering the following questions. For multiple-choice questions, one or more responses may be correct.

1. Which of the following office conditions minimize(s) the health hazard from spilled mercury?
   a. Baseboard heating
   b. Floor carpeting
   c. Tile flooring without seams
   d. Amalgam scrap stored in a closed container

2. By statute, which of the following represents the maximum safe concentration of mercury vapor in the breathing zone for a 40-hour workweek?
   a. 0.05 ng Hg/m^3 of air
   b. 30 ng Hg/m^3 of air
   c. 100 ng Hg/m^3 of air
   d. 0.05 ng Hg/m^3 of air

3. What compound has been eliminated from amalgam to improve corrosion and reduce creep?
   a. Gamma
   b. Gamma-1
   c. Alpha-1
   d. Gamma-2

4. Once amalgamation has occurred, which of the following is/are true of mercury?
   a. It is combined primarily with silver.
   b. It has the toxic properties of unreacted mercury.
   c. It can form at the surface of amalgam restorations if heated to 60° C.
   d. It can never be released from the amalgam.
   e. It can be released in vapor or ionic forms.

5. For each property, list the amalgam type (low-copper, admixed high-copper, and spherical high-copper) that has the highest value.
   a. 1-hour compressive strength _____
   b. Tensile strength _____
   c. Creep _____

6. Which of the following factors is/are important in obtaining a properly triturated dental amalgam?
   a. Speed of the amalgamator
   b. Time of amalgamation
   c. Size of the mix
   d. Manufacturer of the amalgam
   e. Manufacturer of the amalgamator

7. Which of these statements is/are correct in describing a triturated mass of amalgam?
   a. An under-triturated mass is crumbly and dull.
   b. A correctly triturated mass is smooth, homogeneous, and dull.
   c. An overmixed mass is removed readily from the capsule but is soupy in appearance.

8. The objectives during condensation of amalgam are which of the following?
   a. Good adaptation to cavity walls, margins, and matrix
   b. Development of a mass free from voids
   c. Packing to final contour

9. Which of the following statements applies to condensation of amalgam?
   a. Amalgam should be condensed in small increments with uniform force applied.
   b. A condenser is selected on the basis of its ability to apply the pressure needed for adaptation.
   c. Too large a condenser tip results in low condensation pressure and poor adaptation.
   d. A force of 30 to 40 N on a condenser is satisfactory for adequate condensation of admixed and spherical alloys.
   e. Condensation force should be applied laterally as well as vertically.

10. In the finishing of an amalgam restoration, which of the following is/are true?
    a. Final finishing and polishing are done just after the amalgam hardens, regardless of the type of alloy.
    b. Burnishing over margins should not be done because thin areas of amalgam susceptible to fracture can be formed.

c. Polishing should be done in the presence of water.

d. A correct finishing and polishing sequence would include finishing burs, green stone, ilex, and tin oxide.

e. Elevated temperatures during polishing help achieve a high luster on the amalgam surface.

Use short statements to answer the following questions.

11. Which type of amalgam (spherical versus admixed) would you choose for a restoration that had to survive higher occlusal forces shortly after placement, and why?

12. Zinc originally was included in the amalgam alloy to facilitate cutting the amalgam into clean, irregular pieces. Why do most contemporary amalgams not include zinc?

13. Summarize the advantages of precapsulated amalgam.

14. You examine set amalgam under an electron microscope and observe that all the original alloy particles have reacted. What will you predict about the physical properties of this amalgam? Why?

15. You see an old amalgam in a patient's mouth. It is dark and needs polishing. How can you determine if the amalgam has corroded or is just tarnished? If the amalgam has corroded, what is the remedy for this restoration?

16. You are triturating an amalgam in a precapsulated form. The timer on the amalgamator breaks, and you do not know if the amalgam was over-triturated or under-triturated. How will you tell? How do you explain what you see in terms of the amalgamation reaction? Which condition would you rather use clinically?

17. Give the definition of creep, and explain why creep is an important clinical property.

18. A patient arrives at your office and expresses concern about mercury in dental amalgam causing her harm. What will you tell this patient to reassure her about the safety of amalgam?

19. What precautions should be taken to limit the exposure of the dental team and the patient to mercury during the removal of an amalgam?

In the following multiple-choice questions, one or more responses may be correct.

20. Which one of the following is/are *not* true about high-copper dental amalgam restorations?

a. They have better corrosion resistance than low-copper dental amalgams.

b. They contain both tin (Sn) and silver (Ag) in the composition as well.

c. They produce excessive creep.

d. Restorations are brittler than low-copper versions.

21. Dental personnel can do which one of the following to limit their exposure to mercury?

a. Sterilize amalgam scrap

b. Vacuum up a spill immediately

c. Avoid touching freshly mixed amalgam

d. Avoid polishing amalgams

22. The primary difference in the silver alloy between low- and high-copper amalgams is the amount of:

a. Copper

b. Copper and zinc

c. Copper and tin

d. Copper and silver

23. Ideally, the set amalgam should do which of the following?

a. Expand greatly to provide marginal seal against the tooth

b. Shrink significantly to provide space for corrosion products to seal the margins

c. Have little dimensional change

24. Which of the following physical properties are most desirable in set amalgam?

a. High strength, low creep, low corrosion

b. Low strength, low creep, low corrosion

c. High strength, high creep, low corrosion

d. High strength, high creep, high corrosion

25. Higher mercury in an amalgam leads to which of the following?

a. Higher creep

b. Higher strength

c. Lower corrosion

d. Less matrix formation

26. Which of the following occur(s) when dental amalgam is over-triturated?

a. Compressive strength decreases.

b. Corrosion decreases.

c. Tensile strength increases.

d. Only a and b

e. Only a and c

SUGGESTED SUPPLEMENTARY READINGS

American Dental Association Council on Scientific Affairs: Dental amalgam—update on safety concerns, *J Am Dent Assoc* 129:494, 1998.

Fedorowic Z, Nasser M, Wilson N: Adhesively bonded versus non-bonded amalgam restoration for dental caries, *Cochrane Database of Systematic Reviews* 4, 2009. http://dx.doi.org/10.1002/14651858.CD007517.pub2 CD007517.

Ferracane JE, Engle JH, Okabe T, Michem JC: Reduction in operatory mercury levels after contamination or amalgam removal, *Am J Dent* 7:103, 1994.

Fuks AB: The use of amalgam in pediatric dentistry, *Pediatr Dent* 24:448, 2002.

Hörsted-Bendslev P: Amalgam toxicity—environmental and occupational hazards, *J Dent* 32(5):359, 2004.

Mackert JR Jr.: Randomized controlled trial demonstrates that exposure to mercury from dental amalgam does not adversely affect neurological development in children, *J Evid Based Dent Pract* 10(1):25, 2010.

Mackert JR, Bergland A: Mercury exposure from dental amalgam fillings: absorbed dose and the potential for adverse health effects, *Crit Rev Oral Biol Med* 8(4):410, 1997.

Mitchell RJ, Koike M, Okabe T: Posterior amalgam restorations—usage, regulation and longevity, *Dent Clin North Am* 51(3):573, 2007.

Olsson S, Bergman M: Daily dose calculation from measurement of intra-oral mercury vapor, *J Dent Res* 71:414, 1992.

Osbourne JW, Summitt JB, Roberts HW: The use of dental amalgam in pediatric dentistry: review of the literature, *Pediatr Dent* 24:439, 2002.

Roberts HW, Charlton DG: The release of mercury from amalgam restorations and its health effects: a review, *Oper Dent* 34(5):605, 2009.

Setcos JC, Staninec M, Wilson NH: A two-year randomized, controlled clinical evaluation of bonded amalgam restorations, *J Adhes Dent Winter* 1:323, 1999.

Summitt JB, Burgess JO, Berry TG, Robbins JW, Osborne JW, Haveman CW: Six-year clinical evaluation of bonded and pin-retained complex amalgam restorations, *Oper Dent* 29:261, 2004.

Uçar Y, Brantley WA: Biocompatibility of dental amalgams, *Intl J Dent* 2011:981595, 2011. http://dx.doi.org/10.1155/2011/981595.

evolve   Please visit *http://evolve.elsevier.com/Powers/dentalmaterials* for additional practice and study support tools.

6

Finishing, Polishing, and Cleansing Materials

OBJECTIVES

After reading this chapter, the student should be able to:

Abrasion

1. Give the purpose of finishing and polishing techniques and list what may result from a rough surface on a restoration.
2. Define abrasion and contrast abrasive tools or slurries with cutting instruments.
3. Discuss three factors that influence the rate of abrasion, and indicate which factor is easiest to control clinically.
4. Describe surface roughness and gloss.
5. Distinguish finishing, polishing, and cleansing abrasives and techniques and recognize common abrasives.
6. Give two principles of finishing and polishing techniques.
7. List two reasons why an abrasive should not be used in a dry condition.
8. Describe the finishing and polishing of common restorative materials and indicate precautions associated with these techniques. Include dental amalgam, composite, compomer, resin-modified glass ionomer, and acrylic denture resin.

Prophylactic Pastes

9. Give two ideal functions of a dental prophylactic paste.
10. List the major abrasives and therapeutic agents used in prophylactic pastes.
11. Compare cleansing and abrasion of tooth structure by various products.
12. List restorative materials particularly susceptible to wear by a prophylactic paste, and indicate two undesirable results of such wear.

Dentifrices

13. Give the primary function of a dentifrice.
14. Recognize four desirable effects of toothbrushing.

15. List four types of debris in order of increasing difficulty of removal from surfaces of teeth.
16. Recognize the components in a dentifrice, and indicate their function.
17. List several common abrasives used in dentifrices.
18. Give examples of tooth structure and restorative materials particularly susceptible to abrasion by a dentifrice.
19. List four variables of a toothbrush that can influence abrasion caused by a dentifrice.
20. List four guidelines to follow in recommendation of a dentifrice for a patient.

Denture Cleansers

21. List six requirements of an ideal denture cleanser.
22. List three major types of denture cleansers, and identify the active ingredient in each.
23. Describe effective techniques for cleaning dentures, including those with soft liners.
24. Indicate the effects of hot water, hard and stiff bristles, and dentifrices when used to clean dentures.
25. Give the disadvantages of each type of denture cleanser.

Whitening

26. Indicate types of stains for which in-office whitening techniques may be effective.
27. Compare the ingredients of in-office and home whitening agents.
28. Indicate the effect of whitening agents on restorative materials.
29. Give side effects reported for whitening agents.
30. List three major methods of in-office whitening.
31. Describe an in-office whitening gel technique.
32. Describe a home whitening technique.
33. Describe universal whitening guidelines and additional guidelines for in-office whitening gels.

Finishing and polishing techniques are meant to remove excess material and smooth roughened surfaces. A rough surface on a restoration may be uncomfortable and make oral hygiene difficult, because food debris and plaque can cling to it easily. When a restoration is located in proximity to the gingiva, surface roughness can cause painful irritation and eventual recession of the soft tissue. Roughness of metallic restorative materials is responsible for accelerating corrosion. The finishing and polishing of restorative dental materials are important steps in the fabrication of clinically successful restorations.

Cleansing techniques are meant to remove food and other debris from a surface without damaging it. Polishing and cleaning are routine procedures for maintaining the health of the natural dentition. These procedures, however, can lead to roughened enamel surfaces by the use of excessively abrasive dentifrices at home or coarse prophylactic slurries at the dental office. Dentifrices and prophylactic pastes also can abrade some restorative materials during a cleansing procedure.

The materials used for finishing and polishing are primarily abrasives. Most cleansing materials are also abrasives, although many chemical cleansing agents for denture bases exist. An understanding of the properties of these materials and the process of abrasion can improve clinical usage of finishing, polishing, and cleansing materials.

ABRASION

> **! ALERT**
> Abrasion is a wear process.

Abrasion results when a hard, rough surface, such as a sandpaper disk, or hard, irregularly shaped particles, such as those present in an abrasive slurry, plow grooves into a softer material and cause material from such grooves to be removed from the surface. The action of an abrasive is essentially a cutting action. Abrasive tools or slurries, however, differ from dental cutting instruments in that the cutting edges or points of the abrasive are not arranged in any particular pattern. Each point or edge of an abrasive acts as an individual cutting blade and removes some material from the surface being abraded.

The process of abrasion is affected by the physical and mechanical properties of the material being abraded. Properties such as hardness, strength, ductility, and thermal conductivity are important. These properties are discussed later in this chapter with respect to the abrasion of individual restorative materials.

Rate

The rate of abrasion of a given material by a given abrasive is determined primarily by three factors: the size of the abrasive particle, the pressure of the abrasive against the material being abraded, and the speed at which the abrasive particle moves across the surface being abraded. All of these factors can be controlled clinically.

The size of an abrasive particle is an important factor in the rate at which the surface is abraded. Larger particles cause deeper scratches in the material and wear away the surface at a faster rate. The use of a coarse abrasive is indicated on a surface with many rough spots or large nodules. Finer abrasives are then used to remove the scratches caused by the coarse abrasive. New abrasive systems have particles that wear during use, which produces finer particles and an increasingly smooth finish.

A second important factor is the pressure of the abrasive against the surface being abraded. Heavy pressure applied by the abrasive causes deeper scratches and more rapid removal of material. However, heavy pressure also may cause the abrasive to fracture or to dislodge from the grinding wheel and thereby reduce cutting efficiency. Operator control of the abrasion process is lessened when excessive pressure is exerted because material is worn away too rapidly to keep the abrasion from occurring uniformly over the entire surface of the material. Judgment must be exercised in the amount of force applied to the dental handpiece or to the surface that is against a grinding wheel to avoid excessive pressure.

A third factor that controls the rate of abrasion is the speed at which the abrasive travels across the surface being abraded. The higher the speed, the greater is the frequency per unit of time the particle contacts the surface. Increasing the speed increases the rate of abrasion. In a clinical situation, it is easier to control speed rather than pressure to vary the rate of abrasion. Varying the speed has the additional advantage of using low pressure during maintenance of a high cutting efficiency.

Surface Roughness and Gloss

Surface roughness (R_a) is a measure of the irregularity of the finished and polished surface and is measured in micrometers (µm). A smooth surface (R_a less than 0.2 µm) is desirable to reduce retention of bacteria and to have a shiny appearance.

Gloss is a measure of the reflection of light from a surface. A totally nonreflective surface has zero gloss units (GU), and a perfect mirror will read 1000 GU at a measuring angle of 60 degrees. A gloss value of less than 10 is considered to be low in gloss, 10 to 70 is considered semigloss, and greater than 70 is considered high gloss. An ideal restorative material would have high gloss after polishing and would retain its gloss during function in the mouth.

Types of Abrasives

> **! ALERT**
> Finishing abrasives are coarse, hard particles, whereas polishing abrasives are fine particles.

The three types of abrasives used in dentistry can be classified as finishing, polishing, and cleansing abrasives. Finishing abrasives are generally hard, coarse abrasives used primarily for development of desired contours of a restoration or tooth preparation and for removal of gross irregularities on the surface. Polishing abrasives have finer particle sizes and are generally less hard than abrasives that are used for finishing. The polishing abrasives are used to smooth surfaces roughened typically by finishing abrasives or wear particles encountered in the mouth. Cleansing abrasives are generally soft materials with small particle sizes and are intended to remove softer materials that adhere to enamel or restorative material substrates.

Dental abrasives are applied by means of a number of tools. The abrasive particles may be glued onto plastic or paper disks that can be attached to a dental handpiece or attached to strips for finishing of interproximal areas. Paper disks are preferable for finishing contoured surfaces because they are more flexible than plastic disks. The waterproof variety of paper disks is more durable. In the case of diamond rotary instruments, diamond chips are attached to steel wheels, disks, and cylinders. With grinding wheels and dental stones, the abrasive particles are bonded by a matrix material that is molded to form tools of desired sizes and shapes. The abrasive tools just described are used only for finishing.

Abrasives also may be mixed with water, glycerin, or some other medium to produce slurries or pastes. The use of glycerin as a medium prevents the change in consistency that occurs when water, which evaporates, is used to make the slurry. The slurry or paste then is rubbed over the surface of the material being abraded with a cloth or felt wheel, brush, or rubber cup. Abrasive slurries and pastes are used most commonly in dentistry for polishing and cleaning.

The following is a brief discussion of the abrasive agents commonly used for finishing. Values of hardness and grades of abrasives used on some commercial disks are listed in Table 6-1.

Aluminum oxide (Al_2O_3) is an abrasive manufactured from an impure aluminum oxide (bauxite) and produced in various particle sizes. The particles are applied most commonly to paper or plastic disks in coarse, medium, and fine grits. The disks are reddish brown. Aluminum oxide powders (typically 27- and 50-μm particle sizes) are used in air-abrasion units.

Cuttle is an abrasive manufactured from the bones of fish, although this form is no longer used as a dental abrasive. Presently, cuttle is a trade name that refers to a fine grade of quartz (SiO_2). The particles are applied to a paper disk in coarse, medium, and fine grits. The medium cuttle grit is similar in abrasive action to fine sand grit. Cuttle disks are beige.

Diamond is the hardest known substance. Diamond chips normally are impregnated in a binder to form diamond "stones" and disks. Disks, cups, and points with microfine diamonds (PoGo; DENTSPLY Caulk, Milford, DE) are available for polishing resin composite restorations to achieve a high gloss (Figure 6-1).

Garnet is an abrasive that is mined. In pure form, it is composed of oxides of aluminum, iron, and silicon. Garnet is available on paper or plastic disks in extra-coarse, coarse, medium, fine, and extra-fine grits and is red.

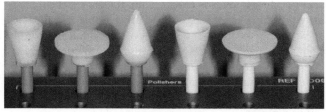

FIG 6-1 Disks, cups, and points for polishing composite restorations. The various shapes allow access to different anatomical conditions. For example, disks are useful for polishing embrasures, whereas points are more useful for polishing pits. (Courtesy Y-W Chen, University of Washington Department of Restorative Dentistry, Seattle, WA.)

Sand is a form of quartz (SiO_2) used as an abrasive agent. It is available on plastic or paper disks in coarse, medium, and fine grits and is beige. Sand disks should not be used interchangeably with cuttle disks, although they are also of quartz, because the particle sizes of the coarse, medium, and fine grits are not the same for both abrasives.

Silicon carbide (SiC) is the second hardest of the dental abrasives and usually is applied to paper or plastic disks. The disks are available in fine, extra-fine, and double extra-fine grits and are black.

The abrasive agents commonly used in dentistry for polishing and cleansing follow. Calcite is a form of calcium carbonate ($CaCO_3$). It is available in various grades as used in prophylactic pastes. Another physical form of calcium carbonate is chalk, which is used in dentifrices as a polishing agent.

Kieselguhr is a polishing agent and is composed of the siliceous remains of minute aquatic plants known as diatoms. The coarse form of kieselguhr is known as diatomaceous earth.

Pumice is a highly siliceous volcanic glass that when ground is useful as a polishing agent in prophylactic pastes and for finishing acrylic denture bases in the laboratory.

Rouge is a fine red powder composed of iron oxide (Fe_2O_3) that usually is used in cake form. It may be impregnated in

TABLE 6-1   Hardness and Grade of Various Types of Finishing Disks

Product*	Abrasive	MOHS value	Knoop (kg/mm^2)	Grade
Waterproof, fine waterproof, extra fine waterproof, double extra fine	Silicon carbide	9+	2480	320 400 600
Adalox, coarse Adalox, medium	Aluminum oxide	9	2100	150 220
Adalox, fine garnet, coarse garnet, medium garnet, fine garnet, extra fine	Garnet (a silicate)	6.5–7	1360	60 80 120 180 240
Cuttle, coarse cuttle, medium cuttle, fine	Flint (quartz, silicon dioxide)	7	820	150 220 400
Crocus	Iron oxide			

*E.C. Moore Co., Inc., Dearborn, MI.
From Charbeneau GT: Unpublished data, University of Michigan School of Dentistry, Ann Arbor, MI.

paper or fabric known as crocus cloth. It is an excellent laboratory polishing agent for gold and other noble metal alloys.

Silex refers to siliceous materials such as quartz or tripoli, which are used as polishing abrasives in the mouth.

Tin oxide (SnO_2) is a pure white powder used extensively as a final polishing agent for teeth and metallic restorations in the mouth. It is mixed with water, alcohol, or glycerin and used as a paste.

Tripoli is a polishing agent that originates from certain porous rocks found in North Africa. It often is confused with kieselguhr.

Zirconium silicate ($ZrSiO_4$) is a hard abrasive that, in small particle sizes, is used as a polishing agent.

In addition to the abrasive agents already cited, several other abrasives are found in prophylactic pastes, including quartz, anatase (TiO_2), feldspar, montmorillonite, aluminum hydroxide, kaolinite, and talc. Further information on prophylactic materials is presented later in this chapter.

The abrasives found in dentifrices include calcium carbonate, dibasic calcium phosphate dihydrate, anhydrous dibasic calcium phosphate, tricalcium phosphate, calcium pyrophosphate, sodium metaphosphate, hydrated alumina, and silica. These are mainly cleansing and polishing abrasives not meant to abrade enamel severely.

Finishing and Polishing Techniques

The finishing and polishing techniques for most restorative dental materials follow similar principles. Initial contouring and smoothing of the surface are done with a coarse abrasive or bur; increasingly finer abrasives then remove the large scratches produced. The use of too fine an abrasive after a coarse one is time consuming and does not give a properly finished surface. A key to successful finishing and polishing is strict adherence to a recommended abrasive sequence.

With each successive change in abrasive, the area being finished and polished is rinsed to remove the previously used abrasive particles. One remaining particle of coarse abrasive can mar a well-polished surface. The abrasive tool or slurry must not be used in a dry condition. Dry polishing may reduce dramatically the efficiency of the abrasive and increase the danger of overheating the surface.

The abrasives chosen to finish and polish various restorative materials depend to a great extent on the properties of the particular restorative material. The discussion that follows involves consideration of the surface roughness that is caused by various abrasive agents, a recommended finishing and polishing sequence, and the precautions that should be taken in finishing and polishing some common restorative materials.

Amalgam

The average surface roughness produced by various methods of instrumentation on amalgam is listed in Table 6-2. A suggested abrasive sequence for finishing and polishing an occlusoproximal restoration is indicated therein.

When an amalgam restoration has been properly manipulated, it will be hardened sufficiently within a few minutes to

TABLE 6-2 **Average Surface Roughness of Dental Amalgam Produced by Various Methods of Instrumentation**	
Method of instrumentation	Roughness (R_a, μm)
Carved	4.6*
Carved and immediately smoothened (burnished)	0.36*
Condensed against uncontoured matrix band	0.61
Rotating finishing Instruments	
S.S. White green stone	0.64–1.0*
Finishing bur	0.46–0.64*
Waterproof (silicon carbide) fine	0.58*
Rotating polishing Instruments	
Robinson Soft Cup Brushwith extra-fine silex	0.18*
With tin oxide	0.10*
Interproximal finishing strips	
Moyco "Evenwet" extra-fine sand	0.30*
Extra-fine on 1 Dentotape with silex–tin oxide	0.10*

*Suggested abrasive sequence for finishing and polishing an occlusoproximal amalgam restoration.
Modified from Charbeneau GT: A suggested technique for polishing amalgam restorations, *J Mich Dent Assoc* 47: 320, 1965.

permit carving with a sharp instrument. Then the amalgam restoration is carved to the margins to remove all excess amalgam. Then it is burnished with a metal instrument that has a broad surface to smooth the surface. After this initial carving operation, the restoration is left undisturbed for an appropriate period before finishing and polishing with rotating instruments or interproximal strips. Most amalgams can be polished the day after their placement. The time delay allows the amalgams to develop strength. Only amalgams that have high early strengths can be finished and polished at the first appointment.

Polishing, in these cases, is done through the application of a sequence of operations that includes the use of fine stones and abrasive disks or strips. The final polish is developed, as indicated in Table 6-2, by the application of extra-fine silex, followed by the application of a thin slurry of tin oxide, with a rotating soft brush. During this final polishing operation, the restoration should be kept moist to avoid overheating.

Some of the fast-setting high-copper amalgams, as discussed in Chapter 5, can be polished about 8 to 12 minutes after placement because of their rapid development of strength. Polishing is performed with a creamy paste of extra-fine silex and water applied gently in an unwebbed rubber cup with a slow-speed handpiece for 30 seconds per surface.

Composites

The average surface roughness produced by various methods of instrumentation on microhybrid and microfilled composite restorative materials, in addition to a suggested sequence for finishing, is listed in Table 6-3. Some examples of commercial finishing and polishing systems for composites are listed in Table 6-4.

TABLE 6-3   Average Surface Roughness of Composites and Resin-Modified Glass Ionomers Produced by Various Methods of Instrumentation

	ROUGHNESS (R_a, μm)		
Method of instrumentation	**Microhybrid composite**	**Microfilled composite**	**Resin-modified glass ionomer**
Mylar matrix	0.05*	0.02*	0.2*
Carbide finishing burs (12-fluted)	0.3*	0.45	0.62
Enhance cups	0.36	0.54	0.7
Enhance paste	0.20	0.36	0.68
Abrasive disks			
Fine	0.15*	0.18*	0.3*
Extra fine	0.08*	0.11*	0.26*
Glaze			0.23*

*Suggested sequence for finishing and polishing.
From Tate WH, Powers JM: Unpublished data, University of Texas School of Dentistry at Houston, Houston, TX.

TABLE 6-4   Examples of Commercial Finishing and Polishing Systems for Composites and Ceramics

Composite finishing and polishing systems		
Product	**Manufacturer**	**Abrasive**
Super-Snap X-Treme	Shofu Dental Corporation	Aluminum oxide
Gazelle Nano Composite Polisher	Microcopy	Aluminum oxide, diamond
PoGo One Step Diamond Micro Polishers	DENTSPLY Caulk	Diamond
Ceramic finishing and polishing systems		
Product	**Manufacturer**	**Abrasive**
Luster for lithium disilicate	Meisinger USA, LLC	Diamond
Luster for zirconia	Meisinger USA, LLC	Diamond

Composites in the past presented a problem in finishing and polishing because of the hard filler particles in a soft resin matrix. Allowing polymerization of the freshly inserted resin to occur against a Mylar (polyester film) matrix produces the smoothest surface on a composite. An acceptable finishing procedure for current microhybrid, microfilled, or nanofilled composites includes the use of diamond stones or 12-blade carbide burs for removal of gross excesses that are not near enamel margins. This step is followed by the use of abrasive disks for the finishing of accessible areas. White stones of suitable shape are used for the finishing of more inaccessible areas. Fine and microfine diamonds and diamond polishing pastes and disks are suitable for the final finishing of composites to produce low surface roughness and high gloss.

The roughness of finished and polished compomer restorations is similar to that of composites. The technique of finishing of compomer restorations is like that of composites.

Ceramics

Silica-based and zirconia-based ceramics are typically polished using diamond-impregnated instruments. Some examples of commercial finishing and polishing systems for silica- and zirconia-based ceramics are listed in Table 6-4.

Resin-Modified Glass Ionomers

The average surface roughness produced by various methods of instrumentation on a resin-modified glass ionomer, in addition to a suggested sequence for finishing, is listed in Table 6-3.

Resin-modified glass ionomers do not finish as smoothly as microhybrid composites. Like the composites, the best finish is obtained when the restoration hardens against a Mylar matrix. An unfilled resin coating (liquid polish) can be applied to smooth the surface after finishing, but the coating may wear away in the mouth.

Glass Ionomers

The roughness of finished and polished glass ionomer restorations is higher than that of composites and resin-modified glass ionomers, primarily because of the larger particle sizes of the filler. The technique of finishing of glass ionomer restorations is like that of composites, except that some products require a delay of 24 hours before polishing to allow further setting.

Gold Alloy

The average surface roughness produced by various methods of instrumentation on a Type II gold casting, as well as a suggested abrasive sequence for finishing and polishing, is listed in Table 6-5.

Gold restorations made by the indirect technique are finished and polished on the die after the occlusion and margins have been properly adjusted. Finishing of the pickled casting and polishing of proximal surfaces is done in the laboratory. Use of careful control of the direction and force of the polishing action avoids the overfinishing of margins and contours. The casting generally is scrubbed with alcohol to prepare its surface for cementation.

TABLE 6-5   Average Surface Roughness of a Type II Gold Casting Produced by the Suggested Sequence for Finishing and Polishing

Method of instrumentation	Roughness (R_a, μm)
Polished wax, pickled casting	0.43
Finishing instruments	
Moore's fine cuttle	0.23
Polishing instruments	
Disks—Moore's crocus	0.08
Rag wheel—Sureshine	0.05
Chamois with rouge	0.04–0.05

From Charbeneau GT: Unpublished data, University of Michigan School of Dentistry, Ann Arbor, MI.

Denture Bases

> **! ALERT**
>
> A shell blaster sprays finely divided nutshells against the surface under high velocity.

The acrylic denture base is ready for finishing and polishing once it has been processed and deflasked. Any gypsum material that remains on the denture can be removed by light scraping or with a shell blaster. Feathered edges of acrylic can be smoothed and rounded with an acrylic finishing bur. A rag wheel and felt cone with pumice slurry are used to finish the tongue side of a maxillary base. A single-row brush wheel and a rag wheel about 6 mm in width are used with pumice slurry to smooth the labial and buccal surfaces on the tongue side of a mandibular denture without destroying the contour. A final high polish is given to all non–tissue-bearing surfaces by a rag wheel with tripoli, Bendick, or a paste of tin oxide and water.

Overheating during the polishing of an acrylic denture base can occur because of the low thermal conductivity of the acrylic and must be avoided. Overheating affects the appearance of the denture and may cause warpage to occur. Acrylic denture teeth must be protected from the pumice because they are abraded easily. After the polishing, the denture should be washed with soap and water and stored in water until it is delivered to the patient.

To maintain infection control, separate polishing burs, rag wheels, and pumice pans should be used for prostheses. Pumice can be mixed with a liquid disinfectant (5 parts sodium hypochlorite to 100 parts distilled water) and green soap (3 parts) to keep the pumice suspended. Pumice should be changed daily. Rag wheels can be sterilized in a steam autoclave or by ethylene oxide.

PROPHYLACTIC PASTES

Routine dental prophylaxis for the removal of exogenous stains, pellicle, materia alba, and oral debris is a widely used procedure in the dental office. Prophylaxis should precede the application of a fluoride gel or solution to make the enamel accessible and more reactive to the fluoride. Ideally, a dental prophylactic paste should be sufficiently abrasive to remove effectively all types of accumulation from the tooth surface without imparting undue abrasion to the enamel, dentin, or cementum. In addition to acting as a cleansing agent, the paste should have the quality of endowing the hard tissue with a highly polished, esthetic appearance. Certain prophylactic pastes contain sodium fluoride or stannous fluoride either mixed with the abrasive or in a more complex, buffered system.

Composition

The abrasives in various commercial prophylactic pastes are listed in Table 6-6.

Properties

Laboratory and clinical studies of cleaning and polishing have compared the efficiency of various prophylactic pastes. Products that contain predominantly pumice and quartz show higher cleansing values but generally result in a greater abrasion to both enamel and dentin. In fact, abrasion data have indicated that some prophylactic pastes may be unnecessarily destructive to enamel. The products containing coarse pumice are generally the most abrasive. Zirconium silicate is a particularly effective cleansing and polishing agent, but the polishing properties of zirconium silicate are influenced considerably by the distribution of particle sizes of the material in various commercial products. In a clinical study, prophylactic pastes with silicate abrasives produced higher polishing scores for enamel with lower abrasion of enamel than pastes with other abrasives did (see Table 6-6). Abrasion of dentin has been measured to be five to six times greater than abrasion of enamel, regardless of the product used.

One product (Clinpro Prophy Paste; 3M ESPE, St. Paul, MN) contains particles of perlite that wear during use. **Perlite** is a volcanic glass with sheetlike geometry. As the particles wear, they become smaller but continue to abrade, which produces an increasingly smoother tooth surface.

TABLE 6-6   Abrasives in Various Commercial Prophylactic Pastes

Prophylactic paste	Abrasive	Manufacturer
Butler Paste-Free Prophy	Pumice incorporated into the cup	Sunstar Americas (Chicago, IL)
Clinpro	Perlite	3M ESPE (St. Paul, MN)
NUPRO NU Solutions Prophy Paste	NovaMin (calcium sodium phosphosilicate)	DENTSPLY Professional (York, PA)
Zircate	Zirconium silicate	DENTSPLY Caulk (Milford, DE)

Prophylaxis pastes that contain fluoride have been subjected to several clinical trials. Results have varied from no benefit to benefits as high as a 35% reduction in caries after 3 years. The design of some of these studies makes it difficult to assess the effects of the prophylaxis agent alone.

During a prophylactic procedure, excessive abrasion of any restorative material present should be avoided. Polymeric materials such as denture base and artificial tooth resins, laboratory composites, and direct composites are particularly susceptible to wear because of their low hardness. The result of such wear can be possible reduction in contours and increased surface roughness, both of which are undesirable.

DENTIFRICES

The primary function of a dentifrice is to clean and polish the surfaces of the teeth accessible to a toothbrush. In addition to enhancing personal appearance by maintaining cleaner teeth, brushing with a dentifrice may reduce the incidence of dental caries, help maintain a healthy gingiva, and reduce the intensity of mouth odors. During the process of cleaning, extraneous debris or deposits to be removed, given in order of increasing difficulty of removal from the tooth surface, are food debris, plaque (a soft, mainly bacterial film), acquired pellicle (a proteinaceous film of salivary origin), and calculus.

Composition and Role of Ingredients

Dentifrices are prepared primarily in paste and powder forms. Tooth powders contain an abrasive, a surface-active detergent, flavoring oils, and sweetening agents. In addition to the powder ingredients, toothpastes contain water, a humectant (to prevent dehydration), a binder, and a preservative. Many dentifrices contain fluoride (Table 6-7) in the form of sodium fluoride, sodium monofluorophosphate, or stannous fluoride to help prevent dental caries. The composition

TABLE 6-8 Composition of a Therapeutic Dentifrice

Major ingredients	Percentage (wt%)
Abrasives	40
Water	29.6
Sorbitol (70% solution)	20
Glycerin	10
Stannous fluoride	0.4

Modified from Council on Dental Therapeutics: *Accepted dental therapeutics,* Chicago, 1979, American Dental Association.

of a dentifrice containing stannous fluoride is given in Table 6-8. Soluble tetrasodium or tetrapotassium pyrophosphates (3.3%) may be added to reduce the rate of formation of supragingival calculus, thus providing a cosmetic benefit. One antiplaque–antigingivitis toothpaste contains triclosan (0.3%) and sodium fluoride (0.24%).

The abrasives used in various dentifrice preparations are listed earlier in this chapter. Ideally, the abrasive should exhibit a maximum cleansing efficiency with minimum tooth abrasion. In addition, an abrasive should be present to polish the teeth. Some toothpastes advertised as able to whiten or brighten teeth contain the harsher abrasive agents such as silica, calcium carbonate, or anhydrous dibasic calcium phosphate. The only satisfactory method of determining the abrasiveness of a dentifrice appears to be a test on teeth, although laboratory data have been published.

Abrasion of enamel by modern dentifrices is generally not a problem unless unusual oral conditions exist; however, exposed dentin and cementum are susceptible to abrasion. An example of cervical abrasion that results from excessive use of a toothbrush and dentifrice is shown in Figure 6-2.

TABLE 6-7 Examples of Dentifrices That Contain Fluoride Accepted by the Council on Scientific Affairs, American Dental Association

Product	Manufacturer
Antiplaque/Antigingivitis with sodium fluoride	
Colgate Total toothpaste	Colgate-Palmolive (New York, NY)
Sodium fluoride	
Aqua-Fresh All with Tartar Control toothpaste	GlaxoSmithKline (Pittsburgh, PA)
Colgate Tartar Control Formula toothpaste	Colgate-Palmolive
Crest Tartar Control Formula toothpaste	Procter & Gamble (Cincinnati, OH)
Sodium monofluorophosphate	
Aqua-Fresh Fluoride toothpaste	GlaxoSmithKline
Colgate Great Regular Flavor Fluoride toothpaste	Colgate-Palmolive

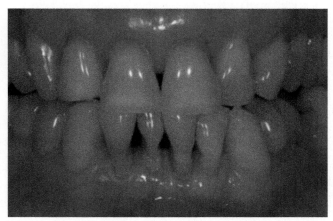

FIG 6-2 Cervical abrasion. The causes of cervical loss of tooth structure is complex but often involves excessive use of toothbrush and dentifrices or use of overly abrasive dentifrices. Repair of these types of lesions is often challenging because of esthetic demands, the proximity of the pulp chamber, and difficulty obtaining good retention form in the cavity preparation. (Courtesy Y-W Chen, University of Washington Department of Restorative Dentistry, Seattle, WA.)

Patients having exposed cementum or dentin should avoid regular use of dentifrice powders or highly abrasive pastes.

Polymeric restorative materials are also susceptible to abrasion from toothbrush and dentifrice use. The patient should be cautioned not to use dentifrices for cleansing denture bases or acrylic denture teeth.

The remaining ingredients in dentifrices increase the effectiveness of the cleansing and polishing agents or to make the dentifrice more appealing to use. A surface-active agent, generally a detergent, is added to improve the wettability of the enamel by the dentifrice, thereby improving contact with enamel by the abrasives. Flavoring oils and sweetening agents, usually saccharin, are added to make the dentifrice more appealing. To keep the paste from drying out, a humectant such as sorbitol, propylene glycol, or glycerin is used. Sorbitol is also a sweetening agent. To help control consistency and to keep the abrasives in suspension, a binder, such as sodium alginate, is used. Sodium carboxymethyl cellulose may serve as a stabilizer for the alginate binder. A foaming agent is added to favor the formation of a stable foam when the paste is used.

Effect of Toothbrush

Many studies have examined the influence of the toothbrush and its variables on abrasion. When compared with the abrasion of common dentifrices, the bristles have little abrasive power. Properties of the bristles, such as configuration, hardness, stiffness, and number, generally do not influence abrasion by themselves, although they do affect the abrasion caused by the dentifrice. Mechanical toothbrushing devices generally cause less abrasion of enamel and dentin than manual brushing does because the force applied to the mechanical devices is usually less.

Selection of Toothbrush and Dentifrice

The best available guidelines to follow in selecting a dentifrice for a patient are based on evaluation of the following four factors:
1. Degree of staining of the dentition
2. Force exerted on the brush
3. Method of brushing
4. Amount of exposed dentin or cementum

Choice of a dentifrice for appropriate abrasion can then be based on the ranking of the abrasivity of dentifrices reported by the American Dental Association. Even so, comparison of products with similar abrasivity scores is not possible because of the experimental error associated with measuring the abrasion data. Selection of a toothbrush should be based on the requirements of the patient's soft tissue. In particular, abrasion of the soft tissue by hard, stiff bristles should be avoided.

DENTURE CLEANSERS

Denture base materials and denture teeth collect deposits in the same manner as natural teeth. Soft food debris that clings to a denture can be removed easily by light brushing followed by rinsing. Hard deposits of calculus and stains, such as those that occur from tobacco tars, are much more difficult to remove. The following two methods are commonly used to remove both stains and calculus:
1. Professional repolishing of the denture
2. Soaking or brushing of the denture on a daily basis at home

The first method, repolishing the surfaces of the denture at extended time intervals, is not suitable for home care of dentures. Repolishing is a technique that follows much the same sequence recommended for the initial finishing and polishing of denture base materials described earlier in this chapter. The technique can alter the surface of a denture made of acrylic polymer appreciably if it is applied too vigorously or too often because acrylic denture bases have relatively poor resistance to abrasion.

The second method, soaking a denture in a solution or brushing it with a powder or paste, is suitable for home care. If denture cleansers are properly used, the accumulation of dental plaque and stains can be controlled effectively.

Requirements

An ideal denture cleanser should meet the following six criteria:
1. Be nontoxic and easy to remove, leaving no traces of irritant material
2. Be able to attack or dissolve both the organic and inorganic portions of denture deposits
3. Be harmless to all materials used in the construction of dentures, including denture base polymers and alloys, acrylic and porcelain teeth, and resilient lining materials
4. Not be harmful to eyes, skin, or clothing if accidentally spilled or splashed
5. Be stable during storage
6. Preferably be bactericidal and fungicidal

Types

Following are three major types of denture cleansers for use at home:
1. Abrasive creams
2. Alkaline hypochlorites
3. Alkaline perborates

Examples of commercial products and their active ingredients are listed in Table 6-9.

Certain denture cleansers contain sodium perborate $NaBO_2 \cdot H_2O_2 \cdot 3H_2O$, which is a source of peroxide (H_2O_2). The decomposition of peroxide in water is favored in a basic solution. The pH of several perborate cleansers ranges from 7 to 11.5. Cleansing presumably results from the oxidizing ability of the peroxide decomposition and from the effervescing action of evolved oxygen. Some of these cleansers also contain chloride ions that can cause corrosion of base metal components.

Effectiveness

The brushing of a denture surface is an effective means of improving denture cleanliness and maintaining a healthy mucosa beneath a removable denture. Chemical cleansers may be useful alternatives to brushing among geriatric or disabled denture patients. Daily overnight immersion of

TABLE 6-9 Types of Commercial Denture Cleansers

Type of cleanser	Product	Active ingredients
Abrasive cream	Dentu-Crème (GlaxoSmithKline, Pittsburgh, PA)	Calcium carbonate
	Fresh N Brite* (Pfizer, Morris Plains, NJ)	Hydrated silica precipitated
Alkaline hypochlorite	Calgon and Clorox	Sodium hypochlorite, trisodium phosphate
Alkaline perborate	Efferdent/Single Layer* (Pfizer)	Sodium perborate or derivative, potassium monopersulfate
	Polident (GlaxoSmithKline)	Citric acid, isopropyl

*Acceptable product of Council on Scientific Affairs.

dentures in an alkaline peroxide solution provides a safe and relatively effective means of cleansing. However, customary 15-minute soaking is neither effective on mature plaque nor completely effective on stains and deposits. Ultrasonic vibration is not an efficient method for removing denture plaque.

Recommended Techniques and Precautions

Several techniques for cleaning dentures can be recommended. One effective technique requires immersion in a solution of one part of 5% sodium hypochlorite in three parts of water followed by light brushing. Another technique for cleaning acrylic dentures is immersion in a solution containing 1 teaspoon of a hypochlorite (Clorox) and 2 teaspoons of a glassy phosphate (Calgon) in one-half glass of water. This cleanser is not recommended for use on prosthetic appliances fabricated from base metals such as cobalt–chromium alloy because chlorine solutions tend to darken these metals. Dentures should never be soaked in hot water because the heat may cause the acrylic to become distorted.

Although light meticulous brushing is a recommended method of cleaning the denture, brushing with hard, stiff bristles should be avoided because these bristles produce scratches on the surface of the denture. Do not use dentifrices to aid in cleaning a denture at home, although pastes with gentle abrasives (acrylic resin, sodium bicarbonate, or a $ZrSiO_4$-ZrO_2 system) can be used. Organic solvents such as chloroform should be avoided because these chemicals may dissolve or craze an acrylic denture. If the denture is not worn after cleaning, it is stored in water to retain its dimensional accuracy. Some soaking types of denture cleansers may cause soft liners to change color. A procedure for cleaning a denture with a soft liner is to clean the external and tooth surfaces of the denture with a soft brush and denture paste and the soft lining material with cotton under cold water. Disadvantages of various types of denture cleansers are summarized in Table 6-10.

WHITENING

In-office whitening (bleaching) techniques may be effective for lightening teeth stained by fluorosis, tetracycline, and acquired superficial discoloration. Recently, whitening techniques have been combined with bonded composites and ceramic veneers as a procedure in esthetic dentistry. Whitening teeth outside the dental office was introduced in 1989.

Composition

Whitening agents used in the office commonly contain 30% to 35% hydrogen peroxide. One system mixes 35% hydrogen peroxide with silica to form a gel. Another system contains calcium, phosphate, and fluoride ions to allow remineralization during treatment.

Home whitening products typically contain 10% to 22% carbamide peroxide or 1.5% to 6% hydrogen peroxide. The pH of these products ranges from 4.6 to 6.7 when undiluted and from 4.3 to 6.6 when diluted 1:2 with water.

Properties

Whitening is often the primary treatment to improve esthetics. The effects may last a year, and retreatment is simple. Yellow, orange, or light brown stains, often associated with aging, are treated most successfully. If no major improvement in color occurs within a reasonable time, bonding or veneering should be considered.

Whitening agents do not adversely affect gold alloys, amalgam, microfilled composites, or porcelain. Some microhybrid composites, resin-modified glass ionomers, and glass ionomers have been roughened slightly by whitening gels. Whitening agents should not come into contact with dentin because some products remove the smear layer, resulting in tooth hypersensitivity.

Side effects are uncommon but include tooth hypersensitivity, soft tissue lesions or sloughing, nausea, temporomandibular joint syndrome from the tray, and sore throats from

TABLE 6-10 Disadvantages of Various Types of Denture Cleansers

Type of cleanser	Disadvantages
Abrasive	Can abrade acrylic dentures and teeth
Alkaline hypochlorite	May cause bleaching, can corrode stainless steel and cobalt–chromium alloys, may leave an odor on denture
Alkaline perborate	Does not easily remove heavy deposits

swallowing the bleach. Gels with a higher viscosity are less likely to be diluted or swallowed during application. It has been shown that hydrogen peroxide is the main cytotoxic component of the peroxide-containing whitening agents, and the extent of cytotoxicity corresponds to the peroxide concentration. Peroxide whitening agents are readily diffused through 0.5 mm of dentin in concentration to produce cytotoxicity.

Techniques

Three major methods of in-office whitening involve the use of heat, light, and gels. Heat and light systems typically use a powerful whitening light or wand that is calibrated to control the temperature. Three in-office treatments or one in-office treatment combined with a home program are needed to produce satisfactory results.

The gel technique is a more conservative chair-side approach. The gel is placed on tooth enamel in a 2-mm-thick layer for 20 to 30 minutes. Patients with dark tetracycline stains usually require three to four 30-minute appointments. The gel technique works faster if combined with the use of a light-curing unit for 10 minutes.

Home whitening techniques require plaque removal followed by use of a tray of gel for 3 to 4 hours once or several times a day. The gel is replenished each hour. Whitening effectiveness is related to the number of hours the tray is worn. Construction of a 2-mm application tray is similar to that of a custom-made mouth protector as discussed in Chapter 3, except that gauze may be used to outline areas of the tray where the whitening agent is to be applied.

Universal whitening guidelines should be followed in the office: comprehensive clinical examination, full-mouth radiographs, photographs, evaluation of existing restorations and pathologic conditions, prophylaxis, rubber dam, eyewear and glove protection, no anesthesia, and constant patient monitoring. Those who use gels must follow additional guidelines: stored 35% hydrogen peroxide activator is refrigerated, anesthesia is never used, the patient is never left unattended, and the patient's eyes are protected.

⟳ QUICK REVIEW

Finishing and polishing techniques are important in preparation of clinically successful restorations. The process of abrasion is affected by properties of the abrasive and the material being abraded. Finishing and polishing begin with coarse abrasives and end with fine ones. Clinically, it is easier to control the rate of abrasion by speed than by pressure. Care must be taken to avoid overfinishing margins and contours of restorations and to avoid overheating denture resins and other restorations. The use of prophylactic pastes and dentifrices also must not unduly abrade tooth structure or restorative materials.

❓ SELF-TEST QUESTIONS

In the following multiple-choice questions, one or more responses may be correct.

1. A rough surface on a restoration is undesirable for which of the following reasons?
   a. Food debris and plaque can easily cling to it.
   b. Irritation and recession of soft tissues can occur in proximity to it.
   c. It is responsible for acceleration of corrosion of metallic restorations.
2. The rate of abrasion is increased by use of which of the following?
   a. A finer particle size
   b. An abrasive tool with rounded cutting surfaces
   c. Greater pressure on the abrasive tool
   d. Greater speed on the tool
3. Which of the following are finishing abrasives, and which are polishing abrasives?
   a. Tin oxide
   b. Sand
   c. Rouge
   d. Alumina
   e. Silicon carbide
   f. Diamond
   g. Silex
   h. Zirconium silicate
4. Final polishing of a dental amalgam to the smoothest surface is achieved by which of the following?
   a. Burnishing
   b. Carving
   c. Use of tin oxide
   d. Use of fine silicon carbide

5. Final polishing of cast gold alloy to the smoothest surface is achieved by which of the following?
   a. Pickling
   b. Electropolishing
   c. Use of rouge on a chamois
   d. Use of fine cuttle
6. Final polishing of non–tissue-bearing surfaces of a denture resin is achieved by which of the following?
   a. Shell blasting
   b. Use of Bendick on a rag wheel
   c. Use of fine pumice
   d. Use of an acrylic finishing bur
7. The best surface for a microhybrid composite resin is achieved by which of the following?
   a. Allowance of polymerization to occur against a Mylar matrix
   b. Use of a greenstone
   c. Use of an extra-fine silicon carbide disk
   d. Use of a white stone
8. Which of the following statements about prophylactic pastes is/are true?
   a. The abrasion of enamel is about twice that of dentin for a given product.
   b. Zirconium silicate is an effective cleansing and polishing agent, independent of its particle-size distribution.
   c. Use prophylactic paste before the application of a fluoride gel to make the enamel accessible and more reactive to the fluoride.
   d. Composites are not susceptible to abrasive wear by a prophylactic paste because of their hardness.

9. Desirable effects of toothbrushing are which of the following?
   a. Reduction of incidence of dental caries
   b. Maintenance of a healthy gingiva
   c. Reduction in intensity of mouth odors
   d. Enhancement of personal appearance
10. The components in a dentifrice may include which of the following?
   a. An abrasive such as insoluble sodium metaphosphate
   b. A therapeutic agent such as stannous fluoride
   c. A humectant such as glycerin
   d. A sweetening agent such as sorbitol
11. Which of the following surfaces is/are particularly susceptible to abrasion by dentifrices?
   a. Cementum
   b. Dentin
   c. Enamel
   d. Gold alloys
   e. Laboratory composites
   f. Acrylic denture resins
   g. Composite resins
12. Which of the following statements about denture cleansers is/are true?

a. Do not soak dentures in hot water because the heat may cause the acrylic denture to become distorted.
b. Use a dentifrice with a stiff-bristled brush.
c. Customary 15-minute soaking of a denture with chemical cleansers is effective neither on mature plaque nor on some stains and deposits.
d. Some chemical denture cleansers may cause corrosion of base metal components of a denture.
   Use short answers to fill in the following blanks.
13. A smooth surface is desirable to _____ retention of bacteria.
14. A gloss value more than 70 GU is considered _____ gloss.

For the following statements, answer true or false.
15. A smooth surface is defined as having a roughness (R_a) of less than 0.2 μm.
   a. True
   b. False
16. As perlite particles wear, they become smaller and no longer abrade the surface.
   a. True
   b. False

SUGGESTED SUPPLEMENTARY READINGS

General Information
Meyer DM: Voluntary programs: ADA Seal program and international implications, *Ann Periodontol* 2(1):31, 1997.

Abrasion, Dentifrices, and Prophylactic Pastes
Berry EA III: Air abrasion in clinical dental practice. In Hardin JF, editor: *Clark's clinical dentistry*, St Louis, 1996, Mosby.

Farah JW, Powers JM, editors: Finishing and polishing, *Dent Advis* 5 (3):1, 1988.

Farah JW, Powers JM, editors: Ceramic finishing and polishing, *Dent Advis* 20(4):1, 2003.

Farah JW, Powers JM: Composite finishing and polishing, *Dent Advis* 20(6):1, 2003.

Gershon SD, Pader M: Dentifrices. In Balsam MS, Sagarin E, editors: ed 2, *Cosmetics science and technology*, vol 1, New York, 1972, John Wiley & Sons.

Hoelscher DC, Neme AML, Pink FE, Hughes PJ: The effect of three finishing systems on four esthetic restorative materials, *Oper Dent* 23:36, 1998.

Hondrum SO, Fernández R Jr.: Contouring, finishing and polishing Class 5 restorative materials, *Oper Dent* 22:30, 1997.

Nygaard-Østby P, Edvardsen S, Spydevold B: Access to interproximal tooth surfaces by different designs and stiffness of toothbrushes, *Scand J Dent Res* 87:424, 1979.

Nygaard-Østby P, Spydevold B, Edvardsen S: Suggestion for a definition, measuring method and classification system of bristle stiffness of toothbrushes, *Scand J Dent Res* 87:159, 1979.

Powers JM, Bayne SC: Friction and wear of dental materials. *ASM handbook: friction, lubrication, and wear technology*, vol 18, Materials Park, OH, 1992, ASM International.

Warren DP, Colescott TD, Henson HA, et al: Effects of four prophylaxis pastes on surface roughness of a composite, a hybrid ionomer, and a compomer restorative material, *J Esthet Restor Dent* 14:245, 2002.

Denture Cleansers
Budtz-Jørgensen E: Materials and methods for cleaning dentures, *J Prosthet Dent* 42:619, 1979.

Whitening
Bunek SS, editor: In-office and take-home whitening, *Dent Advis* 29 (8):1, 2012.

Council on Dental Therapeutics: Guidelines for the acceptance of peroxide containing oral hygiene products, *J Am Dent Assoc* 125:1140, 1994.

Fay R-M, Powers JM: Nightguard vital bleaching: a review of the literature 1994–1999, *J Gt Houst Dent Soc* 71:20, 1999.

Lynch E, Sheerin A, Samarawickrama DY, et al: Molecular mechanisms of the bleaching actions associated with commercially-available whitening oral health care products, *Irish Dent Assoc J* 41:94, 1995.

evolve Please visit *http://evolve.elsevier.com/Powers/dentalmaterials* for additional practice and study support tools.

7

Cements

OBJECTIVES

After reading this chapter, the student should be able to:

Water-Based Cements

1. Do the following when it comes to glass ionomer cements:
   - List the components and indicate their function.
   - Describe the setting reaction, and indicate any variables that may affect the setting.
   - Describe the clinical importance of film thickness, working and setting times, compressive strength, retention and type of bond to tooth structure, and fluoride release.
   - Discuss the properties and biocompatibility.
   - Describe the manipulation.
2. Do the following when it comes to resin-modified glass ionomer cements:
   - List the components and indicate their function.
   - Describe the setting reaction, and indicate any variables that may affect the setting.
   - Describe the clinical importance of film thickness, working and setting times, compressive strength, retention and type of bond to tooth structure, and fluoride release.
   - Discuss the properties and biocompatibility.
   - Describe the manipulation.
3. Define bioceramic cement and discuss its requirements.

Oil-Based Cements

4. Do the following when it comes to zinc oxide–eugenol cements:
   - List the components and indicate their function.
   - Describe the setting reaction, and indicate any variables that may affect the setting.
   - Describe the clinical importance of film thickness, working and setting times, compressive strength, retention and type of bond to tooth structure, and fluoride release.
   - Discuss the properties and biocompatibility.
   - Describe the manipulation.

Resin-Based Cements

5. Do the following when it comes to esthetic resin cements:
   - List the components and indicate their function.
   - Describe the setting reaction, and indicate any variables that may affect the setting.
   - Describe the clinical importance of film thickness, working and setting times, compressive strength, retention and type of bond to tooth structure, and fluoride release.
   - Discuss the properties and biocompatibility.
   - Describe the manipulation.
6. Do the following when it comes to adhesive resin cements:
   - List the components and indicate their function.
   - Describe the setting reaction, and indicate any variables that may affect the setting.
   - Describe the clinical importance of film thickness, working and setting times, compressive strength, retention and type of bond to tooth structure, and fluoride release.
   - Discuss the properties and biocompatibility.
   - Describe the manipulation.
7. Do the following when it comes to self-adhesive resin cements:
   - List the components and indicate their function.
   - Describe the setting reaction, and indicate any variables that may affect the setting.
   - Describe the clinical importance of film thickness, working and setting times, compressive strength, retention and type of bond to tooth structure, and fluoride release.
   - Discuss the properties and biocompatibility.
   - Describe the manipulation.
8. Do the following when it comes to temporary resin cements:
   - List the components and indicate their function.
   - Describe the setting reaction, and indicate any variables that may affect the setting.
   - Describe the clinical importance of film thickness, working and setting times, compressive strength, retention and type of bond to tooth structure, and fluoride release.
   - Discuss the properties and biocompatibility.
   - Describe the manipulation.

High-Strength Bases

9. Do the following when it comes to high-strength bases:
   - Discuss the uses.
   - List the components.
   - Indicate contraindications.
   - Discuss the mechanical properties and biocompatibility.
   - Describe the manipulation.
10. Discuss temporary fillings.

11. Do the following when it comes to low-strength bases:
    - Discuss the uses.
    - List the components.
    - Indicate contraindications.
    - Discuss the mechanical properties and biocompatibility.
    - Describe the manipulation.
12. Discuss the use of modified zinc oxide–eugenol cement.

Cavity Liners and Varnishes

13. Discuss the function of cavity liners and varnishes.

14. Give examples of cavity liners and discuss their composition.
15. Discuss the properties of varnishes and how they can be disrupted and applied.

Special Applications of Cement

16. Describe the type of cement used for special applications, including cementation of orthodontic bands, direct bonding of orthodontic brackets, and root canal sealers.
17. Describe clinically important properties of cements used for special applications.

CEMENTATION

Cements (Figure 7-1) are generally hard, brittle materials formed when a powdered oxide or glass is mixed with a liquid. When mixed to a cementing consistency, dental cements are used to retain restorations such as alloy or ceramic crowns and bridges and esthetic inlays, onlays, and veneers. When mixed to a thicker consistency, some cements can be used as temporary filling materials or to provide thermal insulation and mechanical support to teeth restored with other materials, such as amalgam, composites, or gold. Cements classified as low-strength bases or liners provide protection to the pulp from irritants or serve therapeutically as pulp-capping agents. Varnishes are not cements but are used with cements to provide pulpal protection from irritants. Other cements are used for special purposes in endodontics and orthodontics. Cements are classified according to function in Table 7-1.

The retention of restorations on prepared teeth is a major function of dental cements. Long-term cementation is required for permanent restorations such as crowns and bridges (see Figures 1-7 and 1-9). Strong cements—such as glass ionomer, resin-modified glass ionomer and resin cement—are used for permanent cementation. Often, a bridge must be cemented temporarily to allow adjustments in fit, occlusion, and esthetics, or temporary restorations, such as aluminum, acrylic, or composite provisional restorations, must be cemented for 4 to 8 weeks until the permanent restoration is ready. In these cases, temporary cements are used because of their low strength and good handling characteristics. Cements are classified as water-based, oil-based, or resin-based products. Information on zinc phosphate, zinc polycarboxylate, and compomer cements can be found in Appendix 7-1.

WATER-BASED CEMENTS

Glass Ionomer Cement

Glass ionomer cements are water-based cements used for final cementation of primarily alloy crowns and bridges. A restorative material with a thicker consistency is used for Class V restorations as described in Chapter 4. Examples of commercial products are listed in Table 7-2.

Composition and Reaction

The cement powder is a finely ground aluminosilicate glass, and the viscous liquid is a polycarboxylate copolymer in water. One product (Ketac-Cem Aplicap; 3M ESPE, St. Paul, MN) supplies a powder coated with polyacrylic acid copolymers. It is mixed with a low-viscosity liquid to form the cement. The components of glass ionomer cements react to form a cross-linked gel matrix that surrounds the partially reacted powder particles. Chelation between the polycarboxylate molecules and calcium on the surface of the tooth results in a chemical (adhesive) bond.

Properties

The mechanical properties of glass ionomer cement are compared with other high-strength cements in Table 7-3. Minimum requirements are described by the American National Standards Institute–American Dental Association (ANSI-ADA) Specification No. 96 (ISO 9917 [2000]). The values for compressive and tensile strengths of glass ionomer cements are similar to those of compomer, resin-modified glass ionomer, and zinc phosphate cements. The cement has the irritating qualities of zinc polycarboxylate cements. However, a calcium hydroxide base is recommended for pulpal protection when the ionomer cement is used in a deep cavity. Because of fluoride incorporated in the powder, the cement has an anticariogenic effect as it is leached out. Retention of glass ionomer cements is primarily micromechanical, although some chemical bonding occurs.

Manipulation

Glass ionomer cements are powder–liquid systems packaged in bottles or capsules. The bottle of powder should be tumbled gently before dispensing. The powder and liquid are dispensed onto a paper pad or glass slab. The powder is divided into two equal portions. The first portion of powder is mixed with a stiff spatula into the liquid before the next portion is added. The mixing time should be 30 to 60 seconds, depending on the product. The cement is used immediately because the working time after mixing is about 2 minutes at 22° C. Cooling the mixing slab slows the setting reaction and provides additional working time. The cement should not be used once a "skin" forms on the surface or when the consistency becomes noticeably thicker. During application, contact with water should be avoided; the field is isolated completely. The cement sets in the mouth in about 7 minutes from the start of mixing. Encapsulated products (GC Fuji I

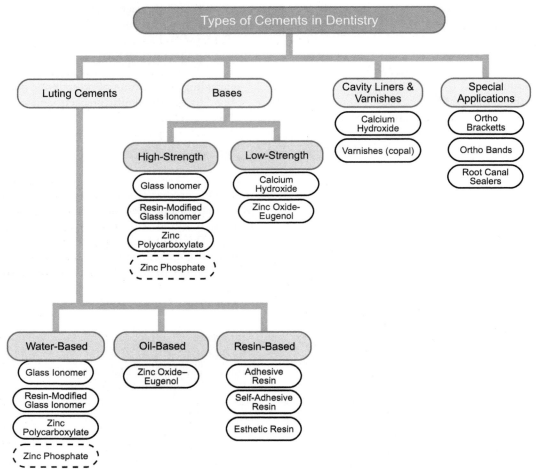

FIG 7-1 As materials, cements serve diverse functions in restorative dentistry. Many are for luting, i.e., retaining indirect restorations in cavity preparations. Cements for crown restorations would be a common example. The luting cements occur in three broad classes: water-based, oil-based, and resin-based. However, cement materials also serve as bases inside cavity preparations under restorations, as cavity liners or sealers over dentin, or in a variety of special applications, such as retention of orthodontic brackets or root canal sealers.

TABLE 7-1	**Summary of Uses of Cements in Restorative Dentistry**
Functions	**Cements**
Cementation of cast alloy crowns and bridges	Adhesive resin (dual cured), bioceramic, glass ionomer, resin-modified glass ionomer, self-adhesive resin, zinc polycarboxylate
Cementation of all-ceramic or indirect composite inlays and onlays	Adhesive resin (dual cured), bioceramic
Cementation of zirconia-based, all-ceramic crowns and bridges	Adhesive resin (dual cured), bioceramic, glass ionomer, resin-modified glass ionomer, self-adhesive resin
Cementation of ceramic veneers	Esthetic resin (dual cured or light cured)
Cementation of resin-bonded bridges	Adhesive resin (dual cured)
Temporary cementation of cast crowns and bridges and cementation of temporary restorations	Zinc oxide–noneugenol, temporary resin
High-strength bases	Compomer, glass ionomer, resin-modified glass ionomer, zinc polycarboxylate
Temporary fillings	Resin-modified glass ionomer, zinc polycarboxylate
Low-strength bases	Calcium hydroxide (self-cured and light cured), glass ionomer, resin-modified glass ionomer
Liners	Calcium hydroxide in a suspension
Varnishes	Resin in a solvent
Special applications	
Cementation of orthodontic bands	Glass ionomer, resin-modified glass ionomer, resin
Direct bonding of orthodontic brackets	Resin
Root canal sealer	Zinc oxide–eugenol

TABLE 7-2 Examples of Traditional Cements Suitable for Final Cementation of Cast Alloy Crowns and Bridges

Cement	Product	Manufacturer
Glass ionomer	GC Fuji I	GC America (Alsip, IL)
	GC Fuji I Capsule	GC America
	Ketac-Cem Maxicap	3M ESPE (St. Paul, MN)
Resin-modified glass ionomer	GC Fuji CEM Automix	GC America
	GC Fuji Plus Capsule	GC America
	RelyX Luting Plus Cement	3M ESPE
Zinc polycarboxylate	Durelon Maxicap	3M ESPE
	Hy-Bond	Shofu Dental

TABLE 7-3 Mechanical Properties of Cements for Final and Temporary Cementation*

Cement	Compressive strength (MPa)	Tensile strength (MPa)	Modulus of elasticity (GPa†)
Cements for final cementation			
Adhesive resin	50–210	40	1.2–10.7
Glass ionomer	90–220	4.5	5.4
Resin-modified glass ionomer	85–120	13	2.5
Zinc polycarboxylate	55–96	3–6	4.4
Cements for temporary cementation			
Zinc oxide–eugenol	2–5	0.4–1.0	0.18
Temporary resin	25–70	14	—

*Properties measured at 24 hours.
†GPa = 1000 MPa.

Capsule, GC America, Alsip, IL; Ketac-Cem Aplicaps, 3M ESPE, St. Paul, MN) require mechanical mixing for 10 seconds. Technique tips for water-based cements are summarized in Box 7-1.

BOX 7-1 Technique Tips for Water-Based Cements

1. Fluff the powder in the container if necessary.
2. Dispense the powder and liquid on a glass slab or paper pad using dispensers provided by the manufacturer.
3. Mix with a spatula using a folding motion for the recommended time.

Resin-Modified Glass Ionomer Cement

Resin-modified glass ionomer cements are water-based cements indicated for permanent cementation of alloy crowns and bridges to tooth structure and core buildups, cementation of posts, and bonding of orthodontic appliances. Resin-modified glass ionomer cements can be used for cementation of zirconia-based all-ceramic crowns and bridges. Examples of commercial products are listed in Table 7-2.

Composition and Reaction

One cement powder contains a radiopaque, fluoroaluminosilicate glass and a microencapsulated catalyst system. The liquid is an aqueous solution of polycarboxylic acid modified with pendant methacrylate groups. It also contains 2-hydroxyethyl methacrylate (HEMA) and tartaric acid. Curing results from an acid–base glass ionomer reaction and self-cured polymerization of the methacrylate groups.

Properties

The values for compressive and tensile strengths of resin-modified glass ionomer cements are similar to those of glass ionomer cements (see Table 7-3). Resin-modified glass ionomer cements have no measurable solubility when tested by lactic acid erosion. The fracture toughness is higher than that of other water-based cements but lower than that of resin cements. Fluoride release is similar to the glass ionomer cements. The early pH is about 3.5 and gradually rises. These cements have minimal postoperative sensitivity. The bond strength to moist dentin is 14 MPa and is much higher than that of most water-based cements.

Manipulation

Resin-modified glass ionomer cements are powder–liquid systems packaged in bottles or capsules or paste–paste systems. With the powder–liquid products, the powder is fluffed before dispensing. The liquid should be dispensed by holding the vial vertically to the mixing pad. The powder is incorporated into the liquid within 30 seconds to give a mousse-like consistency. The working time is 2.5 minutes. The cement is applied to a clean, dry tooth that is not desiccated. No coating agent is needed. HEMA is a known contact allergen; therefore, protective gloves and a no-touch technique are mandatory. A paste–paste product (GC Fuji-CEM; GC America, Alsip, IL) is packaged in an auto-mixed dispenser (Figure 7-2).

Bioceramic Cement

Bioceramic cement (example, Ceramir Crown & Bridge, Doxa Dental Inc., Chicago, IL) is a permanent, radiopaque, luting cement supplied in capsules. It contains glass ionomer and calcium aluminate powder plus water. Activation of the capsule is done prior to mixing in a 4000- to 5000- rpm mixer. Bioceramic cement requires no etching, priming, bonding, or conditioning.

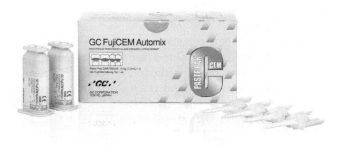

FIG 7-2 Example of paste–paste, resin-modified glass iono-mer cement with dispenser. (Courtesy GC America, Alsip, IL.)

OIL-BASED CEMENTS

Zinc Oxide–Eugenol Cements

Zinc oxide–eugenol cements are oil-based cements that have an **obtundent** (sedative) effect on the pulp and are especially useful for cementation on prepared teeth with exposed **dentinal tubules**. The addition of reinforcing agents to zinc oxide–eugenol cement has resulted in permanent **luting** cements. Temporary cements are not so strong but are useful for short-term cementation of temporary stainless steel crowns and permanent restorations. Zinc oxide–eugenol cements (see Table 7-4) are cements used for short-term cementation of temporary acrylic crowns and completed cast restorations. They are weak and easily cleaned from the casting.

Composition and Reaction

> **! ALERT**
>
> A chelate is a ring-like compound formed from the organic groups and the zinc oxide.

The zinc oxide–eugenol cement powder (Type I) contains zinc oxide (69%); rosin (29%) to reduce brittleness; and zinc acetate, an accelerator. The liquid is eugenol or a mixture of eugenol and other oils. The powder reacts with the eugenol in the presence of moisture to form an amorphous **chelate** of zinc eugenolate. The zinc oxide–eugenol cements (Type I) are formulated with oils other than eugenol for patients sensitive to eugenol.

The polymer-reinforced zinc oxide–eugenol cements (Type II) contain 80% zinc oxide and 20% acrylic resin in the powder and eugenol in the liquid. The ethoxybenzoic acid (EBA)-alumina–reinforced cements contain 70% zinc oxide

TABLE 7-4 **Examples of Cements Suitable for Temporary Cementation of Completed Restorations or Cementation of Temporary Restorations**		
Cement	**Product**	**Manufacturer**
Zinc oxide–noneugenol	Nogenol	GC America (Alsip, IL)
	Temp-Bond NE	Kerr Corporation (Orange, CA)

and 30% alumina in the powder. The liquid is 62.5% EBA and 37.5% eugenol. The EBA in the liquid promotes the formation of a stronger, crystalline matrix. Water and heat accelerate the setting reaction of these cements.

Properties

The moderate strength and low acidic quality of the zinc oxide–eugenol cements are important properties. Minimum requirements are described by ANSI-ADA Specification No. 30 (ISO 3107 [2000]).

The compressive strengths of the permanent and temporary zinc oxide–eugenol cements are listed in Table 7-3. The permanent zinc oxide–eugenol cements are not as strong as other cements but have been shown to be clinically successful for final cementation of crowns and bridges that have good retention. The temporary cements are weaker, a desirable feature for cementation of temporary crowns or for temporary cementation of completed crown and bridge restorations that must be removed easily.

The pH of the zinc oxide–eugenol cements is neutral. Because of the sedative nature of these cements, they do not require a protective varnish or cavity liner. Retention is the result of micro-mechanical interlocking of the restoration and prepared tooth.

Manipulation

The permanent zinc oxide–eugenol cements (Type II) are powder–liquid systems. The powder bottle is shaken gently, and then the powder is dispensed with the supplied scoop and the liquid with a dropper. It is mixed on a glass slab or treated paper pad with a metal spatula. The powder is incorporated into the liquid all at once and mixed for 30 seconds. The mix initially is like putty, but continued mixing for 30 seconds more causes the polymer-reinforced cement mix to become fluid. The EBA-alumina–reinforced cement should be stropped for 60 seconds with broad strokes of the spatula after the initial 30-second mixing to obtain a suitable consistency. The working time of the EBA-alumina cements is long (about 22 minutes), unless moisture is present on the slab. In the mouth, the zinc oxide–eugenol cements set quickly because of the moisture and heat.

The temporary cements (Type I) are typically two-paste systems. Equal lengths of the accelerator and base pastes are dispensed on a paper pad or glass slab. The pastes are colored differently. Mixing is continued until a uniform color is achieved. Some products are available in unit-dose packages.

Zinc oxide–eugenol cements are difficult to remove from the tissues and mixing surfaces after setting. The patient's lips and adjacent teeth are coated with **silicone** grease before application of the cement. Glass slabs and spatulas are wiped clean before the cement sets. Oil of orange is a solvent useful in removal of set cement.

RESIN-BASED CEMENTS

Esthetic Resin Cements

Esthetic resin cements are tooth-colored or translucent resins available in a variety of shades; they are used for bonding of all-ceramic and indirect composite restorations. These

TABLE 7-5 Examples of Resin-Based Cements for Permanent and Temporary Cementation

Product	Manufacturer
Esthetic resin	
Calibra Esthetic Resin Cement	DENTSPLY Caulk (Milford, DE)
RelyX Veneer	3M ESPE (St. Paul, MN)
Variolink Veneer	Ivoclar Vivadent (Amherst, NY)
Adhesive resin	
Multilink Automix	Ivoclar Vivadent
Panavia F 2.0	Kuraray America (New York, NY)
Self-adhesive resin	
Maxcem Elite	Kerr Corporation (Orange, CA)
SpeedCem	Ivoclar Vivadent
RelyX Unicem 2 Automix	3M ESPE
Temporary resin	
Telio Link	Ivoclar Vivadent
Temp-Bond Clear	Kerr Corporation

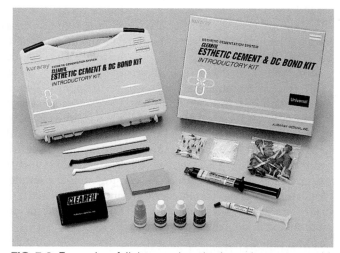

FIG 7-3 Example of light-cured esthetic resin cement with bonding agent and accessories. (Courtesy Kuraray America, New York, NY.)

BOX 7-2 Technique Tips for Resin Cements

1. Resin cements are supplied in automixed syringes and require no mixing by hand.
2. If necessary, be sure to apply a bonding agent to tooth structure.
3. Apply the appropriate primer to the ceramic or metal restoration.
4. Dual-cured resin cements may require activation with a light-curing unit.
5. Clean excess cement before the cement is completely set.

cements require a bonding agent for adhesion to tooth structure and separate primers for bonding to ceramic substrates. Examples of commercial products are listed in Table 7-5.

Composition and Reaction

Esthetic resin cements are composed of dimethacrylate resin and glass filler such as the restorative materials described in Chapter 4. They are light- or dual-cured resins, depending on the application.

Properties

Esthetic resin cements have medium to high strength and low film thickness. Radiopacity is desirable. For cementation of an inlay, the resin cement must be wear resistant at exposed margins. Recent research shows that microfilled resin cements are more wear resistant than microhybrid resin cements. Light-cured resin cements have a long working time, although exposure to operatory light can initiate polymerization. Bond strengths of esthetic resin cements to tooth structure and ceramic substrates are high when these surfaces are treated with a bonding agent or appropriate primer.

Manipulation

Bonding of ceramic and indirect composite restorations requires treatment of the surfaces of the tooth and restorative material. The tooth is etched, and the bonding agent is applied. Ceramic restorations are etched with hydrofluoric acid gel or sandblasted with 50-mm alumina, and then silane is applied. Nonsetting try-in pastes of matching shades are convenient accessories for use with ceramic veneers. Esthetic resin cement (Clearfil Esthetic Cement, Kuraray America, New York, NY) is packaged with bonding agent and accessories as shown in Figure 7-3. Technique tips for resin cements are summarized in Box 7-2.

Adhesive Resin Cements

Adhesive resin cements are used for bonding of most alloy and ceramic restorations, except veneers, implant-supported crowns and bridges, and indirect resin restorations. These cements typically require a separate primer for bonding to tooth, alloy, or ceramic substrates. Examples of commercial products are listed in Table 7-5.

Composition and Reaction

Adhesive resin cements are composed of dimethacrylate resin and glass filler. They are dual- or self-cured resins. One product (C&B MetaBond; Parkell, Farmington, NY) is a **methyl methacrylate** resin with **poly (methyl methacrylate)** filler. These cements are formulated with adhesive monomers that bond well to alloy substrates.

Properties

Adhesive resin cements are radiopaque and have low film thickness. They are characterized by short working times and medium to high strengths. Bond strengths of adhesive resin cements to tooth structure and treated alloy substrates are high (>20 MPa) when these surfaces are treated with a primer.

Manipulation

Bonding of ceramic and indirect composite restorations requires treatment of the surfaces of the tooth and restorative material. Bonding agent is applied to the tooth. The ceramic restoration is etched with hydrofluoric acid gel or sandblasted with 50-mm alumina, and then silane is applied. Before cementation of resin-bonded bridges, the alloy retainers are sandblasted and sometimes treated with a ceramic coating (Rocatec Jr.; 3M ESPE, St. Paul, MN) to improve bond strength. Tooth-colored, translucent, and opaque adhesive resin cements are available. Some adhesive resin cements require a gel barrier to exclude oxygen for complete setting. A dual-cured, paste–paste adhesive resin cement (Panavia F 2.0; Kuraray America, New York, NY) packaged in an auto-mixed dispenser is shown in Figure 7-4.

Self-Adhesive Resin Cements

Self-adhesive resin cements eliminate the need for separate primers for bonding to tooth, alloy, or ceramic substrates. Examples of commercial products are listed in Table 7-5.

Composition and Reaction

Self-adhesive resin cements are composed of diacrylate resins with acidic and adhesive groups and glass filler. They are dual- or self-cured resins.

Properties

Self-adhesive resin cements bond to tooth structure and other materials with low to medium bond strengths. They generally are not as strong as esthetic and adhesive resin cements. Properties measured when these cements are light activated are generally higher than when they are self-cured.

Manipulation

Self-adhesive resin cements eliminate the etching and priming steps. Most products are paste–paste systems with auto-mixed dispensers or encapsulated as shown in Figure 7-5. The capsule has an intraoral tip.

Temporary Resin Cements

Temporary resin cements are used for temporary cementation of crowns and cementation of temporary restorations (see Table 7-4). Temporary resin cements eliminate the problem of potential contamination of teeth by eugenol and other oil-based cements when bonding agents and resin cements are intended for permanent cementation.

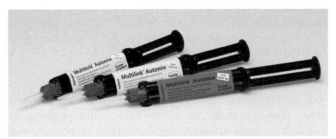

FIG 7-4 Example of dual-cured adhesive resin cement. (Courtesy Ivoclar Vivadent, Amherst, NY.)

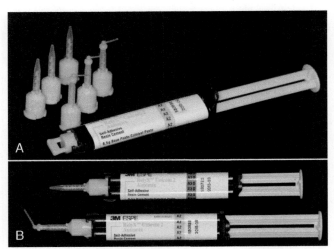

FIG 7-5 A common paste–paste formulation of a self-adhesive resin cement dispensed through automix tips **(A).** The straight tip **(B,** *top*) is used for filling crowns prior to final cementation. The canted thin tip **(B,** *lower*) is used for filling root canals prior to final post cementation. (Courtesy Y-W Chen, University of Washington Department of Restorative Dentistry, Seattle, WA.)

Composition and Reaction

Temporary resin cements are formulated from dimethacrylate resin and radiopaque glass filler, and most are self-cured.

Properties

Temporary resin cements are usually easy to mix and clean up and have low to medium compressive strength (see Table 7-3). Bond strength must be adequate but low enough that the restoration can be removed for permanent cementation.

Manipulation

Temporary resin cements are typically paste–paste systems and are applied without the use of a bonding agent. A product (Integrity TempGrip, DENTSPLY Caulk, Milford, DE) packaged in an auto-mixed syringe is shown in Figure 7-6. Technique tips for temporary cements are summarized in Box 7-3.

HIGH-STRENGTH BASES

High-strength bases are used to provide mechanical support for a restoration and thermal protection for the pulp. Bases may be prepared from glass ionomer, resin-modified glass ionomer, and polymer-reinforced zinc oxide–eugenol products, examples of which are listed in Table 7-6, or from a putty-like consistency of zinc phosphate or zinc polycarboxylate cements.

The composition and reaction of most cements used for high-strength bases are discussed in the "Cementation" section. The composition and reaction of resin-modified glass ionomer high-strength bases are identical to those for the resin-modified glass ionomer restoratives and are described in Chapter 4.

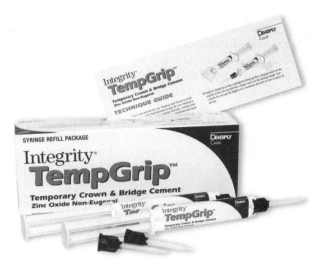

FIG 7-6 Example of paste–paste temporary resin cement in an auto-mixed dispenser. (Courtesy DENTSPLY Caulk, Milford, DE.)

Properties

Some important properties of bases are high strength, moderate modulus of elasticity, and low thermal conductivity.

Compressive and tensile strengths of high-strength bases are listed in Table 7-7. Bases are generally stronger than cements used for retention (see Table 7-3) because the base is mixed at a higher powder-to-liquid ratio. The strength must develop quickly because the base may be required to support the condensation forces during the insertion of a dental amalgam. The ability of the base to resist occlusal forces and to support the restoration is affected by its modulus of elasticity. Zinc phosphate cement provides the best support for amalgam because it has the highest modulus (see Table 7-7).

The base must provide thermal protection to the pulp. As indicated in Chapter 2 (see Table 2-2), the thermal conductivity of metallic restorations is high compared with tooth structure. The thermal conductivity of cement bases is similar to that of tooth structure; thus, the base can protect the pulp from thermal changes. Effective protection requires that the base be at least 0.5 mm thick.

Glass ionomers are used as bases for posterior composites and ceramic or composite inlays and onlays and for crown buildups when adequate tooth support is available. Compomers and resin-modified glass ionomer are used as a base for composites but are not used with traditional ceramics. These bases are viscous and are best placed with a syringe. Several products (Fuji II LC Capsule, GC America, Alsip, IL; Ketac-Bond Aplicap, 3M ESPE, St. Paul, MN) are encapsulated and require mechanical mixing.

BOX 7-3 Technique Tips for Temporary Cements

1. Dispense paste–paste temporary cements in equal lengths and mix on a paper pad with a spatula.
2. Newer temporary cements are supplied in an automixed syringe and require no mixing by hand.
3. Clean excess cement before the cement is completely set.

TABLE 7-6 Examples of High- and Low-Strength Bases

Cement	Product	Manufacturer
High-strength bases		
Bioceramic	Biodentine	Septodont
Glass ionomer	Ketac-Bond Aplicap	3M ESPE (St. Paul, MN)
Resin-modified glass ionomer	GC Fuji II LC Vitremer	GC America (Alsip, IL) 3M ESPE
Zinc polycarboxylate	Durelon Maxicap	3M ESPE
Low-strength bases		
Bioceramic (light-cured)	TheraCal LC	Bisco Dental Products
Calcium hydroxide (light-cured)	Dycal VLC	DENTSPLY Caulk (Milford, DE)
Calcium hydroxide (self-cured)	Dycal	DENTSPLY Caulk
Zinc oxide–eugenol (Type IV)	Alumina Super EBA	Bosworth (Skokie, IL)
	Cavitec	Kerr Corporation (Orange, CA)

TABLE 7-7 Mechanical Properties of High- and Low-Strength Bases*

Cement	Compressive strength (MPa)	Tensile strength (MPa)	Modulus of elasticity (GPa†)
High-strength bases			
Glass ionomer	70–210	3.9–8.3	3.7–9.0
Resin-modified glass ionomer	150–200	20–40	8–20
Zinc polycarboxylate	80	16	5.0
Low-strength bases			
Calcium hydroxide (light-cured)	96	38	—
Calcium hydroxide (self-cured)	12–26	1.0	0.4
Zinc oxide–eugenol (Type IV)	5.5	0.4	0.3

*Properties measured at 24 hours.
†GPa = 1000 MPa.

Manipulation

Glass ionomer and resin-modified glass ionomer bases are mixed directly to their final consistency. Compomers are supplied as single-paste compules and do not require mixing. Zinc phosphate and zinc polycarboxylate high-strength bases are mixed by first reaching the cementing consistency of the cement. Additional powder is then added to achieve the putty-like base consistency.

TEMPORARY FILLINGS

Certain cements mixed to a base consistency may be used successfully as temporary fillings. The temporary filling protects the pulp, reduces pulpal inflammation, and maintains tooth position while restoring esthetics until a permanent restoration can be placed. Zinc oxide–eugenol cements are used most frequently. For shorter-term fillings, an unmodified, zinc oxide-eugenol cement is mixed to a putty-like consistency. Several cotton fibers may be added to the mix. Setting of this mix is accelerated when the surface of the filling is patted with a cotton pellet saturated with hot water. For longer-term fillings, modified zinc oxide–eugenol, resin-modified glass ionomer, or zinc polycarboxylate cements can be used. Resin-based provisional inlay and onlay materials are also available.

LOW-STRENGTH BASES

Low-strength bases harden when mixed and form a cement layer usually with minimum strength and low rigidity. These bases function as a barrier to irritating chemicals and provide a therapeutic benefit to the pulp. Examples of calcium hydroxide, glass ionomer, and zinc oxide–eugenol (Type IV) low-strength bases are listed in Table 7-6. Their properties are summarized in Table 7-7. Low-strength bases are often called "liners" and should be distinguished from the cavity-liner suspensions described in the next section.

Calcium Hydroxide Cement

Calcium hydroxide cement is used for direct and indirect **pulp capping** and as a protective barrier beneath composite restorations. It does not interfere with the polymerization of these materials.

Composition and Reaction

The base paste of one calcium hydroxide cement contains calcium tungstate, calcium phosphate, and zinc oxide in glycol salicylate. The catalyst paste contains calcium hydroxide, zinc oxide, and zinc stearate in ethylene toluene sulfonamide. Setting results from the formation of an amorphous calcium disalicylate. The cements usually contain radiopaque filler.

The light-cured product is a urethane dimethacrylate resin with calcium hydroxide and barium sulfate fillers and a low-viscosity monomer.

Properties

Calcium hydroxide cements have low mechanical properties (see Table 7-7) compared with cements used as high-strength bases, but they are stronger than zinc oxide–eugenol cement (Type IV). The cements have a low thermal conductivity but usually are not used in thick enough layers to provide thermal protection. The cements stimulate the formation of reparative dentin under an indirect pulp cap or at the site of a direct pulp cap. The pH of the cements is basic and varies from 11 to 12. Setting times vary from 2 to 7 minutes, with faster setting cements being more desirable. Solubility in water and in acid varies considerably among products. Products with low acid solubility can be placed with acid-etched composites.

Manipulation

Most calcium hydroxide cements are a two-paste system. Equal lengths of each paste are dispensed onto a paper pad and mixed to a uniform color. The light-cured cement is polymerized by a visible-light source for 20 seconds for each 1-mm layer.

Zinc Oxide–Eugenol Cement

A modified zinc oxide–eugenol (Type IV) cement is used in a deep cavity to retard penetration of acids and reduce possible discomfort to the pulp. Because it is used in thin layers, the base provides little thermal insulation. The strength and modulus of a Type IV zinc oxide–eugenol cement are low (see Table 7-7). The base should be limited to small or nonstress-bearing areas but normally will support forces associated with placement of a restoration. The eugenol has a sedative (obtundent) effect on pulpal tissue.

The cement is supplied as a two-paste system. Equal lengths of the different-colored pastes are dispensed onto a paper pad and mixed to a uniform color. The cement should not be used when a bonding agent and composite are to be placed, because the eugenol inhibits the polymerization. Often a high-strength base is placed over a zinc oxide–eugenol low-strength base to provide strength, rigidity, and thermal protection.

CAVITY LINERS AND VARNISHES

Cavity liners and varnishes function as a protective barrier between dentin and the restorative material, minimize the ingress of oral fluids at the restoration–tooth interface, and may provide some therapeutic benefits to the tooth. They are applied in thin films, and the solvent evaporates. They have no significant mechanical strength and provide essentially no thermal insulation. Recently, bonding agents (Chapter 4) have been used to seal dentin tubules in place of cavity varnishes.

Liners

Cavity liners are suspensions of calcium hydroxide in water or in an organic liquid (Table 7-8). The suspension may be thickened with methylcellulose or ethylcellulose. In addition, some liners contain fluoride. The film serves as a barrier and may neutralize acids. These liners are susceptible to solubility and disintegration in oral fluids and thus should be restricted to coverage of dentin. Some liners may be disrupted by the monomers in composite restorations.

TABLE 7-8	Examples of Calcium Hydroxide Cavity Liners	
Product	Composition	Manufacturer
Hydroxyline	Calcium hydroxide and acrylic polymer in methyl ethyl ketone	George Taub Products & Fusion (Jersey City, NJ)
Hypo-Cal	Calcium hydroxide and barium sulfate in aqueous hydroxyethyl cellulose solution	Ellman (Hewlett, NY)
Pulpdent Liquid Cavity Liner	Calcium hydroxide in aqueous methylcellulose solution	Pulpdent (Watertown, MA)

Varnishes

Cavity varnishes (Copalite; Temrex Corp., Freeport, NY) are solutions of resins, such as copal or nitrated cellulose, contained in organic liquids (chloroform, alcohol). When applied to the tooth, the solvent evaporates, which leaves a porous, resinous film that may be 1 to 40 μm thick, depending on the product. More than one layer of the thinner films may be necessary to act as an effective barrier. Varnishes are insoluble in oral fluids. They reduce leakage around margins and walls of the restoration–tooth interface and appear to prevent penetration of corrosion products from amalgam into dentin. Varnishes may be disrupted by monomers of resin or composite restorations and are not used under a therapeutic base.

Varnish solutions are applied by means of a small cotton pledget. The solvent is evaporated with use of a gentle stream of air.

SPECIAL APPLICATIONS OF CEMENT

Cements have many special applications in dentistry, as indicated in Table 7-9.

Bonding of Orthodontic Brackets

Direct and indirect bonding of orthodontic brackets (Figure 7-7) is accomplished primarily with the use of resin cements, although a light-cured, resin-modified glass ionomer orthodontic cement (Fuji Ortho LC; GC America, Alsip, IL) has been used. The composition of the resin orthodontic cements is similar to that of the esthetic resin cements described earlier in this chapter. The surfaces of the teeth to be bonded are treated with bonding agent. Recently, sixth-generation bonding agents (Transbond Plus; 3M Unitek, Monrovia, CA) have been introduced for direct bonding. These self-etching adhesives eliminate the need for etching with phosphoric acid and rinsing. The cement is applied to the treated enamel and the bracket base positioned. Paste–primer and light-cured resin cements are available (see Table 7-9). With the former cement, the primer is applied to the enamel and the paste to the bracket. Setting

TABLE 7-9	Examples of Cements Used for Special Applications	
Application	Product	Manufacturer
Direct bonding of orthodontic brackets		
Resin (dual-cured)	Phase II	Reliance Orthodontic Products (Itaska, IL)
Resin (paste-primer)	Mono-Lok2	Rocky Mountain (Denver, CO)
Resin (self-cured)	Concise Orthodontic	3M ESPE (St. Paul, MN)
Resin-modified glass ionomer	GC Fuji Ortho LC	GC America (Alsip, IL)
Cementation of orthodontic bands		
Glass ionomer	Ketac-Cem Aplicap	3M ESPE
Resin-modified glass ionomer	GC Fuji Ortho	GC America
Resin	Band-Lok	Reliance Orthodontic Products
Root canal sealers		
Zinc oxide–eugenol	Roth Cements	Roth Drug (Chicago, IL)

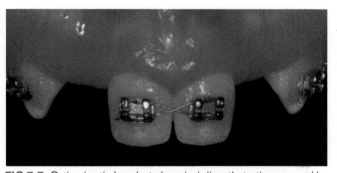

FIG 7-7 Orthodontic brackets bonded directly to the enamel by resin cement. (Courtesy Y-W Chen, University of Washington Department of Restorative Dentistry, Seattle, WA.)

occurs when the bracket is pressed into the primer on the tooth. The film thickness should be less than 0.25 mm to ensure proper setting.

Plastic brackets are bonded successfully with acrylic cements and also with composite cements if conditioned with a bracket primer. Metal and ceramic brackets are bonded successfully with composite cement. When properly applied, the cements bond tenaciously to enamel. Removal of the brackets and cement after treatment requires care to minimize damage to enamel. A 12-fluted finishing bur without water is used and then abraded with pumice for efficient removal of cement.

Cementation of Orthodontic Bands

Orthodontic bands are cemented to the teeth with glass ionomer cements or, less frequently, with zinc phosphate cements. The compositions of these cements were described earlier in this chapter. Some zinc phosphate cements formulated specifically for orthodontics contain fluoride to provide protection from caries. To achieve longer working times, zinc phosphate cement is routinely mixed by use of the cold- or frozen-slab technique. Zinc phosphate cement bonds to the enamel by mechanical interlocking with the surface, whereas the glass ionomer cements have some chemical bonding. Demineralization of the tooth surface, which occurs with zinc phosphate cements, is minimized with the fluoride-releasing glass ionomer cements. Self-cured, fluoride-releasing, resin-modified glass ionomer (Fuji Ortho; GC America, Alsip, IL) and resin cements (Band-Lok; Reliance Orthodontic Products, Itaska, IL) also have been used for cementation of orthodontic bands.

Root Canal Sealers

If the dental pulp is removed, the root canal can be sealed by cementation of a gutta-percha point or by filling with a paste.

Many root canal sealers are formulated from zinc oxide and eugenol. Some important parameters of root canal sealers are working and setting times, flow, film thickness, strength, solubility, and radiopacity. Biologic properties have been studied extensively.

QUICK REVIEW

Cements are used for cementation of restorations and as bases. The most common cements (glass ionomer, resin-modified glass ionomer) are composed of a glass powder and have an acidic liquid. Resin cements are composed of dimethacrylate resin and filler and are used to bond all-ceramic restorations and for special dental applications. Important properties include working time, film thickness, tensile and compressive strengths, modulus of elasticity, and biocompatibility. These properties are best achieved when manipulative techniques are followed precisely.

SELF-TEST QUESTIONS

In the following multiple-choice questions, one or more responses may be correct.

1. Glass ionomer cement is used in which of the following ways?
   a. As a base for thermal and mechanical protection of the pulp under composite restorations
   b. For cementation of orthodontic bands
   c. For retention of cast alloy restorations
   d. For cementation of ceramic crowns

2. Which of the following statements is/are true?
   a. The marginal adaptation of a casting to the tooth is affected by the film thickness of the cement.
   b. Typical values of film thickness and compressive strengths of glass ionomer cements are 25 mm and 90 to 220 MPa, respectively.
   c. The retaining action of glass ionomer cement is primarily one of mechanical bonding between surface irregularities of the tooth and casting by the cement.
   d. Glass ionomer cement is as strong in tension as it is in compression.

3. Which of the following statements is/are true for glass ionomer cements?
   a. The powder is added to the liquid in two portions to control the consistency of the mixture.
   b. Total mixing time varies between 30 and 60 seconds.
   c. Cooling the mixing slab slows the setting reaction.
   d. Once the cementing or primary consistency is obtained, the base consistency is achieved by the addition of powder to the mix.

4. An increased amount of powder in a cementing consistency mix of zinc phosphate cement does which of the following?
   a. Decreases the solubility
   b. Increases the strength
   c. Decreases the film thickness
   d. Increases the setting time

5. The components of zinc oxide–eugenol cement may include which of the following?

   a. Ethoxybenzoic acid (EBA) in the eugenol to improve strength
   b. Alumina or acrylic polymer in the powder to improve strength
   c. Zinc acetate in the powder as an accelerator
   d. Zinc oxide and eugenol formulated as pastes in separate tubes

6. Which of the following statements is/are true for zinc oxide–eugenol cements?
   a. Zinc oxide powder is added to the eugenol liquid on a treated paper pad in six equal increments.
   b. Equal lengths of the base paste and the accelerator paste are mixed together until the mix has a uniform color.
   c. Increases in temperature and humidity shorten the setting time.
   d. A mix appears thick at the start of mixing, but after 30 seconds of additional spatulation it becomes more fluid.

7. Which of the following statements about resin-modified glass ionomer cements is/are true?
   a. Some resin-modified glass ionomer cements are not recommended for cementation of all-ceramic inlays, onlays, or crowns because of their water sorption.
   b. They release more fluoride than glass ionomer cements.
   c. They have no measurable solubility when tested by lactic acid erosion.
   d. The powder is incorporated into the liquid within 30 seconds to give a mousse-like consistency.

8. The components of zinc polycarboxylate cements include which of the following?
   a. Zinc polyacrylate crystals in water
   b. A solution of polyacrylic acid in water
   c. Zinc oxide powder
   d. A paste of zinc oxide and one of acrylic acid

9. Which of the following statements is/are true?
   a. The pH of the mix of zinc polycarboxylate cement is initially acidic, but the acid is weakly dissociated. The pH increases to neutrality in several days.
   b. Resin-modified glass ionomer cements cause minimal postoperative sensitivity.

c. Glass ionomer cement acts as an obtundent like zinc oxide–eugenol cement.

10. Which of the following statements is true for zinc polycarboxylate cements?
   a. The powder is incorporated into the liquid within 30 seconds.
   b. The working time can be extended by use of a cooled glass mixing slab.
   c. After a cement loses its luster and becomes stringy, it is ready to be used.
   d. The correct consistency for cementation is about one and one-half parts powder to one part liquid by weight.
   e. Cementation consistency of zinc polycarboxylate cement is similar to that of zinc phosphate cement.

11. Which of the following statements applies to the comparison of zinc polycarboxylate and zinc phosphate cement?
   a. The viscosity of zinc polycarboxylate cement increases more rapidly with temperature than that of zinc phosphate cement.
   b. Zinc polycarboxylate cements provide superior clinical retention of crowns compared with zinc phosphate cements.
   c. Both cements depend primarily on mechanical bonding for retention clinically.
   d. When first mixed, zinc polycarboxylate cements are slightly more acidic than zinc phosphate cements.

12. Which two of the following are characteristics of light-cured resin cements for cementation of ceramic veneers?
   a. High strength
   b. Variety of stains and shades
   c. Chemical bonding to dentin and ceramics
   d. Fluoride content

13. Which of the following statements about glass ionomer cements is/are true?
   a. The cement powder is an aluminosilicate glass, whereas the liquid is a polycarboxylate copolymer in water.
   b. The cement must be protected from exposure to water during setting.
   c. Pulpal protection is not necessary for use of a glass ionomer cement in a deep cavity.
   d. Components of glass ionomer cements react to form a cross-linked gel matrix that surrounds the partially reacted powder particles.

14. Which of the following cement bases has the highest elastic modulus to best support an extensive amalgam restoration?
   a. Zinc phosphate
   b. Resin-modified glass ionomer
   c. Zinc polyacrylate
   d. Glass ionomer

15. Which of the following materials is/are used over pulp exposures?
   a. Zinc phosphate
   b. Glass ionomer
   c. Calcium hydroxide
   d. Zinc polycarboxylate

16. Which of the following statements is/are true?
   a. Calcium hydroxide bases are supplied with a powder and a liquid catalyst, which is colored.
   b. A small spatula is used to mix equal lengths of the two pastes of a calcium hydroxide base on a paper pad.
   c. Some cavity liners that contain calcium hydroxide harden quickly by evaporation when dried by air.
   d. Varnishes form resin films usually less than 40 mm thick by evaporation of the solvent.

Use short answers to fill in the following blanks.

17. Resin cements used for permanent cementation of all-ceramic restorations are characterized by a(n) _____ working time.

18. Resin-modified glass ionomer cements usually are not recommended for cementation of all-ceramic restoration because their _____ can cause cracking of the ceramic.

For the following statements, answer true or false.

19. Cementation of ceramic and indirect composite restorations requires treatment of the surfaces of the tooth and restorative material with bonding agents.
   a. True
   b. False

20. Demineralization of the tooth surface around a cemented orthodontic band, which occurs with zinc phosphate cements, is minimized with the fluoride-releasing glass ionomer cements.
   a. True
   b. False

SUGGESTED SUPPLEMENTARY READINGS

Berg JH: Glass ionomer cements, *Pediatr Dent* 24:430, 2002.

Bunek SS, editor: Resin cements—Bonding—The end of luting. *Dent Advis* 30(4):1, 2013.

Bunek SS, editor: Provisionalization in restorative dentistry. *Dent Advis* 29(7):1, 2012.

Council on Dental Materials, Instruments and Equipment: Biocompatibility and postoperative sensitivity, *J Am Dent Assoc* 116:767, 1988.

Croll TP, Nicholson JW: Glass ionomer cements in pediatric dentistry: review of the literature, *Pediatr Dent* 24:423, 2002.

Farah JW, Powers JM, editors: Temporary cements, *Dent Advis* 22(6):1, 2005.

Farah JW, Powers JM, editors: Traditional crown and bridge cements, *Dent Advis* 23(2):1, 2005.

Leinfelder KF: Changing restorative traditions: the use of bases and liners, *J Am Dent Assoc* 125:65, 1994.

Powers JM, Craig RG: A review of the composition and properties of endodontic filling materials, *J Mich Dent Assoc* 61:523, 1979.

APPENDIX 7-1 ZINC PHOSPHATE CEMENT

Historically, zinc phosphate cement (Type I) is a water-based cement that has been used for final cementation, although its use today is limited. Because of its acidity at the time of placement into a tooth, pulpal protection is needed. The cement is formed when a powdered oxide is mixed with an acidic liquid.

Composition and Reaction

The zinc phosphate cement powder is primarily zinc oxide with additions of magnesium oxide and pigments. The liquid is a solution of phosphoric acid in water buffered by aluminum and zinc ions to help slow the setting reaction during mixing. A chemical reaction begins when the cement powder is incorporated into the liquid. The surface of the alkaline powder is dissolved by the acidic liquid, which results in an exothermic reaction. The cement is mixed in such a way as to minimize the temperature rise from the heat given off. The set cement is essentially a hydrated amorphous network of zinc phosphate that surrounds incompletely dissolved particles of zinc oxide. The cement is porous.

> **! ALERT**
>
> An exothermic reaction gives off heat as the components react.

Setting of zinc phosphate cement is affected by time and temperature. Cooling the mixing slab increases the working time. The cement normally sets in the mouth within 5 to 9 minutes from the start of mixing. Factors such as a higher powder–liquid ratio, faster incorporation of powder into the liquid, and a warmer slab cause the cement to set faster. Cementation should be completed promptly after mixing; delays can result in larger film thicknesses and insufficient seating of restorations.

Properties

Some important properties of zinc phosphate cement include fast setting, good mechanical properties, low film thickness, low solubility, and low acidity of the set cement. Minimum requirements are described by ANSI-ADA Specification No. 96 (ISO 9917 [2000]).

The compressive strength of zinc phosphate cement is similar to that of glass ionomer cement. Properties of elasticity of zinc phosphate cement can be affected adversely by a low powder-to-liquid ratio, improper mixing, and premature exposure to oral fluids (Table 7-10). The strength develops rapidly, with two thirds of final strength being reached in

1 hour. The low tensile strength of zinc phosphate cement compared with its high compressive strength indicates the brittle nature of this cement.

The film thickness (25 μm maximum) and solubility in water (0.2% maximum weight loss after 24 hours) are within clinically acceptable limits. The pH of zinc phosphate cement is initially low (pH 4.2) but increases to nearly neutral after 48 hours. The initial acidity may have a deleterious effect on the pulp, particularly on one that is traumatized already. Pulpal protection is recommended. The retention of zinc phosphate cement is caused by mechanical interlocking with the surfaces of the tooth and restoration.

Manipulation

The primary instruments for mixing of zinc phosphate cement include a cooled glass slab and a broad spatula. The bottle of powder is shaken gently and the bottle of liquid swirled before dispensing the contents. The cement powder is dispensed with a scoop supplied by the manufacturer. The powder is divided in one corner of the glass slab into four to six portions, depending on the product. The correct amount of liquid is dispensed, given by drops as directed in the instructions, to an area of the slab away from the powder. Before dispensing the powder and liquid, the slab is cooled under cold water to about 21° C and dried. Any moisture left on the slab or condensed onto the slab because it was too cold will have a deleterious effect on the properties of the cement.

The powder is added to the liquid in portions at 15-second intervals for a total mixing time of 60 to 120 seconds, depending on the product. The cement is mixed over a large area of the slab with broad strokes of a flexible metal spatula. The consistency of the cement is tested before adding the last portion of powder. Only part of that portion of powder may be necessary to reach the desired consistency. The cementing consistency strings about an inch above the slab.

ZINC POLYCARBOXYLATE CEMENT

Zinc polycarboxylate cements are water-based cements used as final cements for retention of crowns and bridges. They are not as strong as zinc phosphate cements, but they are less irritating to the pulp. Examples of commercial products are listed in Table 7-2.

Composition and Reaction

Zinc polycarboxylate cements are supplied usually as a powder and a liquid. The powder is mainly zinc oxide, and the

TABLE 7-10	Effects of Manipulative Variables on Selected Properties of Zinc Phosphate Cement				
Manipulative variables	Compressive strength	Film thickness	Initial solubility	Acidity	Setting time
Decreased powder–liquid ratio	Decrease	Decrease	Increase	Increase	Slower
Increased rate of powder incorporation	Decrease	Increase	Increase	Increase	Faster
Increased mixing temperature	Decrease	Increase	Increase	Increase	Faster
Water contamination	Decrease	Increase	Increase	Increase	Faster

liquid is a viscous solution of polyacrylic acid in water. One product (Tylok Plus; DENTSPLY Caulk, Milford, DE) is supplied as a powder to be mixed with tap water. Its powder consists of zinc oxide coated with solid polyacrylic acid. The zinc oxide and the polyacrylic acid react to form a zinc polyacrylate that surrounds the partially reacted zinc oxide powder particles. The reaction is accelerated by heat.

Properties

The important properties of zinc polycarboxylate cements are moderate viscosity, moderate strength, ability to bond to enamel, and mild acidity. Minimum requirements are described in ANSI-ADA Specification No. 96 (ISO 9917 [2000]).

Mixed polycarboxylate cement appears to be too viscous (thick), but it flows readily when applied to the surfaces to be cemented. The compressive strength of polycarboxylate cement (see Table 7-3) is less than that of glass ionomer cement; however, it provides clinically satisfactory retention for well-fitting restorations.

Zinc polycarboxylate cements are slightly acidic (low pH) when first mixed, but the acid is weakly dissociated. Histologic reactions are similar to those of zinc oxide–eugenol cements, but more reparative dentin is observed with the polycarboxylates. Polycarboxylate cements bond well to sandblasted gold alloys, although clinical studies have not demonstrated improved retention with these cements.

Manipulation

The powder bottle is shaken gently. The powder is dispensed with a scoop onto a disposable paper pad or a glass slab, which can be cooled to permit a longer working time. The viscous liquid is dispensed from the dropper bottle in uniform drops. About 90% of the powder is added immediately to the liquid and mixed for 30 to 60 seconds, depending on the product. The remainder of the powder is added to adjust the consistency. A small area of the mixing surface is used, and the cement is mixed with a stiff spatula. The proper consistency is creamy. The cement should be used immediately because the working time is short (about 3 minutes after mixing at 22° C). The cement is no longer usable when it loses its luster and becomes stringy or starts to "cobweb."

Durelon Maxicap (3M ESPE, St. Paul, MN) is supplied in unit-dose capsules.

COMPOMER CEMENT

Compomer cement is a resin-based cement indicated for cementation of cast alloy and ceramic–metal restorations. Cementation of traditional all-ceramic crowns, inlays, onlays, and veneers is contraindicated. The cement should not be used as a core or filling material.

Composition and Reaction

The cement powder contains strontium aluminum fluorosilicate glass, sodium fluoride, and self-cured and light-cured initiators. The liquid contains polymerizable methacrylate-carboxylic acid monomer, multifunctional acrylate-phosphate monomer, diacrylate monomer, and water. The carboxylic acid groups contribute to the adhesive capability of the cement.

Properties

Compomer cement is noted for high values of retention, bond strength (5.3 MPa to dentin), compressive strength, flexural strength, and fracture toughness. The cement has low solubility, has sustained fluoride release, and can be recharged with fluoride by various fluoride treatments.

Manipulation

Paste–paste (Permacem Automix System; DMG AMERICA, Englewood, NJ) and powder–liquid (Principle, DENTSPLY Caulk, Milford, DE) products are available. The paste–paste product is dispensed and mixed by an auto-mixing device. The tooth to be cemented is dried but not desiccated. With the powder–liquid product, the powder is tumbled before dispensing. The powder–liquid ratio is two scoops to two drops. Mixing takes 30 seconds and should be done rapidly. The mixed cement is placed into the crown only, and then the crown is seated. A "gel" state is reached after 1 minute, at which time the excess cement is removed with floss and a scaler. The exposed margins are light cured to stabilize the restoration. Setting occurs 3 minutes after the start of the mixing step. Once set, compomer cement is hard.

8

Impression Materials

OBJECTIVES

After reading this chapter, the student should be able to:
1. Describe the function of an impression material.
2. Describe the relationship between a tooth, an impression of the tooth, and the die.
3. List the requirements for an ideal impression material.
4. List the components in an alginate powder, and describe their function.
5. Describe the properties of alginate substitute impression materials.
6. List the five objectives for alginate impressions.
7. List the factors to be considered when selecting a tray for an alginate impression of the upper and lower arch.
8. Describe how a tray may be modified for an alginate impression.
9. Describe the proper dispensing and mixing of an alginate.
10. Describe the proper loading of alginate into the tray.
11. Describe the procedure for taking an upper and lower impression in alginate.
12. Describe the proper handling and storing of an alginate impression.
13. Compare the properties of hydrocolloid and elastomeric impression materials.
14. Describe the advantages and disadvantages of alginate hydrocolloid impression materials.
15. Describe the setting of alginate impressions.
16. Compare the properties of the four major elastomeric impression materials, and indicate their clinical applications.
17. List which die or model materials are compatible with the various impression materials.
18. Describe the hand mixing of elastomeric impression materials and the auto-mixing of addition silicones and polyethers.
19. List the various methods of disinfection of impressions and their impact on the accuracy.
20. Describe the important properties of elastomeric bite registration materials.
21. Describe the important characteristics of digital impression systems.

The function of an impression material is to record accurately the dimensions of oral tissues and their spatial relationships. In making an impression, a material in the plastic state is placed against the oral tissues to set. After setting, the impression is removed from the mouth and is used to make a replica of the oral tissues. The impression gives a negative reproduction of these tissues. A positive reproduction is obtained by pouring dental stone or other suitable material into the impression and allowing it to harden. The positive reproduction is called a model or cast when large areas of the oral tissues are involved or a die when single and multiple tooth preparations are recorded. Types of impression materials are summarized in Figure 8-1.

The relationships between a tooth, an impression of the tooth, and a die are illustrated in two dimensions in Figure 8-2. When examined from the anterior side, the various parts of the tooth and the impression are in the same relationship to each other, although the highest portions of the tooth are the deepest parts of the impression. When the maxillary die is examined with the occlusal portion downward, the die is a positive reproduction of the tooth preparation. If the die is examined with the occlusal surface upward, the buccal surface (B) is on the left rather than the right. A similar relationship is shown in Figure 8-2 for a cross section of a mandibular left molar, its impression, and the die made from it. The impression of the mandibular molar, when examined from the anterior side, is inverted for ease of examination, and the buccal (B) and lingual (L) surfaces are reversed with respect to the tooth. The cusp (C) is the highest area on the tooth and the lowest area of the impression, and the position of C for the tooth is on the left but on the right for the impression. The die of the mandibular molar, however, is a positive duplication of the tooth.

Impressions may be taken of portions of a tooth, a single tooth, several teeth, a quadrant of the mouth, or an entire dentulous or edentulous arch. Examples of some of these types of impressions and the corresponding dies or casts are shown in Figure 8-3.

A variety of impression materials are described in this chapter, which is indicative of the fact that no single material is ideal for all applications. The list of properties for an ideal impression material presented in Box 8-1 emphasizes the many demands placed on these materials. Not surprisingly, none of the current materials completely satisfies these requirements.

Impression materials can be classified as those that are flexible and those that are rigid at the time of removal from the mouth. A rigid impression material is restricted to applications in areas in

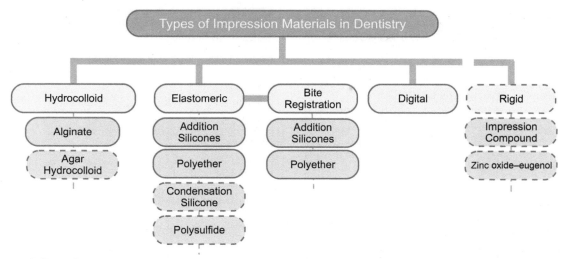

FIG 8-1 Types of impression materials used in contemporary dental practice. Bite registration elastomers are included for completeness. Dashed lines indicate that the material is no longer common in dental practice. Some of these less common materials are discussed briefly in the appendix to this chapter.

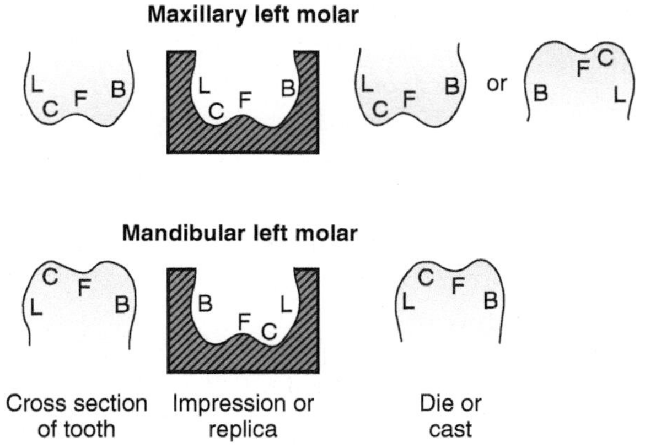

Maxillary left molar

Mandibular left molar

Cross section of tooth   Impression or replica   Die or cast

FIG 8-2 Two-dimensional sketches of a maxillary and mandibular left molar and the corresponding impressions and dies. (*B*, buccal surface; *C*, cusp; *F*, fissure; *L*, lingual surface.)

BOX 8-1 Desirable Properties of Impression Materials

- Ease of manipulation and reasonable cost
- Adequate flow and wetting properties
- Appropriate setting time and characteristics
- Sufficient mechanical strength—elastic recovery and resistant to tearing during removal
- Good dimensional accuracy—stable over time
- Taste and odor acceptable to patient
- Safe—not toxic or irritating
- No significant degradation of properties as a result of disinfection
- Compatibility with all die and cast materials
- Good shelf-life

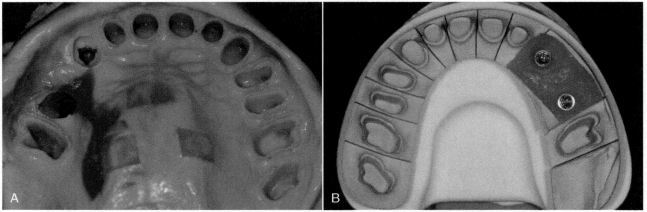

FIG 8-3 Final impression (in addition silicone material, **A**) used to capture fine details needed in a model **(B)** for fabrication of crown restorations and implant placement. (Courtesy Y-W Chen, University of Washington Department of Restorative Dentistry, Seattle, WA.)

TABLE 8-1 Classification of Dental Impression Materials

Rigid	Flexible
Dental compound	*Aqueous*
Zinc oxide–eugenol	Alginate hydrocolloid*
	Elastomeric (incorrectly called inelastic)
	Addition silicone (PVS)*
	Polyether*
	Addition silicone–polyether hybrid
	Condensation silicone
	Polysulfide (rubber base, mercaptan)

*Most commonly used impression materials.

TABLE 8-2 Examples of Alginate Hydrocolloid and Elastomeric Impression Materials

Product	Manufacturer	Packaging
Alginates		
Alginmix	Major Prodotti Dentari (Moncalieri, Italy)	Packet
Hydrogum5	Zhermack (Eatontown, NJ)	Packet
Jeltrate Plus	DENTSPLY Caulk (Milford, DE)	Can, packet
Kromopan 100	Lascod (Firenze, Italy)	Packet
Alginate substitutes		
Alginot	Kerr Corporation (Orange, CA)	AC
Position Penta Quick	3M ESPE (St. Paul, MN)	DMM
Silgimix	Sultan Health Care (Englewood, NJ)	AC, DMM
Status Blue	DMG America (Englewood, NJ)	AC
Addition silicones		
Aquasil Ultra	DENTSPLY Caulk	AC, DMM
Flexitime	Heraeus (Armonk, NY)	AC
Honigum	DMG America	AC, DMM
Imprint 4	3M ESPE	AC, DMM
Polyethers		
Impregum Garant	3M ESPE	AC
Impregum Penta Soft	3M ESPE	DMM
Addition silicone–polyether hybrids		
EXA'lence	GC America	AC
Bite registration materials		
Blu-Mousse	Parkell (Edgewood, NY)	AC
Jet Blue Bite	Coltene/Whaledent	AC
Imprint 4 Bite	3M ESPE	AC, DMM

AC, Automix cartridge; *DMM*, dynamic mechanical mixer.

which no undercuts exist. A rigid impression material could not be used on the teeth shown in Figure 8-2 because, on setting, it would be locked in place and could not be removed over the bulge of the tooth without fracturing. A rigid material can be removed from a tooth prepared for a full crown or from an edentulous arch, as shown in Figure 8-3, *C*, because no undercut areas are present. However, a flexible impression material could make these two impressions, in addition to impressions of single teeth or a full dentulous arch. Not surprisingly, impression materials that are flexible when set are used most frequently. Rigid impression materials (dental compound, zinc oxide–eugenol impression paste) are described in Appendix 8-1.

Impression materials discussed in this chapter are listed in Table 8-1 and are classified as rigid or flexible. An estimate of the usage of impression materials in restorative procedures is 51% for addition silicones, 32% for polyethers, 9% for polysulfides, 6% for hydrocolloids, and 2% for condensation silicones.

ALGINATE HYDROCOLLOID IMPRESSION MATERIAL

Alginate is one of the most widely used aqueous dental impression materials. The wide use of alginates results from (1) the ease of mixing and manipulating them; (2) the minimum equipment necessary; (3) the flexibility of the set impression; (4) their accuracy if properly handled; and (5) their low cost. Their principal disadvantages are that they have low tear strength and they do not transfer as much surface detail to gypsum dies as elastomeric impressions do.

Alginates are used extensively to prepare study models of either the entire dental arch or a segment of it. They also are used to prepare gypsum models for the preparation of athletic mouth protectors. They are not recommended for making impressions of cavity preparations.

Note: Agar hydrocolloid impression materials are described in Appendix 8-1.

Packaging

Manufacturers supply alginate as a powder that is packaged in bulk or in pre-weighed individual packets. Examples of alginate impression materials are listed in Table 8-2. The bulk material is packaged in a sealed screw-top plastic container;

in a hermetically sealed metal can, such as that used to package coffee; or in foil packets as shown in Figure 8-4. The pre-weighed packages are constructed of plastic and metal foil and contain enough material for a single full-arch impression. These packages minimize moisture contact with the powder and extend the storage life of the alginate.

A plastic scoop is provided for dispensing the bulk powder, and a plastic cylinder is supplied for measurement of the water (see Figure 8-4). A wide-bladed, reasonably stiff spatula is used to mix the powder and water. Mechanically driven mixers (Alginator II; DUX Dental, Oxnard, CA) are also available.

Composition

Table 8-3 shows the ingredients in alginate powder and their functions. When water is mixed with the alginate powder, a smooth viscous mass is formed, which becomes an irreversible gel a few minutes after mixing. The overall simplified reaction is as follows:

$$\text{Paste} \rightarrow \text{Gel}$$

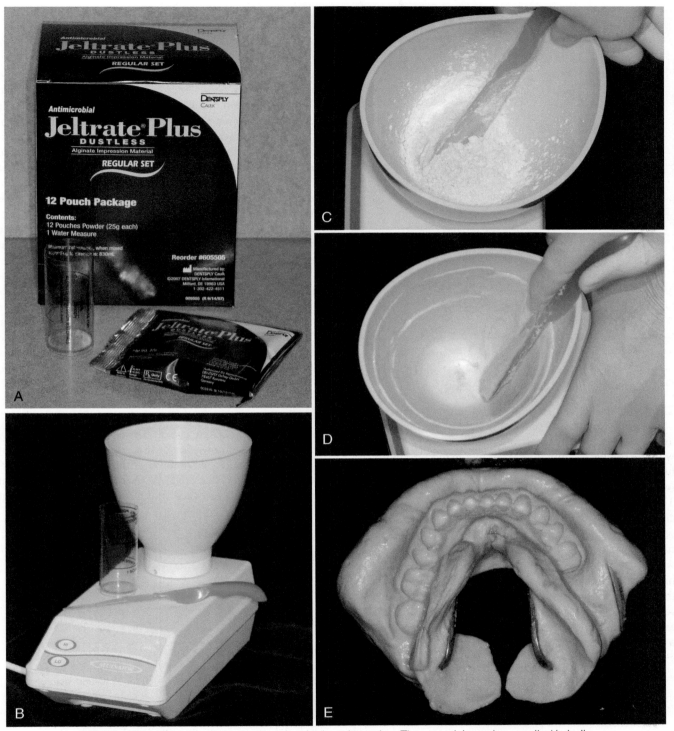

FIG 8-4 Alginate impressions are common in dental practice. The material may be supplied in bulk, but is more commonly supplied in packets **(A)** with a water measure to assure the correct amount of water. Mechanical mixers **(B–D)** are available to mix alginate, although hand-mixing also is common. The resulting alginate impression **(E,** mandibular) must be poured in stone quickly to avoid distortion. (Courtesy Y-W Chen, University of Washington Department of Restorative Dentistry, Seattle, WA.)

TABLE 8-3   Ingredients and Their Function in Alginate Powder

Ingredient	Function
Sodium or potassium alginate salt	To dissolve in water
Calcium sulfate	To react with dissolved alginate to form insoluble calcium alginate
Sodium phosphate	To react preferentially with calcium sulfate and serve as a retarder
Diatomaceous earth or silicate powder	To control consistency of mix and flexibility of impression
Potassium sulfate or potassium zinc fluoride	To counteract the inhibiting effect of alginate on the settling of gypsum model or die material
Organic glycol	To coat the powder particles to minimize dust during dispensing
Pigments	To provide color
Quaternary ammonium compounds or chlorhexidine	To provide self-disinfection
Aspartame	To function as a sweetener

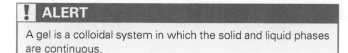

$$\text{Sodium Alginate} + CaSO_4 \bullet H_2O \rightarrow \text{Calcium Alginate}$$
$$\downarrow Na^+ + SO_4^- + H_2O$$

The manufacturer controls the time of setting by the amount of sodium phosphate present in the alginate powder. As long as any sodium phosphate is present, it reacts preferentially with the soluble calcium ions. After all the sodium phosphate has reacted, the soluble sodium alginate reacts with the remaining calcium ions and calcium alginate precipitates. The sodium phosphate therefore is called a *retarder*. The calcium alginate precipitates into a fibrous network; water occupies the intervening capillary spaces. This type of structure is called a *gel*. At least one of the dimensions of the network is colloidal (0.5 μm), and this material traditionally has been named alginate hydrocolloid. The reaction is driven by the lower solubility of calcium alginate compared with sodium alginate. These materials frequently are referred to as irreversible hydrocolloids, because once the paste sets to a gel, the process cannot be reversed.

! ALERT

A gel is a colloidal system in which the solid and liquid phases are continuous.

Properties

American National Standards Institute–American Dental Association (ANSI-ADA) Specification No. 18 (ISO 1563) for alginates established requirements for odor, flavor, lack of irritation, uniformity, mixing and setting times, permanent deformation (alteration in shape) at the time of removal from the mouth, flexibility at the time of pouring the model or die, compressive strength, reproduction of detail, compatibility

with gypsum, and deterioration of the packaged powder during storage.

Mixing and Setting Times

Alginates, when properly mixed by hand, should develop a smooth, creamy consistency free of graininess in less than 1 minute for the normal set material and should be suitable for making impressions in the mouth. The setting time of the alginate is indicated as normal or fast by the manufacturer. An alginate sold as a normal-setting material should set in no less than 2 minutes or more than 4½ minutes after the start of the mix and be workable for up to 2 minutes. The setting time of fast-setting alginate is between 1 and 2 minutes and workable for at least 1¼ minutes. The mixing time of fast-setting alginate is 30 to 45 seconds. In general, the setting time should be no less than that listed by the manufacturer and at least 15 seconds longer than the stated working time.

Because the setting occurs as a result of a chemical reaction, an increase in the temperature of the water used to prepare the mix shortens the working and setting times. The proportions of powder and water also affect the setting times. Thinner mixes increase the time required for the material to set. The usual range of setting times for normal-setting mixes of commercial alginate impression materials is from 2½ to 5 minutes.

Elastic Recovery

Because the set alginate is held between the impression tray and the tissues, knowledge of the extent of any permanent deformation during the removal of the impression is important (Figure 8-5). The ANSI-ADA specification requires at least 95% elastic recovery (no more than 5% permanent

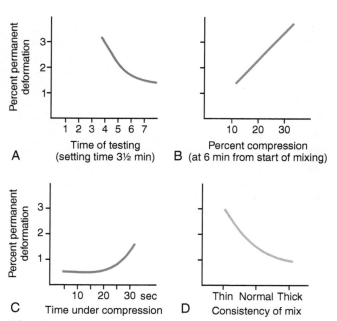

FIG 8-5 Permanent deformation of alginate impressions as a function of time of testing **(A)**, amount of compression **(B)**, time under compression **(C)**, and consistency of mix **(D)**.

BOX 8-2 Permanent Deformation Affected by Manipulation

Permanent deformation increases:
  When the time before testing is shortened
  When the amount of deformation during removal increases
  When the time that it is held under compression increases
  When thinner mixes are used
These effects are shown in Figure 8-4.

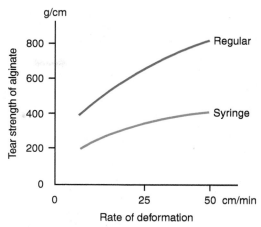

FIG 8-6 Effect of rate of deformation (removal) on the tear strength of alginate impressions.

deformation) when the alginate is compressed 20% for 5 seconds, which simulates removal of the impression from the mouth. Many commercial alginates have actual values of 96% to 98% elastic recovery (2% to 4% permanent deformation). Thus, alginate impression material is flexible but not perfectly elastic (Box 8-2).

Flexibility

The ANSI-ADA specification sets limits of 5% to 20% in compression at the time a model or die is prepared in the impression (10 minutes after the start of mixing). The compression is measured between a stress of 0.01 and 0.10 MPa. Typical values for commercial alginates are between 12% and 18%, but a few manufacturers supply hard-set alginates, which have values of about 5% to 8%.

The relative amounts of water and powder influence the flexibility of the set alginate. Thicker mixes result in lower flexibility.

Strength

The strength of alginates in compression and resistance to tearing are important requirements, although the tear strength is the more critical. The ANSI-ADA specification requires a minimum compressive strength of 0.37 MPa at a time when the material is removed from the mouth. Most commercial products have compressive strengths substantially higher than this limit, with values ranging from 0.5 to 0.9 MPa.

The tear strength of alginates varies from 3.7 to 6.9 N/cm. Because many sections of an impression are thin, tearing may result from a rather small applied force.

The strengths of alginates are a function of the rate at which the impression is deformed; higher rates of deformation (removal) result in higher compressive and tear strengths. An example of the effect of the rate of deformation on tear strength is shown in Figure 8-6, which illustrates that alginate impressions are less likely to tear during removal from the mouth when they are removed rapidly.

The strength of alginate impression materials increases if thick rather than thin mixes are used. The advantage of the use of increasingly thicker mixes is somewhat limited because the consistency becomes too thick, and the flow during seating of the impression is so low that an adequate impression cannot be obtained.

The tear and compressive strengths at the time the impression is removed increase if the time of removal is delayed. The effect of the consistency of the mix and of the time of removal on the tear strength is shown in Figure 8-7. Again, only

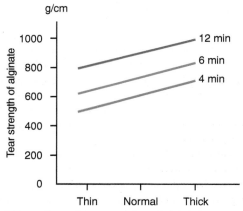

FIG 8-7 Effect of consistency of the mix of alginate and time of testing on the tear strength of alginate impressions.

limited advantage can be taken of the increase in tear strength with time because of the inconvenience of leaving the impression in the mouth for longer periods.

Dimensional Change

> **! ALERT**
>
> Syneresis is the formation of an exudate on the surface of the gel and results in continual shrinkage of the gel.

The accuracy of an impression material is important, and alginates are no exception. A problem with alginate impressions is loss of accuracy with increased time of storage (Figure 8-8). The set alginate is a hydrocolloid gel that contains large quantities of water. This water evaporates if the impression is stored in air, and the impression shrinks. If the impression is placed in water, it absorbs water and expands. Therefore, storage in either air or water results in serious changes in dimensions and a loss of accuracy. Storage in humid air approaching 100% relative humidity results in the least dimensional change. Alginate gels, however, shrink

Dimensional stability of alginates stored
in 100% relative humidity

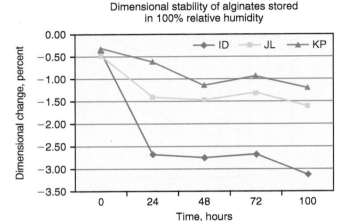

FIG 8-8 Dimensional change of alginate impression materials stored in 100% relative humidity for 100 hours. (Courtesy Lu H, Frey GN, Powers JM: Unpublished data. From Powers JM, Sakaguchi RL, editors: *Craig's restorative dental materials*, ed 13, St Louis, 2012, Mosby.)

even under conditions of 100% relative humidity as a result of a process called syneresis, in which water forms on the surface of the impression. Fortunately, syneresis occurs rather slowly, and alginate impressions prepared from modern products (see Table 8-2) usually can be stored under conditions of 100% relative humidity for up to 5 days without serious dimensional changes.

Studies of the dimensional change of alginates during storage emphasize that they should be stored for as short a period as possible and that the preparation of the model or die should proceed directly after the impression has been made. If the immediate preparation of the model or die is not possible, the next most appropriate procedure is to store the impression in an atmosphere of 100% relative humidity for the shortest possible time.

Reproduction of Detail

The impression material must record the detail of the oral tissues, but this detail also must be transferred to the model or die. The ADA specification recommends that alginates must have the minimum capabilities of transferring a line only 0.075 mm wide to a gypsum model or die material. A number of products have properties that exceed this minimum value.

Disinfection

Guidelines recommend that alginate impressions be rinsed and disinfected. Sodium hypochlorite, iodophor, glutaraldehyde, and phenylphenol solutions have been used, and some manufacturers have added disinfectants to the alginate powder. Studies have shown that test viruses have been inactivated in alginate impressions by (1) a 10-minute soak in 0.5% sodium hypochlorite or a 10-minute wait after spraying the impression with this solution; (2) a 10-minute immersion in an iodophor solution diluted 1:213; (3) a 20-minute immersion in 2% glutaraldehyde diluted 1:4; and (4) a 20-minute immersion in phenylphenol diluted 1:32. The incorporation of disinfectants in the alginate powder also was found to be effective.

Measurements of dimensional changes showed that immersion of alginate impressions for 30 minutes did not affect their clinical accuracy.

Objectives for Taking Alginate Impressions

The objectives are to record the following:
- All teeth in the upper and lower arch
- The entire alveolar process
- The retromolar area of the lower arch
- The area of the hamular notch in the upper arch
- A detailed, undistorted, and bubble-free reproduction of the oral tissues

Selection of the Tray

Criteria for the maxillary tray:
- Completely cover the tuberosity
- Be 4 mm wider than the most apical portion of the alveolar process at the molar region
- Cover the anterior teeth with the incisors contacting the flat arch portion of the tray about 4 mm from the raised palatal part of the tray (Figure 8-9)

Criteria for the mandibular tray:
- Cover all teeth and retromolar pad
- Be 4 mm wider than the buccal and lingual positions of the posterior and the labial and lingual positions of the anterior teeth
- Allow the teeth to be centered and yet comply with the second requirement (Figure 8-10)

Modification of the Tray

To be sure the alginate flows into the labial vestibule when the impression is seated, soft rope wax may be added to the

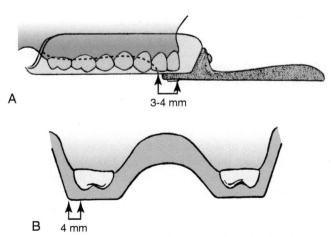

FIG 8-9 Correct tray selection for a maxillary alginate impression. **A,** Side view. **B,** Posterior view. (Modified from Meldrum RJ, Johnson RA, Cheney EA: *Preclinical orthodontics 621/623*, Ann Arbor, 1980, School of Dentistry, University of Michigan.)

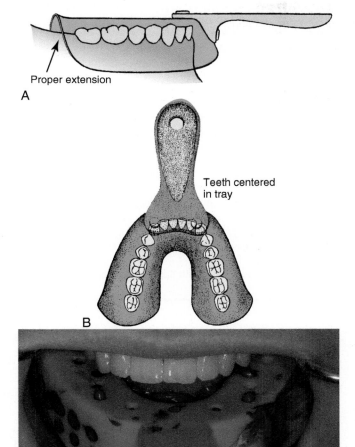

Proper extension

A

Teeth centered in tray

B

C

FIG 8-10 Correct tray selection for a mandibular alginate impression. **A,** Buccal view. **B,** Occlusal view. **C,** View of the loaded impression tray seated in the mouth. (**A, B,** Modified from Meldrum RJ, Johnson RA, Cheney EA: *Preclinical orthodontics* 621/623, Ann Arbor, 1980 School of Dentistry, University of Michigan; **C,** courtesy Y-W Chen, University of Washington Department of Restorative Dentistry, Seattle, WA.)

anterior labial flange of the tray. The rope wax may be added to other borders of either upper or lower tray to make sure that any extensions of the alginate are well supported.

Dispensing the Alginate

The recommended amount of water, for the particular impression, should be measured into the rubber bowl using the manufacturer's liquid dispensing vial. The water temperature should be room temperature (22° to 23° C).

The alginate powder provided in bulk should be aerated (fluffed) by tumbling the container several times before opening. The manufacturer's powder scoop should be dipped lightly into the powder and then tapped lightly with a spatula

to ensure a full measure free from large voids. Finally, the excess powder is scraped off with a spatula.

The powder is sifted into the rubber bowl that contains the water.

Mixing the Alginate

With a stiff, wide-bladed spatula, the alginate powder is stirred with water. The mix is spatulated vigorously against the side of the rubber bowl until a smooth, creamy mix that is free of voids results. Insufficient spatulation results in a grainy mix. Spatulation of an alginate identified by the manufacturer as a regular-set product should be accomplished in about 45 seconds. Fast-set products should be spatulated for about 30 seconds.

Loading the Tray

The spatula is used to transfer the alginate mix from the bowl to the tray. The tray is filled evenly to the top by forcing it firmly into the tray to make sure voids are not trapped. A useful method is to start at the posterior and push the mix anteriorly by adding more and more to the posterior.

Making the Impression

Steps for lower arch impressions:
1. Push the left corner of the mouth away with the side of the tray.
2. Insert the tray with a rotary motion.
3. Place the left heel of the tray in contact followed by the anterior and then the right heel.
4. Have the patient lift the tongue, and with the free hand pull the lip down gently.
5. Seat the tray in the direction of the long axis of the anterior teeth, and the alginate should flow into the vestibules. Apply the seating force moderately slowly to allow the alginate to flow properly.
6. At final seating, the incisal edges and cuspal tips should be about 1 to 2 mm from the metal surface of the tray.
7. The tray is held in position until the alginate has set, which is about 1 minute after it has lost its tackiness, tested by touching a portion with the finger.
8. The set impression is removed with a rapid, firm pull.

Steps for upper arch impressions:
1. Rotate the filled tray into the mouth in a counterclockwise motion while you retract the right cheek of the patient.
2. Start seating the tray by positioning its posterior border, and then continue seating parallel to the axis of the central incisors so that most of the excess alginate flows both in a labial or buccal direction but not in a palatal direction.
3. As with the mandibular impression, hold the tray in position until the alginate sets.
4. Break the peripheral seal by running a finger around the edge, and again remove the impression with a rapid, firm pull.

Steps after Making the Impression

1. Rinse the impression with cool water.
2. Cut away any unsupported alginate.

3. Disinfect the alginate impression. One method is to soak it in hypochlorite bleach diluted 10:1 with water for 10 minutes.
4. Rinse the disinfected impression with cold water.
5. Remove excess water.
6. Proceed to pour the gypsum model (see Chapter 9), or if storage is necessary, wrap loosely in a wet paper towel or seal in a plastic bag for up to 5 days.
7. If stored, the impression should be placed so that the tray supports the alginate. Thus, the tray side of the impression is against the laboratory bench.

Troubleshooting Alginate Impressions

If the alginate set before a satisfactory impression was obtained, several factors could be contributing to this problem:

- Incorrect dispensing of powder and liquid (not aerating the powder before dispensing)
- An unusually high room temperature
- Too much time used in loading the tray and inserting the impression

The best solution for delaying the setting is to reduce the temperature of the mix water rather than to use a thinner mix, which results in lower tear strength.

If the alginate impression contained several large voids in critical areas, what can be done to avoid this problem?

- During the dispensing and mixing of the alginate, the powder is added to the water and often an initial wetting of the powder by water is accomplished by squeezing the alginate between the blade of the spatula and the side of the rubber mixing bowl, which minimizes the incorporation of voids.
- When filling the tray, add alginate at one location, and force the alginate to flow into other portions of the tray.
- As a special precaution, a portion of alginate can be spread over the occlusal surface of the teeth before the loaded tray is inserted.

If the alginate impression had a large amount of material in the posterior palatal area and did not record adequately the area of the vestibule, several factors could be involved:

- The posterior of the tray may not have been seated first followed by the anterior, which allowed a large portion of the alginate to flow into the palatal area (which also could make the patient gag).
- Inadequate alginate may have been placed in the tray.
- The lip may not have been pulled out gently to allow alginate to flow into the vestibule.
- The impression must be seated gradually to give the alginate time to flow.

Technique tips for alginate impression materials are summarized in Box 8-3.

ALGINATE SUBSTITUTE IMPRESSION MATERIAL

Alginate substitute impression materials are addition silicone impression materials that are formulated to provide characteristics similar to alginate impression materials. Examples of alginate substitute impression materials are listed in

---

> **BOX 8-3 Technique Tips for Alginate Impression Materials**
>
> 1. Use prepackaged alginate powder.
> 2. Use correct mixing time to ensure best properties.
> 3. Select proper size of tray—allow a thickness of 3 mm of alginate.
> 4. Apply adhesive to trays if needed and allow it to dry.
> 5. Use a wide spatula and flexible bowl for hand mixing; use a vigorous stropping motion.
> 6. Cool water will extend the mixing time.
> 7. Immerse the impression in a disinfecting solution for 10 to 20 minutes; rinse with water before pouring the gypsum material.
> 8. Pour the impression immediately.
> 9. If necessary, store the impression in a plastic bag with a small amount of water.
> 10. Separate alginate impressions from set gypsum casts within a few hours.
> 11. Clean reusable trays with appropriate cleaners, and then sterilize.

Table 8-2. When compared with alginates, alginate substitutes have improved dimensional stability, accuracy, and elastic recovery; however, the cost of an impression is higher. Products are packaged for auto-mixing or dynamic mixing.

ELASTOMERIC IMPRESSION MATERIALS

Elastomeric impression materials are flexible cross-linked polymers when set. Except for the preparation of study models, elastomeric impression materials dominate the market mainly as a result of their greater accuracy, dimensional stability with time, and ability to record detail as compared with the hydrocolloid materials. The first elastomeric impression materials were polysulfides, followed by condensation silicones, polyethers, and addition silicones. The newest category is the addition silicone–polyether hybrid. Emphasis is placed in this chapter on the most commonly used elastomeric impression materials—addition silicones and polyethers.

Note: Information on polysulfide and condensation silicone impression materials can be found in Appendix 8-1.

ADDITION SILICONE IMPRESSION MATERIALS

Addition silicone impression materials (also known as vinyl polysiloxanes [VPS]) were developed as an alternative to polysulfides and condensation silicones. Examples of addition silicone impression materials are listed in Table 8-2.

Composition and Setting Reaction

The material is supplied as a two-paste or a two-putty system. One contains a low-molecular-weight silicone with terminal vinyl groups, reinforcing filler, and a chloroplatinic acid catalyst, and the other contains a low-molecular-weight silicone with silane hydrogens and reinforcing filler. The two are mixed in equal quantities, and the addition reaction occurs between the vinyl and hydrogen groups with no by-product being formed.

A simplified setting reaction is as follows:

Hydrogen-containing siloxane
+ Vinyl-terminal siloxane
+ Chloroplatinic → Silicone rubber

$$\underset{CH_3}{\overset{CH_3}{\sim\!\!\sim Si}}\!\!-\!\!H + CH_2 = CH\!\!-\!\!\underset{CH_3}{\overset{CH_3}{Si}}\!\!\sim\!\!\sim + H_2PtCl_6 \rightarrow \sim\!\!\sim\underset{CH_3}{\overset{CH_3}{Si}}\!\!-\!\!CH_2\!\!-\!\!CH_2\!\!-\!\!\underset{CH_3}{\overset{CH_3}{Si}}\!\!\sim\!\!\sim$$

The vinyl siloxane is difunctional, and the hydrogen-containing siloxane is multifunctional. Because no volatile by-product (such as water or ethanol) is formed in this reaction, minimal dimensional change occurs during polymerization. Increases in temperature lengthen the rate of reaction and shorten the setting time. If hydroxyl groups are present in the addition silicone, a side reaction occurs that results in the formation of hydrogen. The hydrogen is released gradually from the set impression material and produces bubbles in gypsum dies prepared less than 1 hour, or epoxy dies less than 24 hours, after the impression is taken. Some products permit the immediate pouring of dies by controlling the presence of hydroxyl groups or by the inclusion in the impression material of a hydrogen absorber, such as palladium. Thus, the manufacturer's directions for the time of preparation of dies from a particular addition silicone should be followed.

> **! ALERT**
>
> A hydrophobic surface is poorly wetted by water with a contact angle of 90°.

Nearly all addition silicones contain surfactants and are hydrophilic with contact angles of about 20° to 40°. Hydrophilic silicones wet the oral tissues better than earlier hydrophobic materials and permit gypsum models and dies to be prepared with fewer air bubbles.

> **! ALERT**
>
> A hydrophilic surface is readily wetted by water with a low contact angle.

Consistencies

Addition silicones are supplied as low-, medium-, high-, or very high-viscosity (putty) material. Originally, the addition silicones were packaged in tubes of base and catalyst for hand mixing. Currently, they are supplied in auto-mixing or dual-cartridge systems with the base paste in one cartridge and the catalyst paste in the other and a mixing gun as shown in Figure 8-11. The cartridge is placed in the mixing gun, and ratchet plungers force the pastes through a static mixing

tip. During extrusion through the static mixing tip, the two pastes are folded over each other and exit the tip in a mixed condition. The mixing tip is left on until the next mix, at which time it is replaced by a new tip. The very high viscosity materials are supplied more often as base and catalyst putties in two jars (see Figure 8-11) and are mixed by hand.

Addition silicones also are supplied with the base and catalyst in bulk containers (called sausages) to be mixed in a dynamic mechanical mixer (Dynamix speed; Heraeus, South Bend, Indiana) with a dynamic mixing tip (see Figure 8-11). The dynamic mixer is activated by a switch, and the mixed impression material is dispensed into a syringe or tray.

These automatic mixing systems result in mixes with fewer bubbles than with hand-spatulated mixes. Addition silicones are also available as single-consistency or monophase material that can be used as both a low- and high-viscosity material. They are formulated so that under high shear forces, such as when they are extruded from a syringe, they have a low viscosity. When they are under low shear forces, such as when they are placed in an impression tray with a spatula, they have a high viscosity (shear thinning). Thus, a single mix can be used as a syringe and a tray material. These products are available as an auto-mixed, two-paste system.

Properties

ANSI-ADA Specification No. 19 (ISO 4823) has established requirements for elastomeric impression materials. The properties of the addition silicones are compared with other elastomeric impression materials in Table 8-4. Less dimensional change and higher elastic recovery are noteworthy improvements of the addition silicones over the earlier condensation silicones. The dimensional change in 24 hours of about -0.1% is very low. The elastic recovery at the time of removal from the mouth of about 99.8% (permanent deformation of 0.2%) is the highest of all the impression materials. The percentage flow values of the addition silicones are likewise low. These properties indicate the superior accuracy of the addition silicones.

The working time is short for the addition silicones, and the flexibility is low to moderate. Removal of addition silicone impressions from undercut areas may present difficulties because of this stiffness, and extra space should be provided for the impression material when a custom tray is used.

Tissue culture tests on the base and catalyst pastes have been negative and indicate that addition silicones cause less tissue reaction than the condensation silicones.

Manipulation

The low-, medium-, high-, and very high-viscosity products of one manufacturer's addition silicone are shown in Figure 8-11. A few manufacturers supply the very high viscosity (putty) material for mechanical mixers.

The cartridge is inserted into the gun and the cap on the end removed. The plungers are advanced by the trigger until base and catalyst paste are extruding uniformly. The tip is wiped off, and a static mixing tip is placed on the end of the cartridge. The trigger is used to extrude and mix the base

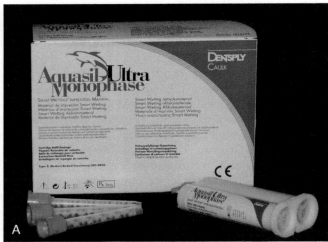
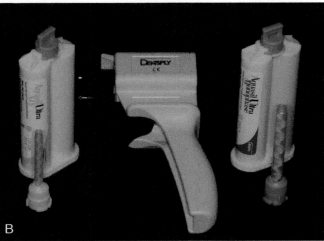
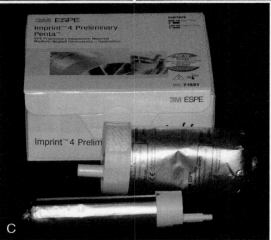

FIG 8-11 Addition silicone impression materials are often supplied in cartridges of base and catalyst **(A)** that are auto-mixed through a dispensing tip and using a mixing gun **(A, B)**. Alternatively, the material may be supplied as "sausages" **(C)** that fit into a power mixer. (Courtesy Y-W Chen, University of Washington Department of Restorative Dentistry, Seattle, WA.)

TABLE 8-4   Qualitative Rating of Physical and Mechanical Properties of Elastomeric Impression Materials

Property	Addition silicones (PVS)	Polyethers	Condensation silicones	Polysulfides
Working time	Short–moderate	Short	Short	Moderate–long
Setting time	Short–moderate	Short	Short–moderate	Moderate–long
Shrinkage on setting	Very low	Low	Moderate–high	High
Elastic recovery after removal	Very high	High	High	Moderate
Flexibility during removal	Low–moderate	Low–moderate	Moderate	High
Tear strength	Low–moderate	Moderate	Low–moderate	Moderate–high
Flow setting under small forces	Very low	Very low	Low	Moderate–high
Wettability by gypsum mixes	Good–very good	Very good	Poor	Moderate
Gas evolution after setting	Yes	No	No	No
Detail reproduction	Excellent	Excellent	Excellent	Excellent

and catalyst through the mixing tip. The material is mixed thoroughly as it exits the tip.

The base and catalyst putties provided in jars are dispensed in equal quantities and are mixed by hand until free from streaks. The two putties should not be mixed when latex rubber gloves are worn because components in the latex rubber will retard or prevent the setting by poisoning the platinum catalyst. Vinyl gloves or bare hands are acceptable. If latex gloves must be worn, they should be washed thoroughly with a detergent and dried just before the putties are mixed.

Low-viscosity addition silicones are also available in unit-dose systems with reusable or disposable syringes. Putties are also available in unit dose. A completed maxillary impression is shown in Figure 8-12.

Technique tips for elastomeric impression materials are summarized in Box 8-4.

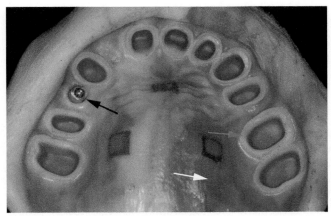

FIG 8-12 Addition silicone impression of crown preparations and an implant *(black arrow)* for final restoration construction. In this impression, a combination of a high viscosity *(white arrow)* and low viscosity *(red arrow)* material has been used. This strategy helps manipulate the material, and the high viscosity phase has the added value of stabilizing the implant impression coping to assure accurate implant positioning. (Courtesy Y-W Chen, University of Washington Department of Restorative Dentistry, Seattle, WA.)

BOX 8-4 Technique Tips for Elastomeric Impression Materials

1. Prepare a custom tray or select a stock tray of an appropriate size and do a try-in.
2. Seated tray should have coverage of the hard and soft oral tissues and without impinging on the soft tissues.
3. Apply adhesive using a brush and let it dry before adding the impression material.
4. Check that openings of auto-mix cartridges are not blocked.
5. Immerse the tip of the syringe in the extruded material to minimize bubbles.
6. Use fast-set/fast-set or regular-set/regular-set materials together.
7. Do not mix VPS putties with latex rubber gloves—components in the latex material will retard the setting.

POLYETHER IMPRESSION MATERIALS

Polyether materials have properties similar to the addition silicones. The polyether polymer is hydrophilic and exhibits good wetting properties, even in a moist field. Polyethers have the disadvantage of limited dimensional stability over time and older materials had poor taste. Examples of polyether impression materials are listed in Table 8-2.

Composition and Setting Reaction

Polyether impression materials are supplied as a base and catalyst system. The base is a moderately low-molecular-weight polyether, containing ethylene imine terminal groups. These terminal groups are reacted together by the action of an aromatic sulfonic acid ester catalyst to form a cross-linked high-molecular-weight elastomer as illustrated by the following figure, in which R is a series of organic groups:

$$CH_3-\underset{\underset{CH_2-CH_2}{|}}{\overset{\overset{H}{|}}{C}}-CH_2-\overset{\overset{O}{\|}}{C}-O-R-O-\overset{\overset{O}{\|}}{C}-CH_2-\underset{\underset{CH_2-CH_2}{|}}{\overset{\overset{H}{|}}{C}}-CH_3 + \quad \rightarrow \text{ Cross-linked rubber}$$

Properties

The properties of polyether impression materials are compared with other elastomeric impression materials in Table 8-4. The consistency is listed as medium viscosity but is high compared with that of other medium-viscosity elastomeric impression materials. It is also available as a low- and high-viscosity polyether system.

The elastic recovery of the polyethers is slightly less than that of the addition silicones. The stiffness of the newer polyethers is indicated by a flexibility of 5% and 7%. With older polyethers, the low flexibility caused problems in the removal of the impression from the mouth, and a 4-mm rather than a 2-mm thickness of impression material between the tray and the teeth was recommended.

The dimensional change of polyethers is higher than that of the addition silicones. The polyether absorbs water and changes dimensions if stored in contact with water until equilibrium is reached. Thus, polyether impressions should not be stored in water and should be washed and dried after removal from the mouth and disinfectants.

The aromatic sulfonic acid ester catalyst can cause skin irritation, and direct contact with the catalyst should be avoided. Thorough mixing of the catalyst with the base should be accomplished to prevent any irritation of the oral tissues.

Manipulation

The polyether materials are supplied in two mixing systems: (1) as a cartridge with a mixing gun and (2) as a sausage with a dynamic mechanical mixer (Figure 8-13). A stock or individual tray may be used, but in either instance an adhesive should

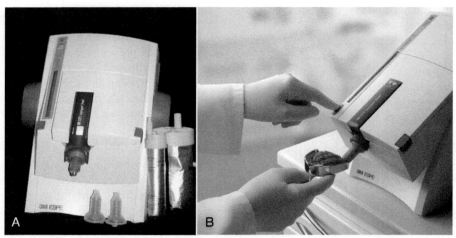

FIG 8-13 Polyether impression materials are commonly mixed in a motorized mixer **(A)** because they tend to be stiffer and harder to manipulate through a mixing gun. Motorized mixing assures precision during dispensing and control of the amount of the material used **(B)**. (Courtesy Y-W Chen, University of Washington Department of Restorative Dentistry, Seattle, WA.)

be used. The material generally is used in a single-mix technique, but a syringe-tray technique may be used. If a syringe-tray technique is desired, it is better to use the low- and high-viscosity product.

The impression should be pulled slowly to break the seal and then removed in a single stroke; it should be rinsed with cold water, disinfected, and blown dry. The impression should not be stored in water or in direct sunlight, and the dies or models should be prepared promptly.

Unreacted polyether may be removed with organic solvents such as acetone or chloroform or with soap and water. The set elastomer may be removed with chloroform or other chlorinated solvents, such as trichloroethylene.

Polyether materials have a good shelf life and should be usable after 2 years of storage at room temperature.

DISINFECTION OF ELASTOMERIC IMPRESSIONS

A variety of disinfectants—including (1) neutral glutaraldehyde, (2) acidified glutaraldehyde, (3) neutral phenolated glutaraldehyde, (4) phenol, (5) iodophor, and (6) chlorine dioxide—may be used to disinfect addition silicone and polyether impressions. The impressions are immersed in appropriately diluted solutions for 10 minutes, except for chlorine dioxide, in which they are immersed for only 3 minutes. The accuracy of high-strength stone dies poured into these impressions was excellent for addition silicones but was unacceptable for polyethers. As a result, disinfection of polyether impressions by immersion is not recommended except for very short (2 to 3 minutes) times in chlorine compound disinfectants. Also, the surface quality of high-strength stone dies poured against the impressions is acceptable. Overall, the selection of the impression material is of greater

importance than the selection of the disinfectant. Times for disinfection vary, so product data should be used to determine the appropriate immersion time.

ELASTOMERIC MATERIALS FOR BITE REGISTRATION

Bite registrations in the past have been taken in wax as discussed in Chapter 10. The following factors limit the accuracy of wax bite registrations: (1) distortion on removal; (2) release of internal stress on storage; (3) high flow properties; and (4) large dimensional change from mouth to room temperature. Elastomeric bite registration materials ideally should (1) be fast setting; (2) be mousse-like in the tray; (3) have no taste or odor; (4) be rigid when set; and (5) be easy to trim.

Addition silicone and polyether materials are now commonly used to take bite registrations. Examples of bite registration materials are listed in Table 8-2. Most of the products are addition silicones supplied as auto-mixing systems. The addition silicones are noted for their short working times of 1.5 to 3 minutes, low strain in compression (high stiffness) of 1% to 2%, no measurable flow of 0.01%, and low dimensional change at 1 day of about -0.08% and at 7 days of about -0.13%. The properties of the polyether bite registration material are similar, except for a higher dimensional change at 1 and 7 days of about -0.3%. Based on these properties, the elastomeric bite registration materials are superior to waxes for taking bite registrations. Elastomeric bite registration materials should not be used for crown and bridge impressions because they have less elastic recovery than corresponding impression materials.

DIGITAL IMPRESSIONS

Several digital impression systems that allow the dentist to take a digital impression in place of a traditional elastomeric

TABLE 8-5 Digital Impression Systems

Product	Manufacturer	Type of imaging	In-office milling	Laboratory milling
3M ESPE Lava Chairside Oral Scanner C.O.S.	3M ESPE (St. Paul, MN)	LED–continuous video	No	Yes
CEREC AC	Sirona Dental Systems (Charlotte, NC)	Bluecam LED	Yes	Yes
E4D Dentist	E4D Technologies (Richardson, TX)	Laser	Yes	Yes
iTero	Cadent (Carlstadt, NJ)	Laser	No	Yes

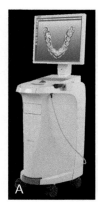
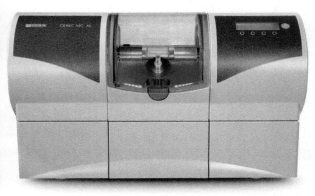
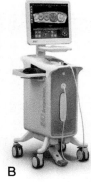
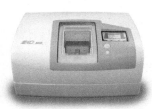

FIG 8-14 In-office CAD/CAM systems. **A,** CEREC AC. **B,** E4D Dentist. (**A,** Courtesy Sirona Dental Systems, Charlotte, NC. **B,** Courtesy D4D Technologies, Richardson, TX.)

impression are currently on the market (Table 8-5). Two of these systems (CEREC AC, Figure 8-14, *A*, and E4D Dentist, Figure 8-14, *B*) offer the option of in-office design and milling but also allow design and milling by dental technicians. Several other systems also produce digital impressions that require design and milling at a dental laboratory or milling center.

Milling centers and dental laboratories can use computer-aided design/computer-aided manufacturing (CAD/CAM) to produce restorations directly from the digital impression data (Figure 8-15). Restorations can be milled from a variety of materials such as composites, feldspathic porcelain, leucite-reinforced ceramic, lithium disilicate ceramic, and zirconia. Wax patterns and acrylic provisional restorations can also be milled. The digitally produced models can be used to produce restorations by traditional methods in the dental laboratory.

Digital impressions offer a precise fit with fewer incidents of remakes and shorter seating/adjustment time (Figure 8-15).

Models for orthodontics and crown and bridge can be produced from digital impressions using 3-D printing. Three-D (dimensional) printing uses a process similar to ink-jet printing to produce a plastic model that is accurate.

QUICK REVIEW

Elastomeric impression materials are distinguished from alginate impression materials by their stability in air after setting, their excellent reproduction of surface detail, and their higher tear strengths. The addition silicones have very low shrinkage on setting, low flow, and high elastic recovery, which makes them the most accurate impression material. Polyether impression materials have excellent wettability. Addition silicones can be disinfected by immersion. The accuracy and dimensional stability of addition silicone bite registration materials make them the preferred material for recording occlusal relationships. Digital impressions offer a precise fit with fewer incidents of remakes and shorter seating/adjustment time.

Alginate is an irreversible hydrocolloid impression material that owes its wide use to the simplicity of the system and technique of use combined with adequate flexibility, strength, and clinical accuracy for study models of dentulous patients. Alginates do not yield adequate surface detail on high-strength stone models to be used to make highly precise crown and bridge restorations. Alginate impressions should be poured promptly because they change dimensions when stored in air and water. When stored in 100% relative humidity, some alginates can be stored for up to 5 days before significant changes take place. Alginate impressions may be disinfected by immersion without clinically significant dimensional changes.

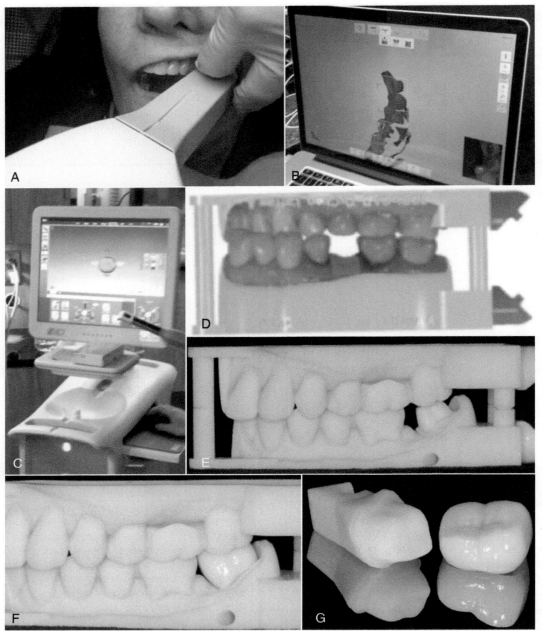

FIG 8-15 Digital impressions are emerging as a major method of capturing intra-oral information and have the potential to eliminate the traditional impression altogether. A digital "wand" **(A)** is inserted into the mouth and manipulated to capture the information on a computer **(B).** Once the file is captured, the computer and software **(C)** create a virtual model **(D)** of the teeth of interest as well as the opposing dentition. The computer directs a three-dimensional printer to print a physical model out of resin **(E),** and the restoration (#18, **F, G**) is constructed and delivered to the patient. In some applications, the restoration can be milled via the computer file with no physical model at all. The accuracy and success of the traditional impression are still currently the gold standard against which these new technologies are measured. (Courtesy Y-W Chen, University of Washington Department of Restorative Dentistry, Seattle, WA.)

⚡ SELF-TEST QUESTIONS

In the following multiple-choice questions, one or more responses may be correct.

1. Which of the following statements is/are true?
   a. An impression gives a negative reproduction of a tooth.
   b. An impression gives a positive reproduction of the soft tissue.
   c. The die of a mandibular molar is a positive duplication of the tooth.
   d. The die of a maxillary molar is a negative duplication of the tooth.
   e. When an impression rests on its tray, the lowest area of the impression is the cuspal surface.

2. Indicate whether the following impression materials are classified as rigid or flexible:
   a. Polyether
   b. Zinc oxide–eugenol
   c. Alginate hydrocolloid
   d. Polysulfide
   e. Addition silicone
   f. Dental impression compound
   g. Addition silicone–polyether hybrid

3. Indicate which of the functions listed in the right-hand column correspond to the components of alginate impression material listed in the left-hand column.

a. Calcium sulfate	1. Soluble alginate
b. Sodium alginate	2. Retarder, reacts first with CaSO₄
c. Water	with $CaSO_4$
d. Sodium phosphate	3. Insoluble alginate
e. Calcium alginate	4. Gel formation
f. Diatomaceous earth	5. Provides soluble calcium ions
g. Quaternary ammonium flexibility of impression compounds or chlorhexidine	6. Controls consistency of mix
h. Glycols	7. Makes the powder dustless
	8. Provides disinfection quality

4. The alginate hydrocolloid:
   a. Consists of calcium alginate that has precipitated into a fibrous network with water occupying the intervening capillary spaces
   b. Is a reversible hydrogel
   c. Sets by a double decomposition–precipitation reaction
   d. Usually contains salts to counteract the inhibiting effect of alginate on the setting of gypsum model material

5. Regular-setting alginate should do which of the following?
   a. Develop a smooth, creamy consistency free of graininess in less than 30 seconds
   b. Set within 2 to 4½ minutes
   c. Set more slowly if mixed with cold water
   d. Set more slowly if mixed to a thin consistency

6. The elastic recovery of alginate can be maximized clinically by which of the following?
   a. Increasing the time in the mouth before removal of the impression
   b. Using a mix of thinner consistency
   c. Decreasing the percentage of deformation during removal of the impression
   d. Using more material between the tray and the teeth

7. Which of the following statements is/are true?
   a. Alginate impressions should be stored for as short a period as possible.
   b. Alginate gels expand when stored in water.
   c. Alginate gels shrink when stored in air or 100% relative humidity.
   d. Modern alginate impressions can be stored in 100% relative humidity without serious dimensional changes for up to 5 days.

8. Which of the following statements is/are true for alginate?
   a. The can of alginate should be aerated, or fluffed up, before dispensing the powder for each mix.
   b. The powder-dispensing cup should be overfilled slightly to allow the powder to fill the cup after compaction.
   c. The powder should be added to the water and initially stirred to wet the particles.
   d. Graininess in the mix and poor detail in the impression can result from insufficient mixing.
   e. Alginate should be mixed with a vigorous stropping or wiping action against the side of the rubber bowl.

9. Which of the following statements is/are true with respect to alginates?
   a. Mixed alginate generally is added to the anterior portion of the tray and pushed toward the posterior part.
   b. Patient gagging can be minimized by reducing the amount of alginate in the posterior palatal area.
   c. The posterior portion of the tray usually is seated first.
   d. Sufficient alginate should be present in the anterior part of the tray to record the soft tissues.
   e. The clinical setting time is reached when the surface is no longer tacky.

10. Which of the following statements is/are true for alginate impressions?
    a. The impression should be rinsed with cool water to remove any saliva or blood and then disinfected.
    b. Excess water that collects in the cuspal areas of the impression causes the gypsum model to be weak in these areas.
    c. The impression should be placed face down on the bench to allow excess water to drain.
    d. The impression can be stored for a short period if tightly wrapped in a damp towel.
    e. Alginate not supported by the tray need not be cut away because it is away from the area of interest.

11. Indicate which of the elastomeric impression materials listed in the right-hand column contain the components listed in the left-hand column, and indicate the function of each component in the left-hand column by selecting the matching item in the right-hand column.

a. Polymer containing ethylene imine terminal groups	1. Polyether
	2. Addition silicone
b. Vinyl-terminated siloxane	3. Addition silicone–polyether hybrid
c. Siloxane with ethylene imine side groups	4. Base
d. Sulfonic acid ester	5. Catalyst
e. Chloroplatinic acid	

12. A comparison of the properties of elastomeric impression materials would indicate which of the following?
    a. Addition silicones show less dimensional change than polyethers.
    b. Polyethers are stiffer than addition silicones.
    c. Polyethers show less flow than addition silicones.
    d. Addition silicones show less permanent deformation than polyethers.
    e. Addition silicones show less working time than polyethers.

13. Which of the following properties applies to a regular-consistency addition silicone impression material?
    a. Dimensional change at 24 hours of about −0.1%
    b. Elastic recovery on removal from typical undercuts of more than 99%
    c. Positive tissue culture tests on mixed material
    d. Requires special gypsum die material
    e. Highly flexible
    f. High flow under low forces

14. Which of the following statements apply to polyether impression materials?
    a. Polyether impressions are inaccurate because they absorb water and change dimensions.
    b. Soft polyether products are stiffer than addition silicones.
    c. Polyethers exhibit less elastic recovery than addition silicones.
    d. The products with higher stiffness can be compensated for by an increase in the thickness of impression material between the impression area and the tray.

15. The impression material that shows the least dimensional change as a result of disinfection by immersion is which of the following?
    a. Alginate
    b. Addition silicone
    c. Polyether

16. Which of the statements is/are true for addition silicones?
    a. Many products release hydrogen after setting, and high-strength stone models should not be poured until 1 hour after setting.
    b. Most products are all hydrophilic because of the addition of surfactants.
    c. They are available only as monophase systems.
    d. They are available as auto-mixing systems.
    e. The putties should be mixed while latex gloves are worn to protect the operator from the catalyst.

17. Which statement(s) is/are true for immersion disinfection of impression materials?
    a. The accuracy of polyether impressions is the least affected.
    b. Selection of the type of disinfectant is more important than selection of the impression material.
    c. Addition silicones are the least affected by disinfection.
    d. None of the above.

18. Which of the following statements is/are true for elastomeric bite registration materials?
    a. They are highly flexible.
    b. They have very low flow once set.
    c. They are addition silicones or polyethers.
    d. They have long working times.
    e. They usually are supplied as auto-mixing systems.

Use short answers to fill in the following blanks.

19. _____ impression materials are restricted to use in areas in which no undercuts exist, whereas _____ impression materials can be used to make impressions of both undercut and nonundercut areas.

20. _____ describes the formation of an exudate (liquid) on the surface of set alginate on standing, even if stored in a moist environment.

21. Alginate is called a(n) _____ hydrocolloid.

22. The only suitable model materials for pouring into alginate impressions are _____ products.

23. An elastomeric impression material that is readily wetted by water or saliva is a _____ material.

24. Elastomeric impression products that are suitable for use as a syringe material as well as a tray material are identified as _____ materials.

Use short statements to answer the following questions.

25. You have taken an alginate impression that has acceptable qualities except the alginate tore. What could have caused the problem, and how might a satisfactory impression be made?

26. You have taken an alginate impression and find you have a number of voids in critical areas. What are the possible causes, and what should be corrected in retaking the impression?

27. You made a mix of alginate impression material, and it set before you could fully seat the impression. What are the possible causes for this problem, and how would you avoid it when retaking the impression?

For the following statements, answer true or false.

28. Manufacturers produce regular-set and fast-set alginates by adjusting the amount of sodium phosphate in the powder, which reacts preferentially with calcium sulfate compared with the sodium alginate when water is added.
    a. True
    b. False

29. All of the following shorten the setting time of alginate impression materials: (1) increased temperature of the mix water; (2) decreased water-to-powder ratio; and (3) increased room temperature.
    a. True
    b. False

30. The manipulation of regular-setting-time alginate impression materials includes the following: (1) adding the powder to the water; (2) stirring to wet the powder with water; and (3) spatulating for 30 seconds.
    a. True
    b. False

31. Alginate impression materials are set completely when they lose their tackiness, and therefore waiting an extra 1 to 2 minutes before removal does not improve the tear strength.
    a. True
    b. False

32. Rapid removal of set alginate impressions decreases the chance of tearing the impression but does not increase its accuracy.
    a. True
    b. False

33. Large portions of set alginate unsupported by the tray should be cut away because its weight can distort the impression.
    a. True
    b. False

34. Rinsing the alginate impression is unnecessary because the powder contains disinfectants such as quaternary ammonium or chlorhexidine compounds.
    a. True
    b. False

35. Alginate gels are irreversible with respect to heat.
    a. True
    b. False

36. The advantages of an elastomeric impression compared with alginate are the following: (1) better dimensional stability on storage; (2) higher tear strengths; and (3) better surface detail transferred to dental stone models.
    a. True
    b. False

37. Addition silicone impression materials are noted for the following: (1) short–medium setting times; (2) high tear strengths; and (3) excellent recovery of deformation on removal.
    a. True
    b. False

38. Soft polyether impression materials are noted for (1) being very stiff when set; (2) having high tear strengths; and (3) having long setting times.
    a. True
    b. False

39. Addition silicone impression materials are noted for (1) their high accuracy and stability with time and (2) being available in auto-mixing systems.
    a. True
    b. False

40. If the instructions for an addition silicone material say you should wait an hour before pouring a stone model, pouring at 15 minutes will probably result in surface bubbles in the model from the release of hydrogen.
    a. True
    b. False

41. The easier the wetting of an elastomeric impression by a mix of dental stone, the greater chance of bubbles in the model.
    a. True
    b. False

42. Digital impressions can only produce restorations that are milled in the dental office.
    a. True
    b. False

43. Digital impressions offer a precise fit with fewer incidents of remakes but longer seating/adjustment time.
    a. True
    b. False

SUGGESTED SUPPLEMENTARY READINGS

Baumann MA: The influence of dental gloves on the setting of impression materials, *Br Dent J* 179:130, 1995.

Bunek SS, editor: Impression materials, *Dent Advis* 31(2):1, 2014.

Bunek SS, editor: Digital dentistry, *Dent Advis* 30(9):1, 2013.

Council on Dental Materials, Instruments and Equipment, Council on Dental Practice, and Council on Dental Therapeutics: Infection control recommendations for the dental office and the dental laboratory, *J Am Dent Assoc* 116:241, 1988.

Drennon DG, Johnson GH: The effect of immersion disinfection of elastomeric impressions on the surface detail and reproduction of improved gypsum casts, *J Prosthet Dent* 63:233, 1990.

Drennon DG, Johnson GH, Powell GL: The accuracy and efficacy of disinfection by spray atomization on elastomeric impressions, *J Prosthet Dent* 62:468, 1989.

Farah JW, Powers JM, editors: Alginate and alginate substitutes, *Dent Advis* 24(2):1, 2007.

Farah JW, Powers JM, editors: Impression and bite registration materials, *Dent Advis* 28(2):1, 2011.

Farah JW, Powers JM, editors: Digital impressions, *Dent Advis* 27(6):1, 2010.

Johnson GH, Drennon DG, Powell GL: Accuracy of elastomeric impression materials disinfected by immersion, *J Am Dent Assoc* 116:525, 1988.

Look JO, Clay DJ, Gong K, et al: Preliminary results from disinfection of irreversible hydrocolloid impressions, *J Prosthet Dent* 63:701, 1990.

evolve Please visit *http://evolve.elsevier.com/Powers/dentalmaterials* for additional practice and study support tools.

APPENDIX 8-1: AGAR HYDROCOLLOID IMPRESSION MATERIAL

Agar hydrocolloid was the first successful flexible aqueous impression material used in dentistry. The flexibility of the material at the time it is removed from the mouth allows impression of undercut areas and thus fully dentulous impressions of the entire arch. Although agar hydrocolloid is an excellent impression material and yields accurate impressions, alginate hydrocolloid and elastomeric impression materials have largely replaced it. The preference for alginates has been a result of the minimum equipment required in their clinical application, and the advantage of elastomeric impressions has been their greater dimensional stability and the improved quality of gypsum models.

Agar impression material is supplied as a gel in a collapsible tube or as a number of cylinders in a glass jar. The first form is used with a water-cooled impression tray and the second with a syringe. The syringe material may be used in combination with a tray material.

The gel of the tray material consists of 12% to 15% agar, 0.2% borax as a strength improver, 1% to 2% potassium sulfate to ensure proper setting of the gypsum model and die materials against the agar, 0.1% benzoates as preservatives, other additives to control the flow of the material when heated, the flavoring, and 80% to 85% water as the balance. The syringe materials have the same components but a lower concentration of agar (approximately 6% to 8%).

> **⚠ ALERT**
>
> A sol is a colloidal system in which the dispersed phase is solid and the continuous phase is liquid.

The agar gel is converted to a sol by heating in water, usually boiling, 100° C, and becomes a gel again by cooling to 43.3° C. Once the gel has been converted to a sol, it remains fluid for extended periods (all day) by being stored at 65.7° C. The gel has a liquefaction temperature different from its solidification temperature of the sol; this is termed hysteresis and has important clinical significance. Agar hydrocolloid impression material is called a reversible hydrocolloid because the transformation of the gel to the sol is reversible with respect to heat.

Agar impressions are highly accurate at the time of removal from the mouth but shrink when stored in air or 100% relative humidity and expand when stored in water as with alginate. The least dimensional change occurs when the impressions are stored in 100% humidity; however, prompt pouring of plaster or stone models is recommended.

More information on the properties and manipulation of agar hydrocolloids is presented in earlier editions of this textbook.

CONDENSATION SILICONE IMPRESSION MATERIALS

Condensation silicone impression materials are not used commonly in the dental office but rather are used as an accurate duplicating material in the dental laboratory. This impression material is supplied as a base and an accelerator (or catalyst). The base paste contains a moderately low-molecular-weight silicone liquid, called a dimethylsiloxane, which has reactive -OH groups. Reinforcing agents such as silica are added to give the proper consistency to the paste and stiffness to the set elastomer. The accelerator usually is supplied as a liquid but may be provided as a paste by the use of thickening agents. The accelerator consists of a tin organic ester suspension and an alkyl silicate such as ortho-ethyl silicate.

The multifunctional ethyl silicate produces a network or cross-linked structure that partly accounts for the low values of permanent deformation and flow. The ethyl alcohol produced as a by-product in the reaction gradually evaporates and contributes to the rather high shrinkage during the first 24 hours after setting. The setting reaction is sensitive to moisture and heat, with increases in either resulting in shorter setting and working times.

Manufacturers typically supply condensation silicones in a putty-wash (very low viscosity) combination. The putty-wash system increases the accuracy of the impressions because the putty has a lower dimensional change than the wash material. Also, the dimensional change of the putty affects accuracy little because it occurs before the final impression is taken, and the dimensional change of the thin layer of wash material is small. Now some products are supplied as a low-viscosity material in an auto-mixed cartridge system.

The qualitative ratings of the physical and mechanical properties of condensation silicones are presented in Table 8-4. The dimensional change during 24 hours after setting is relatively high. About 50% of the dimensional change occurs during the first hour after setting, and the remaining 50% occurs between 1 and 24 hours.

More information on the properties and manipulation of condensation silicones is presented in earlier editions of this textbook.

POLYSULFIDE IMPRESSION MATERIALS

The polysulfide impression materials (also called rubber base or mercaptan) are supplied as two pastes, with one tube labeled catalyst or accelerator and the other marked base. Three types are available and are classified as low, medium, and high viscosity. The low-viscosity class is used as a syringe material in combination with a tray material, and the medium material is used alone. The low-viscosity material also is used for denture impressions in combination with a custom-made tray.

The base material consists of about 80% low-molecular-weight organic polymer and contains reactive mercaptan groups (-SH) and 20% reinforcing agents, such as titanium dioxide, zinc sulfate, copper carbonate, or silica. The accelerator, or catalyst, tube contains a compound that causes the mercaptan groups to react to form a polysulfide elastomer. The catalyst is carried by an inert oil such as dibutyl or dioctyl phthalate. The most common catalyst is lead dioxide, with or without manganese dioxide; using it results in the paste being dark brown to dark gray. Another catalyst system is copper hydroxide, and when mixed with the white base paste a blue-green color results.

A qualitative ranking of physical and mechanical properties for polysulfide impression materials is given in Table 8-4. The permanent deformation values of 2% to 3% (elastic recovery of 97% to 98%) indicate that compression during removal of the impression material should be kept to a minimum.

Polysulfide impression materials shrink 0.3% to 0.4% during the first 24 hours, and thus models and dies should be prepared promptly. Studies indicate that accuracy is improved slightly if the models or dies are prepared 30 minutes after removal, but certainly no long delays should occur. Materials with a dimensional change of 0.4% or less have been clinically successful.

More information on the properties and manipulation of polysulfide impression materials is presented in earlier editions of this textbook.

RIGID IMPRESSION MATERIALS

Impression Compound

The principal application of impression compound is for a check impression to determine whether the cavity preparation contains undercuts that would cause problems in cast gold alloy restorations. Impression compound is composed of resins, waxes, organic acids, fillers, and coloring agents and is supplied as sticks or cones (Figure 8-16).

Impression compound is heated cautiously over a flame or in hot water until thoroughly softened and then pressed into the cavity preparation and held firmly until it cools thoroughly. A water spray of 16° to 18° C may be used to aid in the cooling. It is then removed and the impression checked for indications of fracture or deformation, which would indicate undesirable undercut areas in the cavity preparation.

Zinc Oxide–Eugenol

Elastomeric impression materials almost have eliminated the use of zinc oxide–eugenol impression pastes for edentulous impressions. It is supplied in two tubes: one contains zinc oxide, oils, and additives, and the other contains eugenol, oils, resin, and additives. Equal lengths of the two pastes are mixed with a spatula, and the material initially sets in 3 to 5 minutes with a final setting time of less than 10 minutes. The reacted

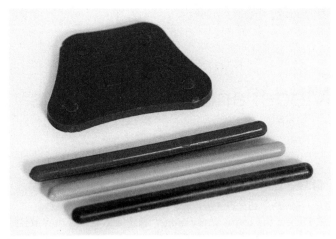

FIG 8-16 Examples of types of impression compounds.

material consists of a matrix of amorphous zinc eugenolate that holds the unreacted zinc oxide particles together. The dimensional change during setting is about 0.1%. The material is not strong and thus must be supported by an impression tray. No separating medium is needed before a stone model is poured, and after the stone has set it can be separated from the impression by immersion in hot water at 50° to 60° C for 5 to 10 minutes.

9

Model and Die Materials

OBJECTIVES

After reading this chapter, the student should be able to:

1. Define the terms *study model, cast,* and *die* as they relate to model and die materials.
2. Describe the physical properties important to model and die materials, and explain why they are important.
3. Compare the advantages and disadvantages of the different model and die materials in terms of abrasion resistance, ease of use, time and equipment required, and other relevant properties.
4. Describe the physical and chemical difference between model plaster, dental stone, and high-strength dental stone.
5. Describe the setting reaction of gypsum materials and the effect of excess water on the set mass.
6. Name accelerators and retarders that affect the gypsum setting reaction.
7. Define water–powder ratio, its values for the various types of gypsum, and its effect on the physical properties of gypsum materials.
8. Describe the differences between initial and final setting times and their chemical relevance, and explain how each can be determined.
9. Describe the factors that influence the ability of gypsum to reproduce detail in an impression.
10. Explain the concept of wetting and why it is important to gypsum materials.
11. Define the properties strength, hardness, abrasion resistance, and dimensional accuracy, and explain why they are important clinically to gypsum materials.
12. Describe the general procedure for measuring, mixing, and pouring an impression with a gypsum material.
13. Describe the various methods of spatulation of gypsum materials.
14. Give a specific method for disinfecting gypsum models, and state whether it is better to disinfect an impression or a model.
15. Describe the general setting reaction of epoxy model materials.
16. Describe the general manipulation properties of epoxy model materials.

In dentistry, replicas of the hard and soft tissues are used for diagnosis and treatment of oral disease. These replicas are called *study* models, casts, or dies. Each of these replicas has a specific purpose in dental practice. Study models are used to observe the patient's oral structures. For example, orthodontists use study models to evaluate the crowding of the teeth or progress in correction of that crowding. A cast is a working model. Casts of teeth are used to make orthodontic retainers, and casts of the remaining ridges in the edentulous patient are used to make dentures. Dies are highly accurate replicas of a single tooth and generally are used to make metal crowns or inlays.

Models, casts, and dies always are made from an impression of the soft and hard oral tissues. The accuracy of the model therefore depends on the accuracy of the impression, and any flaws present in the impression are reproduced in the model (see Chapter 8). However, the accuracy of a model also depends on the materials used to pour the impression. The ability of the material to flow into details of the impression and its expansion or contraction during setting are two properties that influence the accuracy of the model. The relationship between the impression and model can be confusing (see Figure 8-1 and Figure 9-1) because the impression is an inverse negative of the mouth. The right side of the impression becomes the left side of the model, and low points in the impression become high points in the model. Models and dies can also be prepared from digital impressions.

DESIRABLE QUALITIES AND TYPES OF PRODUCTS

> ! **ALERT**
>
> The desirable qualities of model materials depend on the dental application.

A number of qualities are required of materials to be used for making models, casts, or dies. These qualities are accuracy, dimensional stability, reproduction of fine detail, strength and resistance to abrasion, ease of adaptation to the impression, color, and safety, among others. To a large extent, the desired qualities depend on the application. For example, dentists do not require the same dimensional accuracy for a

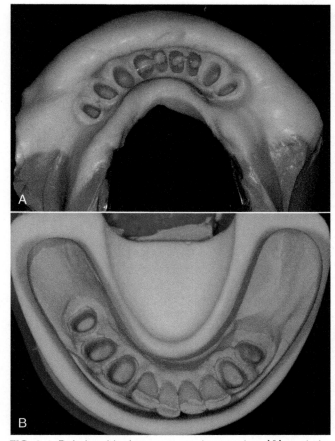

FIG 9-1 Relationship between an impression **(A)** and the replica of the patient's teeth **(B)** that came from pouring the impression. (Courtesy Y-W Chen, University of Washington Department of Restorative Dentistry, Seattle, WA.)

TABLE 9-1	Compatibility of Die Materials with Impression Materials	
Material	**Compatible with**
Gypsum products	Agar
	Alginate[†]
	Condensation silicones
	Addition silicones (PVS)[†]
	Polysulfides
	Polyethers[†]
Epoxy resin products	Condensation silicones (some require separator)*
	Addition silicones (PVS) (some require separator)*[†]
	Polyethers[†]
	Polysulfides (with separator)

*A separator is a material that is applied to the impression material before pouring with the die material. It prevents the die material from bonding or otherwise reacting with the impression material.
[†]Most commonly used impression materials.

TABLE 9-2	Comparison of Gypsum and Epoxy Materials	
Property	**Gypsum**	**Epoxy**
Abrasion resistance	Poor	Good
Ease of use	Easy	Moderately difficult
Time required	Minimal	Several hours
Equipment required	Minimal	Minimal
Harmful chemicals	None	Some (allergy)
Compatibility with impression materials	Excellent (see Table 9-1)	Limited (see Table 9-1)
Dimensional change	Slight expansion	Slight contraction
Accuracy	Good	Good

Modified from Sakaguchi RL, Powers JM, editors: *Craig's restorative dental materials,* ed 13, St Louis, 2012, Mosby.

study model as for a die. Because a die is used to make a precision crown or inlay, it must be dimensionally accurate.

Of the desirable properties mentioned previously, accuracy and dimensional stability are paramount because models, casts, and dies must reproduce an intraoral structure accurately and must remain the same size, or they are of little use to the dental team. Strength and abrasion resistance are necessary for applications such as dies, in which a wax pattern of the restoration is made on the die, and the die must not wear away, even though instruments rub against it. The color of the material may be important to provide contrast when pouring impressions. The most appropriate material varies with each application; the practitioner must therefore select the material with properties that are most desirable for the application at hand.

Two common materials are used to pour impressions: gypsum materials and epoxy materials. This chapter focuses primarily on the gypsum materials because they are by far the most common. However, epoxy materials are discussed briefly. Electroplated metal dies are used rarely and are not discussed. Information about these materials is presented in the seventh edition of this textbook. Not all materials can be poured into all impression materials. The problem of

model material–impression compatibility can be significant, but it is primarily a problem for the epoxy materials. As Table 9-1 shows, gypsum products can be poured into almost all impression materials used in practice today. Epoxy materials are compatible with most of the elastomeric impression materials, but they cannot be used with the alginates or agar impression materials.

Table 9-2 shows the major advantages and disadvantages of each model material. For most applications, the gypsum materials are easy to use with excellent impression material compatibility. However, they are abraded easily during manipulation. Epoxy materials have fair compatibility with impression materials and have good abrasion resistance, but most set slowly. When digital crown and bridge or orthodontic impressions are made, plastic models can be printed using stereolithography or 3-D printing. Thus, each type of material has advantages and disadvantages, and the proper material must be selected for each application.

GYPSUM PRODUCTS

Of all model materials, gypsum materials are the most common. Five types of gypsum products are available in dentistry: impression plaster, model plaster, dental stone, high-strength/low-expansion dental stone (also called die stone), and high-strength/high-expansion dental stone. Model plaster is used for study models that do not require abrasion resistance. Model plaster should not be confused with orthodontic plaster, which is a mixture of model plaster and dental stone. Impression plaster is used primarily to mount casts on an articulator. It differs from model plaster in that the setting time has been shortened to 3 to 5 minutes and the dimensional change on setting reduced to 0.06%. Dental stone (also called simply stone) is stronger and more resistant to abrasion than plaster and is used for casts that need abrasion resistance. Casts made of dental stone are durable enough to be used for forming mouth protectors. Dies require the highest abrasion resistance and strength and usually are made of high-strength dental stone.

Chemical and Physical Nature
Physical Form

> **! ALERT**
>
> The use of excess water in the gypsum mix increases setting time, reduces strength, reduces expansion, and reduces hardness of the set gypsum.

The physical forms of model plaster, dental stone, and high-strength dental stone are different, but they are made of the same chemical: calcium sulfate hemihydrate ($CaSO_4 \cdot \frac{1}{2} H_2O$). All of these forms are manufactured from the mineral gypsum, which is calcium sulfate dihydrate ($CaSO_4 \cdot 2H_2O$). The only difference between the model materials and gypsum is the amount of water in the crystal. During the manufacture of model materials, water is driven out of the dihydrate gypsum to form the hemihydrate. The differences between plaster, stone, and high-strength stone are the physical forms of the hemihydrate formed when the water is driven out, not its chemical makeup.

Plaster is produced by heating the gypsum (dihydrate) in an open kettle at about 115° C (Figure 9-2). The hemihydrate produced is a porous powder called β-calcium sulfate hemihydrate. This hemihydrate has relatively small, irregular crystals. Dental stone is produced by heating the gypsum under pressure in the presence of steam at 125° C. The hemihydrate produced under these conditions is called α-calcium sulfate hemihydrate (see Figure 9-2). This hydrate has larger, denser, more regular crystals than the β-calcium sulfate hemihydrate of plaster. Boiling gypsum in a 30% solution of calcium chloride produces high-strength dental stone. The hemihydrate crystals produced in this case are the least porous, most regular, and largest of all of the hemihydrates.

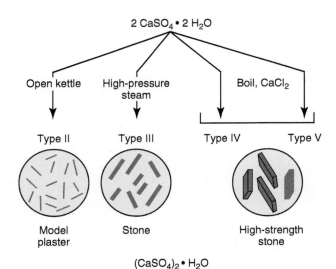

FIG 9-2 Manufacture of gypsum crystals. The size and density of the crystals depend on the conditions of heating of the dihydrate starting product. High-strength stone is composed of the largest, densest crystals, whereas model plaster has the smallest, most porous crystals. In general, larger, denser crystals require less excess water to wet them and form a mix with a consistency appropriate for manipulation.

Chemical Reaction and Excess Water

All forms of calcium sulfate hemihydrate react with water to form the dihydrate (gypsum) as shown in the following reaction:

$$CaSO_4 \cdot \frac{1}{2}H_2O + 1\frac{1}{2}H_2O \rightarrow CaSO_4 \cdot 2H_2O + heat$$
Hemihydrate · · · · · · · · · · · Dihydrate (gypsum)

Thus, model plaster, dental stone, and high-strength stone revert to the gypsum dihydrate when combined with water. It is this setting reaction that occurs when the model material sets into a hard mass. This reaction gives off heat and is therefore exothermic. Theoretically, if 100 g of any hemihydrate were combined with 19 mL of water, all of the hemihydrate would be converted to the dihydrate; that is, sufficient water would exist for all of the hemihydrate to react. However, in practice, this amount of water does not produce a mass that can be manipulated and poured into an impression. If mixed, this mass would be dry and crumbly. Therefore, in practice, excess water must be added when mixing to produce a workable mass that can be poured into an impression.

> **! ALERT**
>
> Plaster has the most excess water in the set mass; high-strength stone has the least.

Because of their different crystal sizes and porosity, the hemihydrates of plaster, stone, and high-strength stone require different amounts of excess water to produce a workable mass. High-strength stone, with its large, dense crystals, requires the least excess water. Dental stone requires somewhat more water, and plaster requires the most excess water. In general,

TABLE 9-3   Amount of Water Needed to Mix Gypsum Materials*

Gypsum	Mixing water (mL/100 g of powder)	Excess water[†] (mL/100 g of powder)
Model plaster	37–50	18–31
Dental stone	28–32	9–13
High-strength dental stone (Types IV, V)	19–24	0–5

*Recommended water–powder ratio varies with each product.
[†]Assumes required water is 19 mL/100 g of powder.

the larger and denser the crystal size of the hemihydrate, the less excess water is required to get a workable mass. With any of these materials, the excess water does not react but simply is trapped in the mass when it sets. Thus, plaster has the most excess water in the mass, and high-strength stone has the least (Table 9-3). The presence of excess water has significant consequences on the physical properties of gypsum, as discussed later. After the material sets completely, any excess water eventually evaporates and leaves voids in the mass. These voids reduce the overall density of the material. Therefore, set plaster has the lowest density (most porosity) because it had the most excess water and the most voids in the mass. Set high-strength dental stone has the highest density.

Accelerators and Retarders

The rate of the gypsum reaction can be altered by chemicals that the manufacturer adds to the hemihydrate powder. Accelerators are chemicals that increase the rate of setting, and retarders have the opposite effect. Some accelerators and retarders work by changing the solubility of the hemihydrate and dihydrate forms of the calcium sulfate. Accelerators make the dihydrate less soluble than the hemihydrate, so the reaction is moved toward the dihydrate because the dihydrate assumes its solid form rapidly. Potassium sulfate is an effective accelerator acting by this mechanism. A 2% water solution of potassium sulfate substituted for pure water reduces the setting time of model plaster from 10 minutes to 4 minutes. Retarders make the hemihydrate only slightly less soluble than the dihydrate. Therefore, the reaction proceeds more slowly toward the dihydrate. Borax, a chemical with the formula $Na_2B_4O_7 \cdot 10H_2O$, will extend the setting time of some gypsum products to several hours if added to the powder at a concentration of 2%.

Other chemicals act as accelerators or retarders by different mechanisms. Set gypsum particles (dihydrate) accelerate the reaction by acting as nucleation sites on which new dihydrate particles can form. These particles also are called terra alba, and concentrations of 0.5% to 1.0% added to the water are effective. A practical way of using terra alba is to use the slurry water (water containing particles of dihydrate) from the model trimmer to mix the gypsum. However, the user should be warned that the setting time using this method is extremely short. Colloidal particles, such as blood, saliva,

agar, or unset alginate, retard the setting reaction of gypsum. Colloids are fine particles of protein or other chemicals suspended in a liquid. These colloids bind to the hemihydrate and interfere with the addition of water to form the dihydrate. The result is a soft, easily abraded surface on the gypsum cast. To avoid this problem, impressions should be rinsed thoroughly in cold water to remove traces of blood and saliva before the impression is poured.

Water–Powder Ratio

The water–powder ratio for a material is defined as the amount of water in milliliters added to 100 g of powder. By convention, the water–powder ratio generally is expressed as a fraction, such as 45/100 or 0.45. This fraction means that 45 mL of water is added to 100 g of powder. For a given type of stone, the higher the water–powder ratio is, the soupier the consistency of the mix. Table 9-3 shows the water–powder ratios for model plaster, dental stone, and high-strength dental stone. Some variation occurs, depending on the manufacturer; therefore, ranges are given in the table. However, model plaster generally has the highest water–powder ratio, and high-strength stone will have the lowest. Because all model materials require about 19 mL of water for every 100 g of powder for the conversion of the hemihydrate to the dihydrate, any water over 19 mL is excess. This fact also is demonstrated in Table 9-3. Therefore, model plaster has the most excess water (18 to 31 mL). The excess water required for mixing is a function of the particle size of the hemihydrate as described previously.

> **! ALERT**
> The physical forms of model plaster, dental stone, and high-strength dental stone are different, but they are all made of calcium sulfate hemihydrate.

The water–powder ratio influences the physical properties of set gypsum materials. The use of excessive water lengthens the setting time and reduces the strength (Table 9-4). The reduced strength is a result of the excess water used in the mix that leaves voids on evaporation. Increased water also reduces the setting expansion of set gypsum materials. Although it is tempting to increase setting time by using more water, it is not advisable because the strength of the material will be reduced and the expansion of the material will not be

TABLE 9-4   Effect of Water–Powder Ratio on Setting Time and Compressive Strength of Model Plaster with Hand Spatulation

Water–powder ratio (mL/g)	Initial setting time (min)	1-Hour compressive strength (MPa)
0.45	8	12.5
0.50	11	11.0
0.55	14	9.0

Modified from Sakaguchi RL, Powers JM, editors: *Craig's restorative dental materials*, ed 13, St Louis, 2012, Mosby.

appropriate. Therefore, following the recommendations of the manufacturer is important in a decision regarding the water–powder ratio. Manufacturers offer different products with different setting times that have been adjusted by the use of accelerators or retarders.

Temperature and Humidity

The temperature of the water used for mixing and the temperature of the environment affect the setting reaction of gypsum materials. If the room temperature (20 to 25° C) is raised up to body temperature (37.5° C), the setting time decreases. The temperature of the mixing water has a similar effect. However, if the water temperature is raised above 37.5° C, the setting time will increase, because the dihydrate becomes more soluble in the water. In fact, the hemihydrate will not set at all as the mixing water reaches 100° C.

Gypsum materials are hygroscopic (absorb water from the air) to some extent. If model plaster, stone, or die stone is left in an open container for several days, it absorbs water from the air, and the surface of the particles will convert to the dihydrate. The net effect during mixing is an increased setting time because of the low solubility of the surface dihydrate. Although it would seem the dihydrate would act as an accelerator (as terra alba), experience shows that this is not true. To avoid changes in the rate of the setting reaction, gypsum materials should be kept in a closed container to protect them from humidity.

Hardening Solutions

Commercial solutions are available that, when mixed with gypsum materials in place of water, harden the gypsum and also increase its abrasion resistance. Increased hardness and abrasion resistance are especially important for die materials, in which extreme accuracy is needed to ensure the proper fit of crowns and inlays. These solutions are composed of water, 30% colloidal silica, and other chemical modifiers. The liquid–powder ratios of these solutions may be different from the water–powder ratios, because the modifiers reduce the amount of excess water needed to wet the hemihydrate particles and give a workable consistency to the mix. The amount of hardening obtained depends on the impression material that is used. Hardeners increase the hardness only 2% if silicone impression materials are used, but they increase hardness 110% for polyether materials.

Properties of Gypsum Materials
Setting Time

The total setting time for gypsum materials can be divided into the initial setting time and the final setting time. The initial setting time is the interval between the time the water and powder are mixed and the time that the mix can no longer be poured into a mold or impression. Therefore, the initial setting time is identical to the working time of the material. Clinically, the initial setting time can be observed when the freshly mixed material loses its gloss. Chemically, this loss of gloss occurs because the chemical reaction of the

hemihydrate uses up the water and the surface water is drawn into the bulk of the material. Gypsum should not be manipulated after the initial setting time because it is still weak and often fractures. The initial setting time should be within 8 to 16 minutes from the start of mixing according to American National Standards Institute–American Dental Association (ANSI-ADA) Specification No. 25 (ISO 6873 [2000]).

The final setting time is defined as the time at which the conversion of the hemihydrate to dihydrate is essentially complete. Clinically, this means that the gypsum then can be removed from its impression or otherwise manipulated without distortion or fracture. The final setting time is hard to discern clinically but can be detected roughly by the dissipation of the heat of reaction. Traditionally, the gypsum is allowed to set 45 to 60 minutes as an arbitrary time, although some die materials may reach final set in as little as 20 minutes. The final set is measured arbitrarily by the ability of a needle (Gilmore needle) to penetrate into the material. By definition, the material reaches final set when the Gilmore needle cannot penetrate into the set mass under a defined load.

Reproduction of Detail

> **! ALERT**
>
> Reproduction of detail of an impression depends on the compatibility and interactions between the model material and the impression material.

Gypsum materials must be able to reproduce fine details in impressions so that the gypsum models will be as accurate as possible. For high-strength die materials, reproduction of detail is especially critical because a precision casting will be fabricated on the gypsum die. As Figure 9-3 shows, the microscopic surface of gypsum is inherently porous. Therefore,

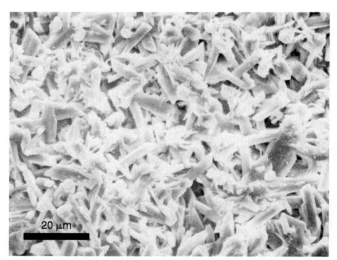

FIG 9-3 Scanning electron micrograph of the surface of set high-strength dental stone (die stone). The surface is porous with many interlocking crystals of calcium sulfate dihydrate. To the naked eye, this surface would appear smooth.

TABLE 9-5   Knoop Hardness and Surface Roughness of Gypsum and Epoxy Dies

Die material	Knoop hardness (kg/mm^2)	Surface roughness (μm)
Epoxy	25	0.05
High-strength stone without hardener	77	0.41
High-strength stone with hardener	79	0.28

Modified from Fan PL, Powers JM, Reid BC: Surface mechanical properties of stone, resin, and metal dies, *J Am Dent Assoc* 103:408, 1981.

TABLE 9-6   Relationship between Contact Angle of High-Strength Stone on Various Impression Materials and Number of Bubbles on Poured Cast

Materials	Contact angle of high-strength stone (degrees)	Number of bubbles on cast
Agar	40	—
Alginate	44	—
Polyether	49–51	9–28
Polysulfide	>67–77	39–43
Silicone (hydrophilic)	>50	—
Silicone (hydrophobic)	>92–98	56–69

Modified from Lorren RA, Salter DJ, Fairhurst CW: The contact angles of die stone on impression material, *J Prosthet Dent* 36:176, 1976.

the surface of a gypsum die is relatively rough compared with other types of model and die materials, such as epoxy materials (Table 9-5). This inherent roughness limits the ability of gypsum materials to capture the finest details of impressions, although from a practical standpoint the reproduction of detail is sufficient for most applications. Reproduction of detail is measured by pouring the gypsum material against a metal die with lines of decreasing depth scribed on it. The ability of the material to flow into and register finer and finer lines is used to rate its detail of reproduction. The use of hardening solutions reduces the porosity of die materials and thus increases their detail reproduction somewhat (see Table 9-5).

The type of impression material plays a big role in the detail reproduction of model and die materials. To capture the most detail, the die material must be chemically compatible with the impression, and it must also "wet" the impression material readily—that is, the die material must not "bead up" or resist flowing onto the impression material (see Chapter 2). Chemical compatibility is a function of how the material and the impression interact (or do not interact) chemically. Table 9-1 lists the compatibility of the major types of model and die materials. Wetting is a function of surface interactions of the model material with the impression. Gypsum is essentially a water-based material. Impression materials may also be water based, such as alginates or agar materials; or they may be nonwater-based, such as addition silicones or polyethers. When gypsum is poured against a water-based impression material such as alginate, good wetting occurs, and the detail of reproduction is good. However, when gypsum is poured against a nonwater-based material such as an addition silicone, the wetting may be reduced. The reduced wetting limits the ability of the gypsum to flow into all details of the impression and increases the risk of bubble formation in the gypsum. The effect is similar to that of a bead of water asked to flow onto a highly waxed car—the water cannot flow well. Improved wetting in this situation can be achieved by use of a surfactant (a special chemical that acts like a soap) either in the impression material or sprayed onto the impression material. Effective vibration of the stone can reduce the number of bubbles and improve reproduction of detail.

Wetting of impressions by gypsum or other materials is expressed quantitatively by the contact angle of the gypsum on the impression material (Table 9-6). The larger the contact angle, the worse the wetting is and the more difficult it will be to pour a bubble-free impression with good detail reproduction. Surfactants act by reducing the contact angle of the gypsum on the impression material. The reader is referred to Chapter 2 for further discussion about contact angle.

Strength

The strength of gypsum materials is indicative of the ability of the material to resist fracture. Compressive strengths of gypsum materials vary significantly by type. Plaster has the lowest compressive strength because it has the most excess water (see Tables 9-3 and 9-7). High-strength die stone, on the other hand, is almost four times as strong in compression because of the amount of excess water that is minimized. The compressive strength is one factor that contributes to the hardness and abrasion resistance of materials. The ADA specifications require that a material reach a minimum

TABLE 9-7   Strength and Dimensional Change of Gypsum Products

Gypsum	ADA Type*	Minimum 1-hour compressive strength (MPa)	Maximum setting expansion at 2 hours (%)
Model plaster	II	9	0.30
Dental stone	III	20	0.20
High-strength/ low-expansion dental stone	IV	35	0.15
High-strength/ high-expansion dental stone	V	35	0.30

*Note that Type I gypsum is reserved for impression gypsum, which is now used to mount casts on articulators.

compressive strength 1 hour after setting (ANSI-ADA Specification No. 25 [ISO 6873 (2000)], see Table 9-7).

Tensile strength is important for gypsum materials because it is a measure of the ability of the material to resist fracture during bending forces that occur during the removal of an impression from a model. Because gypsum materials are brittle, they will tend to fracture rather than bend if the tensile strength is insufficient. Although the tensile strengths of the different types of gypsum materials are significantly lower than their compressive strengths (2.3 MPa for plaster versus 40 MPa for its compressive strength), the high-strength stone and model stone have higher tensile strengths than model plaster.

When a model or die is wet, its compressive and tensile strength is approximately half that of its strength when dry (excess water evaporated). For this reason, many practitioners wait for models and dies to dry before they use them. However, accelerated drying at high temperatures in ovens is not recommended because it removes the water bound in the dihydrate and weakens the gypsum crystalline structure.

Hardness and Abrasion Resistance

The surface hardness and abrasion resistance of gypsum materials are important because the practitioner wants little or no loss of shape to occur on the model during its manipulation to study occlusion or fabricate a restoration. Both hardness and abrasion resistance are related to compressive strength, although these relationships are complex. As compressive strength increases, hardness and abrasion resistance increase. As with compressive strength, hardness and abrasion resistance increase when the gypsum material is in the dry condition. Hardening solutions also improve the abrasion resistance of gypsum materials because they increase compressive strength and reduce surface roughness. Gypsum materials are significantly harder than their epoxy counterparts, but this increased hardness does not necessarily translate into better abrasion resistance because epoxy materials are generally more abrasion resistant.

> **! ALERT**
>
> Compressive strength is an important factor in hardness and abrasion resistance of gypsum materials.

Dimensional Accuracy

Ideally, a model and die material should neither expand nor contract so that the size of the oral structure captured in the impression is reproduced accurately. However, gypsum materials expand slightly on setting. The amount of expansion depends on the type of gypsum material and a number of other factors. Model plaster generally expands the most, whereas die materials generally expand the least (see Table 9-7). The expansion means that models and dies will be slightly bigger than the size dictated by the impression. The expansion of gypsum in an impression is complex and is not uniform in every direction. Therefore, for a die, the

buccal–lingual expansion may not equal the vertical expansion. Setting expansion also is affected by the water–powder ratio; a high ratio (more water) causes less expansion. Manufacturers can use chemicals such as sodium chloride and potassium sulfate to alter setting expansion.

The addition of water to gypsum materials after the initial mixing can increase setting expansion. This type of expansion is called hygroscopic expansion. The water can be added in discrete amounts, or the mixed gypsum material can be submerged in water. Hygroscopic expansion can be significant; high-strength stone can increase from 0.05% expansion without added water to nearly 0.1% with added water. Hygroscopic expansion of gypsum is important in casting investment materials and when the gypsum is poured into a water-based impression material such as alginate or agar. In the latter case, the water in the impression can be taken up by the gypsum to increase expansion of the model or die.

Manipulation

The proper manipulation of gypsum materials is critical to their performance. Manipulation can be divided into several phases: the measurement and combination of powder and liquid, spatulation, pouring, and disinfection (Figure 9-4).

Measurement and Combination of Powder and Water

As discussed earlier, every gypsum material has a recommended water–powder ratio (see Table 9-3). The water–powder ratio affects the consistency of the mix, the strength of the material, and its expansion and setting time. Therefore, proportioning the water and powder correctly is critical. The amount of water is measured with use of a small graduated cylinder in milliliters, and the powder is measured on a scale by mass and not by volume. Many companies have apportioned the powder into single-mix packets that eliminate the need for the user to weigh the powder. However, many offices buy the powder in bulk to save money, so weighing the mass of the powder is recommended in this case. Experienced users often do not measure the powder and water but add powder to the water until the correct consistency is obtained. Although less accurate, this method is probably adequate for plaster and stone if the strength and dimensional change are not critical to the application. However, the proportions of powder and water are almost always measured for high-strength die stone because its physical properties are critical to the accuracy of the final restoration. Inexperienced users would be well advised to measure all materials until they become calibrated to the proper consistency of correctly mixed materials.

> **! ALERT**
>
> Accurate measurement of the powder and water is essential when using high-strength dental stone.

When the powder and water are added to the mixing bowl (see Figure 9-4), the water should be added first, then the

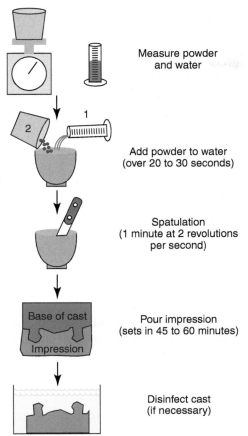

Measure powder and water

Add powder to water (over 20 to 30 seconds)

Spatulation (1 minute at 2 revolutions per second)

Base of cast

Impression

Pour impression (sets in 45 to 60 minutes)

Disinfect cast (if necessary)

FIG 9-4 Diagram of the steps involved in the proper manipulation of gypsum products. The mass of powder is weighed on a scale, and the volume of water is measured in a graduated cylinder. Experienced users often do not measure the powder and water. However, powder and water used for pouring dies always should be measured. The powder should be added to the water over a period of 20 to 30 seconds to allow air in the powder to escape. The mix should then be spatulated for about 1 minute at two revolutions per second. Alternatively, a power mixer can be used, and spatulation times will be shorter (15 to 20 seconds). The impression is then poured, and sufficient material is added above the impression to form a base. After 45 to 60 minutes of setting time, the impression is removed. At this point in time, the model may be disinfected if necessary.

powder sprinkled into the water slowly over a period of about 30 seconds. This technique allows any air entrapped in the powder to escape, which reduces the number of bubbles in the final mix. Even when a mechanical mixer with a vacuum is used, adding the powder to the water is advisable. Most beginning students have such anxiety about the material setting too quickly that they tend to add the powder all at once in their zeal to get the material mixed quickly. In reality, the reaction of the powder with the water will not occur to a great extent without spatulation, so these fears are largely unwarranted. The risks of bubbles in the mix far outweigh the risk of the material setting too quickly.

An easy-to-mix, fast-set specialty stone (HandiMix, Whip Mix Corp., Louisville, KY) is now available in unit-dose

packaging for custom trays, mouthguards, and study casts. An activator liquid (30 mL) is added to a jar of powder (120 g) and shaken by hand. Models are ready for separation in 10 minutes. This material is not recommended for crown and bridge master models.

Spatulation

> **! ALERT**
>
> Spatulation is mixing the powder and water together and is done mechanically or by hand.

The act of mixing the powder and water together is called spatulation. Spatulation of gypsum material is done either by hand or mechanically. Plaster materials typically are mixed by hand in a flexible rubber bowl (Figure 9-5). Stone may be mixed either mechanically or by hand, but high-strength die stone is almost always mechanically mixed.

When gypsum is mixed by hand, the mass of powder and water is stirred using a spatula at a rate of about two revolutions per second for about 1 minute. Many users of gypsum materials do not spatulate the gypsum adequately, and the physical properties such as strength suffer as a result. Inadequate spatulation often is caused by a fear that the material will set before pouring, although this fear is unfounded unless accelerators such as terra alba have been used in the mix. When mixing, the operator should scrape the sides of the bowl with the spatula to ensure that the water wets all of the powder.

When gypsum is mixed by a power mixer, the operator should stir slightly the powder and water together by hand for a few seconds to ensure that the mechanical mixer will work effectively (Figure 9-6). Mechanical mixers are power driven and are connected to a vacuum line during mixing, which reduces the air in the bowl and the number of bubbles in the mix. Power-driven mixers commonly are used to mix die materials and rotate at a high rate of speed. Thus, following the manufacturer's directions for time of mixing exactly is imperative because even a second more or less of mixing can alter significantly the physical properties of the gypsum or its setting time.

Regardless of the method used to mix the material, a vibrator almost always is used to help remove any bubbles that formed during mixing. Typically, the mix is vibrated for 10 to 15 seconds to force bubbles to the top of the mix. Vibration also is used to facilitate moving the gypsum into an impression or other container. Vibration effectively reduces the consistency of the material and allows it to flow.

Technique tips for mixing gypsum material are summarized in Box 9-1.

Pouring the Model

Several common methods exist for pouring a model or cast. In the first method, strips of soft wax called boxing wax are wrapped around the impression to form a mold for the gypsum (Figure 9-7). Generally, the wax is extended

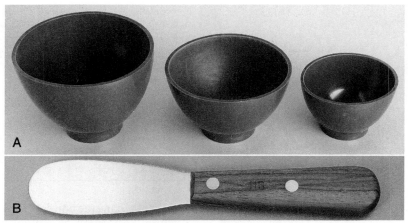

FIG 9-5 Flexible rubber mixing bowls **(A)** and metal spatula with a stiff blade **(B)** used for mixing gypsum by hand. (From Boyd LRB: *Dental instruments: a pocket guide,* ed 4, St Louis, 2012, Saunders.)

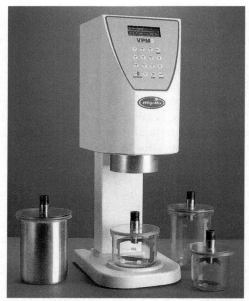

FIG 9-6 Programmable, power-driven vacuum mixing unit. The unit is designed for vacuum mixing all types of gypsums, plasters, and investments. Utilizing multiple stages, the VPM2 can be programmed for time, speed, and paddle direction. A twin-chamber, oil-less vacuum pump offers a powerful vacuum quickly, removes air, and reduces the risk of bubbles, providing a bubble-free mix. (Courtesy Whip Mix Corp, Louisville, KY.)

BOX 9-1 Technique Tips for Mixing Gypsum Materials

1. Disinfect the impression before pouring the model.
2. Use prepackaged gypsum products.
3. Measure the water in a graduated cylinder.
4. Add prepackaged powder to water to minimize bubbles.
5. Spatulate with a clean stiff spatula for 60 seconds until a smooth, uniform mix is achieved.
6. Use a laboratory vibrator once a uniform mix has been achieved to remove bubbles.

---

approximately 1 cm beyond the tissue side of the impression to provide a base for the model. In manipulation of the wax, care must be taken not to deform the impression material. The mixed gypsum then is placed into the impression in increments with a spatula, with the use of vibration to enhance the flow of the material into the impression. Care should be taken to allow the material to flow across the impression and avoid the entrapment of air that results in bubbles. Increments of gypsum are added until the mold is filled completely with gypsum. Alternatively, the teeth and soft tissues may be poured in stone or die stone and allowed to set, with a second pour of plaster or stone added to complete the base at a later time. The advantage of having the base in the softer plaster is that it is easier to trim it on a model grinder.

A second method for pouring a model begins by pouring the teeth and soft tissue surfaces in gypsum as already described. The filled impression then can be inverted and placed on a pile of freshly mixed gypsum placed on a nonabsorbent surface such as a glass slab. This pile will form the base. With this method, the consistency of the base material must be thick enough that the impression will not sink into the base. Most beginning students overmanipulate the inverted impression on the base, thereby causing a "vibration" of the impression into the base. Thus, manipulation of the inverted impression as little as possible once it is placed on the base is important. Before the base sets, shaping the base with a spatula is recommended to reduce the time required for model trimming once the model is set. The third method for pouring a model is similar to the second method but uses a container called a model former to form the base for the impression (Figure 9-8).

Regardless of the method used to pour the impression, the impression should not be removed from the gypsum for 45 to 60 minutes to allow the final set to occur. Early removal often fractures the model, which therefore requires a new impression. One indication that the final set has started occurs when the model becomes warm. The heat is a result of the

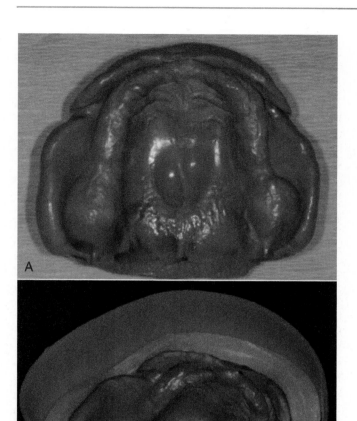

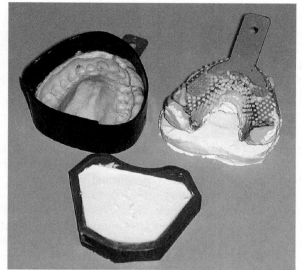

FIG 9-8 Pouring the cast by boxing can be done with a model former *(bottom)* or inversion on a patty base *(top right)*. A flexible rubber model former is used to contain a mix of gypsum and establish a base for a model. If the correct consistency of gypsum is mixed and the operator avoids too much manipulation and vibration, the freshly poured impression can be placed (inverted) on the model former without risk of the impression "sinking" into the base. Alternatively, the model former may be used after the material in the impression has set. (From Hatrick CD, Eakle WS, Bird WF: *Dental materials: clinical applications for dental assistants and dental hygienists,* ed 2, St Louis, 2011, Saunders.)

FIG 9-7 Impressions are sometimes "boxed" to facilitate pouring and construction of the model. Here, an impression of a maxillary edentulous arch **(A)** must be poured in gypsum to fabricate the master cast needed for denture construction. However, containing and supporting the gypsum is difficult. The cast is boxed using waxes **(B)**; this strategy makes pouring easier. The model will also be more accurate, and ultimately the fit of the denture will be improved. (Courtesy Y-W Chen, University of Washington Department of Restorative Dentistry, Seattle, WA.)

exothermic reaction as the hemihydrate converts to the dihydrate. Ensuring that the alginate does not dry out before it is poured is also important. Aside from distorting the impression, the quality of the gypsum poured into a dry impression is poor because the alginate robs the gypsum mix of some of its water. Furthermore, an alginate impression should be rinsed completely and disinfected before pouring. Any residual water in "low" places of the impression should be removed, or the gypsum will be weakened because of too much water. Finally, the edges of the alginate impression should not be allowed to dry out after it is poured with

gypsum because they become hard and inflexible, which increases the risk of fracturing the teeth when the impression is removed. The poured impression may be kept moist by storing it in a humid environment, such as a humidor or wet paper towel, after the initial set.

Technique tips for loading a tray with gypsum material are summarized in Box 9-2.

BOX 9-2   Technique Tips for Loading a Tray with Gypsum Material

1. Add a small amount of mixed gypsum material in one corner of the impression.
2. Place the impression gently on a vibrator to remove bubbles and then continue to add gypsum material.
3. Use a model former or use boxing wax to obtain the proper shape of the arch.
4. Add gypsum to the model former, and invert the filled impression and place in the gypsum base. Do not trap the tray in set gypsum.
5. Allow gypsum material to set for 60 minutes until cool, and dry before removing the model.
6. Separate the model from the impression.
7. Immediately clean the tray unless it is disposable.

Disinfection

Models, casts, and dies may be disinfected with a spray of iodophor used according to the manufacturer's instruction or by immersion in 1:10 dilution of a 5% sodium hypochlorite solution for 30 minutes. A disinfected model should be inspected closely for damage to its surfaces, because not all disinfectants are compatible with gypsum products. For models that require complete sterilization, a gypsum model can be sterilized in ethylene oxide. Autoclaves and chemiclaves cannot be used because they damage the model. In general, disinfecting the impression rather than the model is preferable because it is easier and prevents transfer of contaminated items into the dental laboratory.

EPOXY PRODUCTS

Dies of epoxy for use in fabrication of crowns, bridges, and inlays can be poured into polyether, polysulfide, or silicone elastomeric impression materials, although a separator must be used with polysulfide impressions to prevent the epoxy from bonding to the impression (see Table 9-1). Epoxy dies are tougher and more abrasion resistant than high-strength stone dies, but they are not as accurate or as stable dimensionally.

Epoxy die materials are two-component systems that include a resin and a hardener. This system is similar to systems used for epoxy glues sold commercially. The resin is a viscous material known as a monomer, and an example of a resin monomer molecule is shown here.

$$CH_2-CH-R-CH-CH_2$$

with epoxide (O) groups bridging CH_2-CH and $CH-CH_2$

The hardener is another chemical called a polyamine that causes the resin monomer molecules to link together into large networks of molecules. This linking process is called polymerization. As the polymerization occurs, the mix becomes thicker and thicker and gradually hardens completely. The setting reaction is generally slower, and it may take several hours for the polymerization to be complete. The hardener is toxic and allergenic and should not come into contact with the skin during manipulation of the unset material.

Epoxy die materials have a working time of about 15 minutes and set within 1 to 12 hours depending on the product. Although epoxy dies are not as hard as gypsum dies, they have superior compressive strength and abrasion resistance. Epoxy materials shrink 0.03% to 0.3% during setting, in contrast with gypsum materials that expand slightly on setting. The shrinkage of epoxy materials may continue up to 3 days after mixing. Because the epoxy materials are so viscous when poured, porosity can occur easily. One manufacturer minimizes porosity by centrifuging the impression after the epoxy has been poured. Another manufacturer supplies the epoxy in an auto-mixing system similar to addition silicone impression materials that minimizes porosity. Most epoxy dies should not be used until 16 hours after pouring, because they set slowly. However, newer fast-setting epoxy materials have been developed that are slightly flexible and allow chair-side fabrication of composite inlay and onlay restorations.

DIES FROM DIGITAL DATA

In the current era of computer-aided design (CAD)/computer-aided manufacturing (CAM) dentistry, dies can be prepared from digital impressions scanned directly from the mouth or scanned from an elastomeric impression. One type of die can be prepared by stereolithography or 3-D printing, in which a laser or UV light polymerizes the plastic die from a vat of monomer. Another type of die can be milled from a block of plastic. Both types of dies are highly accurate.

In some cases, a gypsum die is prepared from an elastomeric impression and is scanned by the dental laboratory or milling center for subsequent milling of the restoration. One company has introduced a scannable Type IV die stone (GC FUJIROCK EP OptiXscan, GC America, Alsip. IL).

❓ SELF-TEST QUESTIONS

In the following multiple-choice questions, one or more responses may be correct.

1. The amount of water that reacts chemically with 100 g of a dental gypsum product is which of the following?
   a. Dependent on the water–powder ratio of the product
   b. 50 mL
   c. 30 mL
   d. 19 mL
2. Excess water mixed with model plaster does which of the following?
   a. Wets the hemihydrate particles so that they can react
   b. Is bonded to the precipitated dihydrate crystals
   c. Is eventually lost by evaporation once the gypsum is set
   d. Improves the ease of mixing the powder particles
3. Which of the following statements is/are true with respect to gypsum products?
   a. The amount of excess water necessary to mix the hemihydrate powder depends on the size, shape, and porosity of the particles.
   b. Dental stone requires more excess water to mix than does model plaster.
   c. The set mass will be denser and stronger if the excess water for a particular product is increased.
   d. The rate of growth of the dihydrate crystals will be reduced if the hemihydrate crystals are mixed in more excess water than recommended.
4. Which of the following statements is/are true?
   a. The initial setting time characterizes the start of the chemical reaction of model plaster.
   b. The initial setting time of model plaster can be detected clinically by the phenomenon known as loss of gloss.
   c. Common practice allows the model plaster to harden for 45 to 60 minutes before removal of it from the impression.
   d. The setting time of gypsum can be altered easily by the operator with the use of accelerators or retarders.
5. Which of the following statements is/are true?
   a. The strength of gypsum materials is indirectly related to the density of the set mass.
   b. Because high-strength stone is mixed with the least amount of excess water, it is the strongest of the gypsum materials.
   c. The wet strength of gypsum is about twice the dry strength.
   d. The wet strength is a measure of strength of gypsum before all the water has reacted.
6. Which of the following statements is/are true?
   a. All gypsum materials show a measurable linear expansion during setting that results from the growth of calcium sulfate dihydrate crystals.
   b. Model plaster develops a maximum setting expansion of 0.3%.
   c. Dental stone develops a maximum setting expansion of 0.2%.
   d. High-strength, high-expansion stone develops a maximum setting expansion of 0.3%.
7. Increasing the water–powder ratio of high-strength stone would do which of the following?
   a. Lengthen the initial setting time
   b. Increase the 1-hour compressive strength
   c. Increase the setting expansion
   d. Increase the amount of excess water used to mix the material
8. Which of the following statements is/are true for manipulation of model plaster?
   a. The powder is added to the water in the mixing bowl.
   b. Spatulation can be described best as a whipping action.
   c. Hand mixing should be done in a rigid plastic bowl.
   d. The average time of hand spatulation is 1 minute.
9. Indicate which of the following are retarders and which are accelerators for the setting of model plaster, dental stone, or high-strength stone.
   a. 2% solution of K_2SO_4
   b. Slurry water from model trimmer
   c. $CaSO_4$ dihydrate crystals
   d. Saliva
   e. Agar
   f. Alginate
   g. Borax
10. Which of the following statements is/are true?
    a. It is common practice to pour the teeth of an impression in model plaster and the base in dental stone.
    b. In manipulation of boxing wax to form a mold around an impression, care must be taken not to deform the impression.
    c. To minimize the difficulty of removing the impression from the set gypsum, model plaster should not be allowed to extend over the impression tray.
    d. Before the model plaster sets, it is practical to shape and smooth the base with a spatula to reduce time at the model trimmer.
    e. An alginate impression poured with gypsum should be stored in an atmosphere of high relative humidity for short periods.
11. Which of the following statements is/are true?
    a. Epoxy dies are less resistant to abrasion than stone dies.
    b. Epoxy dies expand about 0.1% during hardening.
    c. Polysulfide impression materials require a separator with epoxy die materials.
    d. Epoxy dies are stronger than stone dies.

Use statements to answer the following questions.

12. An assistant pours an alginate impression with an epoxy material. What will you predict about the quality of the cast, and why?
13. An assistant pours an impression with white-colored stone thinking that it is model plaster. He finds that the material sets very rapidly. What may be wrong?
14. In error, a dentist mixes yellow dental stone with the water–powder ratio of plaster. How much water did the dentist add to 100 g of stone, and what are the likely effects on the physical properties of the set stone?
15. An office dental lab is very messy, and the plaster mixing bowl has old, set plaster in it. A hygienist in a hurry uses the dirty bowl to mix some model plaster. She finds that the setting time of the mix is very short. What may have happened?
16. A dental office buys high-strength die stone in bulk to save money. The container is left open to the air for weeks. On mixing some stone to pour an impression for a crown, the material is very slow to set. What is the likely cause?

17. An assistant fails to add surfactant to a silicone impression before pouring in high-strength die stone. What is a likely problem with the cast? Why?

18. A dentist uses a power mixer to mix high-strength dental stone. Instead of mixing for 15 seconds, the dentist does not time the mix and mixes 20 seconds in error. What is likely to happen?

19. A hygienist pours an impression in stone and makes the base simultaneously. Although the stone is mixed correctly in all regards, the inverted impression sinks into the base as the hygienist manipulates the base. What is the problem?

20. On removal of an alginate impression from its poured model, a dentist discovers several fractured teeth on the model. What are possible causes, assuming that the dentist used the correct removal technique?

In the following multiple-choice questions, one or more responses may be correct.

21. Which type of gypsum product has the most water added?
    a. Model plaster
    b. Dental stone
    c. High-strength stone
    d. All are equivalent.

22. If one gypsum model (A) has a compressive strength twice that of model B, which will have the higher surface hardness or abrasion resistance?
    a. A
    b. B
    c. They will be the same.

23. A loss of gloss at the surface of gypsum materials indicates which of the following?
    a. The final set of the material.
    b. The initial set of the material.
    c. It is not indicative of any physical property of the material.
    d. The material is ready to be disinfected.

24. Aside from disinfection, an impression material should be rinsed thoroughly before pouring for which of the following reasons?
    a. Colloids on the impression will make the gypsum weak.

b. The additional water on the surface of the impression will strengthen the gypsum.
    c. The water will cool the impression and give a faster set to the gypsum.
    d. None of the above

25. When mixing gypsum, add which of the following?
    a. The water to the powder
    b. Water and powder at the same time
    c. The powder to the water
    d. It makes no difference.

26. Increasing the water–powder ratio of a gypsum mix will cause the expansion of gypsum to do which of the following?
    a. Increase
    b. Decrease
    c. Have no effect

27. You are in a gypsum mine, and you take a shovelful of the material into a bucket. What do you have?
    a. Calcium chloride dihydrate
    b. Calcium sulfate dihydrate
    c. Calcium chloride hemihydrate
    d. Calcium sulfate hemihydrate

28. The setting reaction of a plaster material is characterized by which of the following?
    a. The release of heat (it is exothermic)
    b. The formation of titanium sulfate
    c. The formation of a hemihydrate crystal structure
    d. None of the above

29. If one adds too much water to a gypsum material when it is mixed, one gets a material that has which of the following?
    a. A shorter setting time
    b. A higher compressive strength
    c. A higher expansion
    d. A softer surface

30. The appropriate water–powder ratio for high-strength stone is which of the following?
    a. 50 mL/100 g
    b. 30 mL/100 g
    c. 24 mL/100 g
    d. 15 mL/100 g

SUGGESTED SUPPLEMENTARY READINGS

Anusavice KJ, editor: Gypsum products. In *Phillip's science of dental materials*, ed 11, Philadelphia, 2003, Saunders, p. 255.

Fan PL, Powers JM, Reid BC: Surface mechanical properties of stone, resin, and metal dies, *J Am Dent Assoc* 103:408, 1981.

Garber DK, Powers JM, Brandau HE: Effect of spatulation on properties of high-strength stones, *J Mich Dent Assoc* 67:133, 1985.

Sakaguchi RL, Powers, JM: Gypsum products and investments. In *Craig's restorative dental materials*, ed 13, St Louis, 2012, Mosby.

evolve Please visit *http://evolve.elsevier.com/Powers/dentalmaterials* for additional practice and study support tools.

Waxes

After reading this chapter, the student should be able to:

1. Describe the difference between pattern waxes and processing waxes.
2. Define the properties of melting range, excess residue, flow, thermal expansion, and residual stress as they apply to dental waxes, and cite the clinical relevance of these properties.
3. Describe the composition and use of inlay wax, casting wax, and baseplate wax. Explain the properties that make these waxes unique and clinically useful.
4. Describe the common properties of pattern waxes that are important clinically.
5. Describe the composition and important physical properties of the various processing waxes used in dentistry.

Waxes are used in many aspects of dentistry in the clinic and the laboratory. Although not used in the final dental restoration, waxes are often important in the fabrication and success of the final metal or ceramic restoration. The use of wax in dentistry dates back 200 years to the taking of impressions of the teeth with beeswax.

Dental waxes are always a mixture of various components. These components may be natural waxes from minerals, plants, or animals, or they may be synthetic waxes. Gums, fats, fatty acids, oils, and various resins also may be added to modify the properties. Dental waxes may have pigments for color. The mixing of components allows manufacturers to create a wide variety of properties useful to dentistry, but it also makes waxes complex.

Component waxes in dental waxes are usually organic molecules with high molecular weights as shown in the following structures:

$$CH_3\text{-}(CH_2)_{15\text{-}42}\text{-}CH_3 \quad \text{and}$$

$$CH_3\text{-}(CH_2)_{13}\text{-}CH_2\text{-}\overset{\displaystyle O}{\overset{\displaystyle \|}{C}}\text{-}O\text{-}CH_2\text{-}(CH_2)_{28}\text{-}CH_3$$

Organic molecules in waxes are composed primarily of long chains containing carbon, hydrogen, and oxygen. The top structure is a hydrocarbon (from paraffin), and the bottom structure is a high molecular weight ester. The parentheses in the structures indicate repeating units of carbon and hydrogen. The long chains allow waxes to be flexible at room temperature or sticky as solids or as liquids. Properties such as hardness, melting range, and flow depend on the amounts of the various waxes and the molecular structure of the organic molecules in the mixtures.

> **! ALERT**
>
> The lost-wax technique is a method of using a wax pattern to define a space within a stonelike material, which eliminates that pattern (hence the name "lost wax") and then casts the space into metal.

Waxes can be classified broadly as pattern waxes and processing waxes. Pattern waxes include casting waxes, baseplate wax, and inlay wax. They are used to fabricate a restoration using the lost-wax technique (Figure 10-1). Details of the lost-wax technique are described in Chapter 12. A model of an inlay pattern is shown in Figure 10-2. Processing waxes include boxing, beading, utility, and sticky wax. These waxes are used as auxiliary materials. For example, these waxes aid in the making of castings or impressions or during soldering. Self-cured and light-cured resins also have been used as pattern "waxes" or as "processing waxes."

With the increasing use of digital impressions, waxes are available that can be milled or printed.

IMPORTANT PROPERTIES OF WAXES

Because of their complex composition, waxes have properties unlike any other dental material. Some properties are especially important for pattern waxes used to fabricate dental restorations. American National Standards Institute–American Dental Association (ANSI-ADA) Specification No. 122 (ISO 15854) describes minimum requirements. However, the following descriptions of properties apply to all waxes and are useful in understanding properties of most waxes.

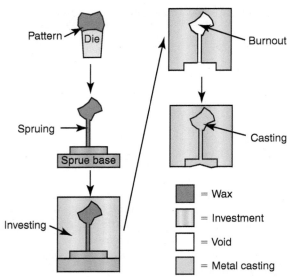

FIG 10-1 Lost-wax technique. A wax pattern of the restoration is made on a die with a pattern wax (usually inlay wax). A sprue, sprue base, and casting ring are added, and then the sprue and pattern are invested (filled) with a gypsum-based material. After the investment sets, the base of the sprue holder is removed, and the invested pattern and sprue are placed into an oven to burn out the wax (hence the name "lost wax"). Once the wax is burned out, a space remains where the sprue and wax pattern were. The molten metal is cast into this space.

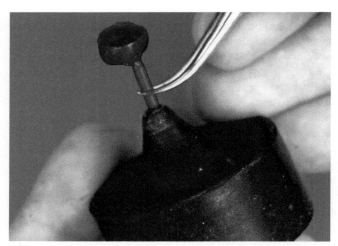

FIG 10-2 Wax pattern of a crown restoration attached to a sprue and ready for investing. The crown pattern is upside down to facilitate placement of the sprue and casting. (From Rosenstiel SF, Land MF, Fujimoto J: *Contemporary fixed prosthodontics,* ed 4, St Louis, 2006, Mosby.)

Melting Range

Because waxes are mixtures of different components, they do not melt at a single temperature and do not have a melting point. Rather, they have a melting range. At the low end of the range, some but not all of the components melt, which causes the wax, still solid, to flow much more (see the discussion of flow). As the temperature increases through the melting range, more of the components melt and the wax flows severely, and eventually all components become a liquid.

Excess Residue

Because wax patterns used in the lost-wax technique are melted or burned to remove them from the casting mold, the wax must not leave a residue, which would affect the quality of the final restoration (see Figure 10-1).

Flow

> **! ALERT**
>
> Flow is a change in shape or dimension in response to an applied force.

Flow is the change in shape under an applied force. It is caused by the slippage of the long-chained wax molecules over each other. Flow is highly dependent on temperature and time. At low temperatures, waxes hardly flow at all, but as the temperature approaches the melting range of the wax, the flow increases dramatically (Figure 10-3). For pattern waxes, flow is generally not desirable at room or mouth temperature, because it results in a permanent distortion of the wax pattern. For processing waxes, flow is a highly desirable property because these waxes need to be pliable at room temperature.

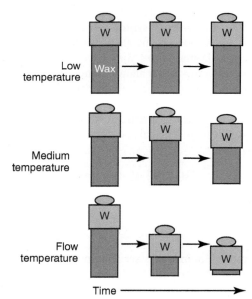

FIG 10-3 Flow of wax. Flow is a function of time and temperature. If a small weight, W, is placed on top of a cylindrical wax sample *(shaded area)*, no change in height occurs if the wax is at a low temperature relative to its flow temperature *(top row)*. As the temperature approaches the flow temperature, some change in dimension occurs over time, medium temperature *(second row)*. At the flow temperature, large changes in dimension occur, flow temperature *(bottom row)*. In all cases, the amount of flow is time dependent and usually is expressed as a percentage of the original height.

Thermal Expansion

When waxes are heated, they expand significantly. This expansion can be quantified as a percentage of the original dimension of the specimen. It usually is reported as parts per million of expansion per Celsius degree of the rise in temperature of the specimen (Figure 10-4). This number is called the "coefficient of thermal expansion of the wax," and the higher this coefficient is, the greater the expansion as the wax is heated. In general, waxes have the highest coefficients of thermal expansion of any dental material. For example, the coefficient of thermal expansion of a typical pattern wax is $323 \times 10^{-6}/°C$, but that of dental ceramic is 20 times less at about $14 \times 10^{-6}/°C$. For pattern waxes, the thermal expansion is critical. Small changes in temperature can cause a sufficient change in dimension to make the pattern inaccurate.

Residual Stress

Residual stress is stress remaining in a wax as a result of manipulation during heating, cooling, bending, carving, or other manipulation. Manipulation of wax puts molecules of the wax into positions that they do not like but cannot change because of their solid state. These stresses that are present in wax generally are released as the temperature of the wax increases, and the wax molecules can move more freely.

A pattern wax is used to create a model of a dental restoration that will be cast using the lost-wax technique.

The release of residual stress at higher temperatures causes an irreversible deformation that can destroy the fit of a wax pattern. For this reason, techniques that prevent the formation

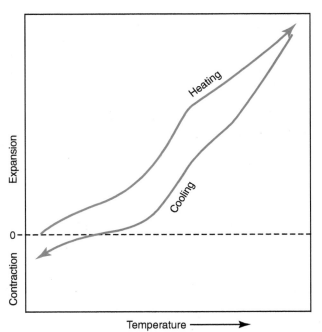

FIG 10-4 Thermal expansion of wax. As wax is heated, a significant expansion occurs but may not be linear with the increase in temperature. As the wax cools, contraction occurs but not reversibly. Thus, a wax pattern that goes through a heating-and-cooling cycle may have dimensions different from what it had originally.

of the stresses and keep those that have formed from being released have been developed in the manipulation of wax. To prevent residual stresses from forming, waxes should not be carved or burnished at temperatures well below their melting range. Wax patterns are carved with warm (37° C) instruments, and melted wax is added in small increments to prevent rapid or uneven cooling, which promotes residual stress. To prevent the release of stress already created, wax patterns should not be subjected to temperature changes or should not be stored at high temperatures. The time between finishing and investing the pattern (see Figure 10-1) should be minimized (less than 30 minutes) because longer storage times allow time for stresses to be released. If conditions of time or temperature of the storage of the pattern are suspect, details of the pattern such as proximal contacts and margins should be refinished.

PATTERN WAXES

As previously described, pattern waxes are used to create a model of a dental restoration such as a crown or partial denture that eventually is cast using the lost-wax technique.

Inlay Wax

Inlay waxes generally are used to fabricate wax patterns for crowns, inlays, or bridges. These waxes generally are available in round sticks (7.5 cm long and 6 mm in diameter) of several colors such as red, yellow, blue, and green. They are also available in various hardnesses for different casting applications. The hardness is controlled by adjustment of the components. The composition of inlay wax is complex, and it may contain five or six different waxes, such as paraffin, carnauba, ceresin, and beeswax. Paraffin and ceresin are mineral waxes, carnauba is a plant wax, and beeswax is an insect wax.

Casting Wax

These waxes are used to form the wax pattern of the metallic framework of removable partial dentures (Figure 10-5). They are available in sheets and in ready-made shapes, which are convenient for making the wax pattern of the partial denture. Little information is available about their composition, but casting waxes are believed to contain many of the same components as inlay waxes. Many casting waxes possess a slight tackiness to help hold them in position on the gypsum cast before investing and casting.

Baseplate Wax

Baseplate wax derives its name from its use on the baseplate of a denture. Baseplates (or record bases) are used to build the contours of a denture and hold the position of the denture teeth before the denture is processed in acrylic. Baseplate wax is pink or red, which provides some esthetic quality during the construction of a denture (Figure 10-6). It is available in sheets 7.5 cm wide, 15 cm long, and 0.13 cm thick.

Baseplate wax typically contains ceresin, beeswax, carnauba wax, and various synthetic waxes. Its composition can be altered to give various hardnesses. Three common

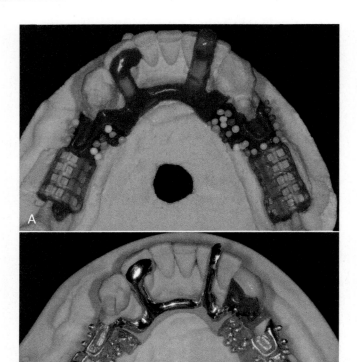

FIG 10-5 Casting waxes are commonly used to construct the wax patterns for partial denture frameworks **(A)**. The wax is applied to a refractory cast, and the framework is invested and cast **(B)** using the lost-wax technique. The size of the appliance makes achieving an accurate casting more complex than for smaller prostheses such as crowns. (Courtesy Y-W Chen, University of Washington Department of Restorative Dentistry, Seattle, WA.)

hardnesses of baseplate wax are available (ISO 15854, Table 10-1), each with separate flow requirements. Type I wax is soft at room temperature and is used for contouring dentures. Type II is a medium wax to be used for patterns that will be placed into the mouth in a temperate climate. Type III waxes are hardest and are for mouth use in tropical climates. The flow qualities as a function of temperature of Type III wax are similar to inlay wax. As with all waxes, residual stress can easily be incorporated and, if released, will move teeth and change the occlusion of the denture. When dentures are being fabricated, steps must be taken to limit this distortion (see the earlier discussion of residual stress).

Resins

Although different from waxes, resins have been used as patterns for dental restorations. Resins offer higher strength and lower flow than pattern waxes and burnout without residue. Chemically cured acrylic resins and light-cured composite resins are available. Light-cured resins offer more working time to build the pattern than self-cured resins. The curing can be accomplished in a "light oven" or with a handheld light unit.

Important Properties of Pattern Waxes

All pattern waxes and resins must possess low flow at their working temperature to prevent distortion of the wax pattern. The melting range of the wax also must be higher than the environment in which the pattern is made. This fact is especially important for so-called direct wax patterns, which are made directly in the mouth. On the other hand, too high of a melting range may make development of residual stresses a problem or may make working with the wax difficult. Finally, all pattern waxes and resins must burn out with no residue because the residue would interfere with the casting of the pattern (see Figure 10-1).

PROCESSING WAXES

Processing waxes are used in various auxiliary roles in the fabrication of models and impressions and in soldering. Several processing waxes deserve special comment because they are widely used.

Boxing and Utility Waxes

> **! ALERT**
>
> Processing waxes are used in auxiliary roles in the fabrication of models, impressions, and during soldering.

Boxing and utility waxes are soft, pliable waxes used primarily in taking and pouring impressions. The waxes are usually dark in color and have a slight tackiness, which allows them to be attached to each other or to stone models or impression trays. In orthodontics, waxes of this type may be white and are called periphery wax. They also can be melted easily to seal them to these surfaces. Their soft nature allows them to be adapted to impression materials that are easily distorted, such as alginate.

These waxes are made primarily from beeswax, paraffin, and other soft waxes. Boxing wax is supplied as long (40 cm) strips that are 4 to 5 cm wide and 0.1 cm thick. These strips are molded around an unpoured impression (see Figure 10-6) to help contain the stone when it is vibrated into the impression. Utility and periphery wax are long beads (40 cm or more) about 0.5 cm in diameter. These may be used in combination with boxing wax, as just described, during the pouring of impressions. Additionally, they are used around the periphery of an impression tray to reduce irritation of the tray on the soft tissues or to extend the tray before the impression is taken (see Figure 10-6).

Sticky Wax

Sticky wax is actually a somewhat misleading name for this wax because it is hard and brittle at room temperature. However, when heated, it is sticky and will adhere tenaciously to dry stone or other dental materials. It is used commonly to assemble metallic or resin pieces temporarily in position or to seal a plaster splint to a stone cast in the process of forming

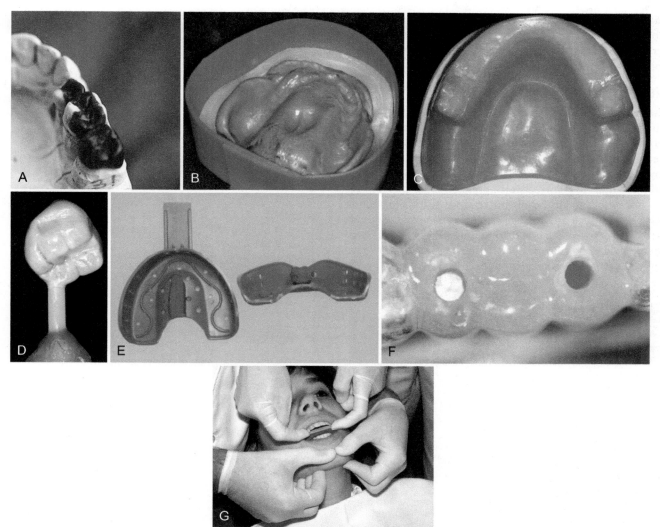

FIG 10-6 Applications of waxes in dentistry. **A,** Inlay pattern wax. **B,** Boxing wax. **C,** Baseplate. **D,** Casting wax. **E,** Utility wax. **F,** Sticky wax. **G,** Bite wax. (**A,** From Hatrick CD, Eakle WS, Bird WF: *Dental materials: clinical applications for dental assistants and dental hygienists,* ed 2, St Louis, 2011, Saunders; **B–D,** courtesy Y-W Chen, University of Washington Department of Restorative Dentistry, Seattle, WA; **E,** From Tsu Y-T: A technique of making impressions on patients with mandibular bony exostoses, *J Prosthet Dent* 93[4]:400, 2005; **F,** from Arfai NK, Kiat-Amnuay S: Radiographic and surgical guide for placement of multiple implants, *J Prosthet Dent* 97[5]:310, 2007; **G,** from Dawson PE: *Functional occlusion: from TMJ to smile design,* St Louis, 2007, Mosby.)

TABLE 10-1 Flow Requirements for Dental Baseplate Wax			
	FLOW (%)		
Wax	**23° C**	**37° C**	**45° C**
Type I	Max. 1.0	Min. 5.0; max. 90.0	Not applicable
Type II	Max. 0.6	Max. 10.0	Min. 50.0; max. 90.0
Type III	Max. 0.2	Max. 1.2	Min. 5.0; max. 50.0

Modified from International Organization for Standardization: ISO 15854: 2005. *Dentistry-casting and baseplate waxes,* Geneva, Switzerland, 2005, ISO.

porcelain facings (see Figure 10-6). Because it is brittle at room temperature, sticky wax will break rather than become distorted if the assembled pieces move. The pieces can then be rejoined in their proper relationship, rather than unknowingly used in a distorted relationship.

Corrective Impression Wax

Corrective impression wax is used as a wax veneer over an original impression to register the detail of soft tissues in a functional state (see Figure 10-6). Corrective waxes probably are formulated from hydrocarbon waxes such as paraffin and ceresin. Some may contain metallic particles. Most of these waxes also contain castor oil to provide adequate flow at mouth temperature. The flow of these waxes at mouth temperature (37.5° C) is 100%. Thus, they are distorted easily immediately after removal from the mouth.

Bite-Registration Wax

Bite-registration wax is used for accurate articulation of certain models of opposing arches. Specially formulated bite waxes are made from beeswax or paraffin or ceresin and oils. Some products contain aluminum or copper particles. The flow of these waxes at 37.5° C is from 2.5% to 22%, which indicates that, like corrective impression wax, these waxes are susceptible to distortion on removal from the mouth. Other waxes, such as 28-gauge casting or baseplate wax, also have been used as bite-registration materials. To a large extent, addition silicone and polyether materials have replaced waxes for bite registration.

QUICK REVIEW

Dental waxes are complex mixtures of natural and synthetic components, many of which are organic molecules. Although dental waxes are not used as the final restoration in dentistry, they are critical to the success of many dental restorations. Dental waxes are divided into pattern waxes, which are used to make a model of the final restoration, and processing waxes, which are used in auxiliary roles. The lost-wax technique is commonly used with pattern waxes to convert the wax pattern accurately into metal or ceramic. Waxes can also be milled or printed. The physical properties of waxes are diverse, but all waxes share the properties of having a melting range, the tendency to flow, the ability to harbor residual stresses, and the largest thermal expansion of any dental material. The proper manipulation of waxes is critical to ensure that these properties do not interfere with the success of the final dental restoration.

SELF-TEST QUESTIONS

In the following multiple-choice questions, one or more responses may be correct.

1. Which of the following is approximately the coefficient of thermal expansion of a dental inlay wax?
   a. $-50 \times 10^{-6}/°C$
   b. $20 \times 10^{-6}/°C$
   c. $80 \times 10^{-6}/°C$
   d. $200 \times 10^{-6}/°C$
2. Which of the following is/are true of residual stress?
   a. Is developed in wax when it is cooled under stress
   b. Results in a uniform dimensional change that can be compensated for in the casting process
   c. Can be minimized by the manipulation of a wax at a temperature as high as is practical
   d. Can cause warpage that increases at higher storage temperatures and during longer storage times
3. A pattern wax might be used to do which of the following?
   a. Make a corrective impression
   b. Form a mold around an impression
   c. Form the general size and contour of a restoration
4. Casting waxes possess useful properties, such as which of the following?
   a. Tackiness
   b. No residue other than carbon
   c. Minimum values of flow at mouth temperature
   d. Specified values of coefficient of thermal expansion
5. Which of the following statements is/are true?
   a. Boxing wax is used for forming a mold around an impression before a gypsum cast is poured.
   b. Utility wax must stick to itself.
   c. Sticky wax must have less than 0.2% residue on burnout.
   d. Utility wax is used to prevent sag and distortion of an alginate impression in a tray.
   e. Sticky wax is used to assemble metallic or resin pieces in a fixed temporary position and is brittle at room temperature.
6. Which of the following statements apply to bite-registration waxes?
   a. They are used to articulate models of opposing quadrants accurately.

b. Formulations are made from carnauba wax.
c. The flow of these waxes at 37° C is from 5% to 80%.
d. These waxes may distort when removed from the mouth.

Use short statements to answer the questions.

7. You are treating a patient on a hot day, and the office temperature is significantly higher than normal. You notice that when you use a wax bite record to mount casts on your articulator, the occlusal relationship is not correct. Which properties of wax were most likely responsible for this problem? What precautions could you take to prevent this problem?
8. A pattern wax is used to make a pattern for a crown on tooth number 30. The technician makes the pattern at the end of the day and plans to invest it for casting the next morning. Unknown to the technician, the heat fails in the laboratory overnight but returns to its original temperature by morning. Ultimately, the casting made from this wax pattern does not fit the die. Why did this problem occur? What properties of the wax used for the wax pattern are responsible? How could the technician have decreased the chances of this problem occurring?
9. In error, a denture is made with Type I baseplate wax rather than Type II. What is the likely result? If Type II wax were used, what would have happened?
10. You secure two gypsum casts together with sticky wax. On setting the casts on the counter just before mounting them on an articulator, a coworker bumps the casts, and the sticky wax fractures. Why should you be glad that you used sticky wax?
11. Describe the techniques that can be used to limit the problem of residual-stress incorporation in wax.

Use short answers to fill in the following blanks.

12. Sticky wax is _____ at room temperature.
13. Bite-registration waxes have been replaced clinically by _____ bite-registration materials.

For the following statements, select true or false.

14. The flow of a dental wax increases as the temperature increases.
    a. True
    b. False

15. As wax is heated, a significant expansion occurs, but on cooling, contraction occurs reversibly.
    a. True
    b. False

16. Warm temperatures and long storage times increase the possibility of release of residual stress in wax patterns.
    a. True
    b. False

17. The release of residual stresses in a wax pattern will result in distortion of the wax pattern.
    a. True
    b. False

18. During burnout of a wax pattern, it is essential that the wax decompose and leave no residue.
    a. True
    b. False

19. If a wax pattern cannot be invested promptly, readapt the margins before investing the pattern.
    a. True
    b. False

20. Residual stresses in a wax pattern can be minimized by manipulating the wax at temperatures below room temperature.
    a. True
    b. False

SUGGESTED SUPPLEMENTARY READINGS

Craig RG, Eick JD, Peyton FA: Properties of natural waxes used in dentistry, *J Dent Res* 44:1308, 1965.

Craig RG, Eick JD, Peyton FA: Strength properties of waxes at various temperatures and their practical applications, *J Dent Res* 46:300, 1967.

Craig RG, Powers JM, Peyton FA: Differential thermal analysis of commercial and dental waxes, *J Dent Res* 46:1090, 1967.

Craig RG, Powers JM, Peyton FA: Thermogravimetric analysis of waxes, *J Dent Res* 50:450, 1971.

Powers JM, Craig RG: Penetration of commercial and dental waxes, *J Dent Res* 53:402, 1974.

Powers JM, Craig RG: Thermal analysis of dental impression waxes, *J Dent Res* 57:37, 1978.

evolve   Please visit *http://evolve.elsevier.com/Powers/dentalmaterials* for additional practice and study support tools.

11

Casting Alloys, Wrought Alloys, and Solders

OBJECTIVES

After reading this chapter, the student should be able to:

1. Describe how dental casting alloys are categorized by the American Dental Association (ADA), and explain the extent to which this classification is important to clinical performance and patient safety.
2. Describe the general composition and properties of high-noble, noble, and base-metal casting alloys.
3. Describe the properties of alloys that affect ceramic–alloy bonding and the clinical consequences of poor ceramic–alloy bonding.
4. Define wrought alloys, and describe how they are used in dentistry and how they differ from cast alloys.
5. Explain how solders are used in dentistry, and list properties important to their successful use.
6. Explain what properties of alloys are most important to alloy biocompatibility.

Alloys have been used in dentistry for thousands of years to replace natural tooth structure. The earliest restorations used pure gold because it was easy to purify, melt, and manipulate. Gold in foil form probably was used first as a dental restorative material several thousand years ago. Gold foil is unique because it can weld to itself under hand pressure into a solid mass at mouth temperature (Figure 11-1). This restorative strategy is still used but is not common in clinical practice. Other pure metals such as platinum also are used in dentistry, but pure metals, including gold and platinum, generally lack appropriate properties to be used for large dental restorations. For this reason, metals and nonmetals are mixed together to form alloys to restore damaged teeth.

> **! ALERT**
>
> Alloys are mixtures of metallic or nonmetallic elements; alloys have better properties for dental restorations than any single element.

Alloys have physical and chemical properties more appropriate to dental applications than pure metals. Some alloys are formed into restorations by casting. A wax model of the restoration is made, and an alloy is melted and cast into the shape of the wax (Chapters 10 and 12). Thus, these alloys are referred to as dental casting alloys, and the restorations made from these alloys are castings. For anterior or posterior restorations, ceramic can be bonded over the alloy to provide an esthetic result. Alloys used for this purpose are called ceramic-bonding alloys or ceramic-fused-to-metal alloys. Other alloys are first cast but are then shaped by mechanical force (e.g., machining) into their final forms. These alloys are referred to as wrought alloys and include wires, files, and dental implants. Still other alloys are used to join alloys together. These types of alloys are solders, and they must be melted without distorting the alloys they join. Finally, alloy composites are formed by sintering (Chapter 14) and are used as metal substructures for ceramic–alloy restorations.

Alloys play critical roles in dentistry (Figure 11-2). Some alloys are used for inlays, onlays, crowns, or fixed and removable partial dentures. Orthodontic wires have special bending properties that permit controlled application of forces to teeth and bone. Endodontic files used to shape root canals are made from stainless steel or titanium-based alloys. Endosseous dental implants are made from titanium-based alloys (Chapter 15). This chapter introduces several principles about dental alloys and solders and surveys the composition, physical properties, and biologic properties of alloys that are most important to clinical success in dentistry. Casting and soldering are discussed in Chapter 12.

The manipulation of alloys is generally not the purview of the dental auxiliary. However, a basic knowledge of these important materials is critical to appropriate clinical care, communication with patients, coordination with laboratory personnel, and appropriate financial considerations, particularly insurance coverage and claims.

FUNDAMENTAL CONCEPTS ABOUT METALS AND ALLOYS

Noble Metals, Base Metals, and Nonmetals

Metals are elements that tend to react by donating electrons to other elements. Nearly two-thirds of the periodic table of the

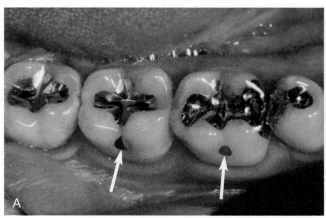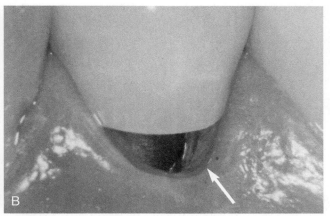

FIG 11-1 A and B, Gold foil restorations *(arrows)*. The foil, which is gold in nearly pure form, is placed piece by piece into the restoration. If uncontaminated, the pieces weld together into a single mass under hand pressure at mouth temperature. In previous times, this technique was used to restore tooth lesions of significant size, but today its use is restricted to small pit lesions, usually in the posterior teeth. The gold foil technique is technically demanding, but quality restorations last for decades. (Courtesy Richard D. Tucker, University of Washington Department of Restorative Dentistry, Seattle, WA.)

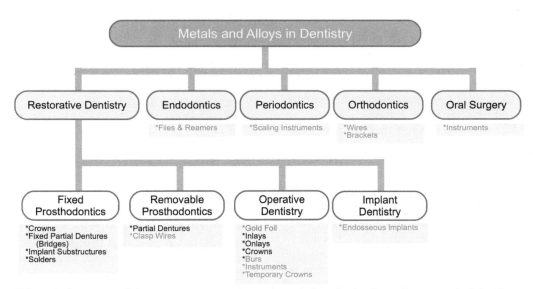

FIG 11-2 Summary of the common uses of metals and alloys in dentistry. Pure metals *(blue)* have limited use in dental restorations but commonly are combined with other metals or nonmetals to form alloys. Alloys have diverse uses in nearly all dimensions of dentistry, including solders, wires, instruments, crowns, bridges, implants, and removable partial dentures. The alloy end product may be formed by mechanical force *(wrought alloys, shown in red text)* or by casting *(casting alloys, shown in black text)*.

elements is composed of metals. Most elements used in dental alloys or solders are metals, but nonmetals also play important roles. For example, carbon is sometimes added to alloys in small amounts (<1 wt%) to strengthen the alloy significantly (e.g., "carbon-steel").

> **! ALERT**
>
> Noble metals such as gold, platinum, and palladium resist corrosion, even under the harsh, corrosive conditions of the oral cavity. Metals that are not noble are called base metals.

In dentistry, metals are subdivided into two major groups: noble metals and base metals (Figure 11-3). **Noble metals** are defined by their resistance to corrosion even under extreme conditions that occur in the oral cavity. There are seven noble metals in the periodic table, but only three are common in dental casting alloys: gold (periodic table symbol Au), palladium (Pd), and platinum (Pt). Some metallurgists also consider silver (Ag) a noble metal, but because of its tendency to corrode in the oral environment, silver is not considered a noble metal in dentistry. Noble metals are expensive simply because they are rare. For this reason, noble metals

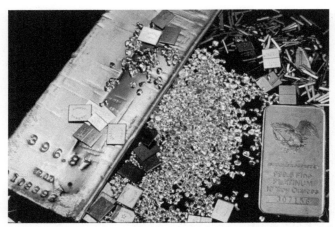

FIG 11-3 Gold *(left)*, palladium *(middle)*, and platinum *(right)* are three noble elements commonly used in dental alloys. Gold and platinum also have been used in pure form in dentistry. These three metals are classified as noble because they show little tendency to corrode in the oral environment. The larger number stamped on the gold indicates the mass in grams.

are traded as precious metals in commodities markets. However, the term *precious* should not be used to describe dental metals or alloys as this term indicates only costs on the commodities market. Furthermore, there are precious metals that are not noble. The term *noble* is preferred because it describes an important physical property of the metal or alloy.

In dentistry, base metals are metals that are not noble metals. In dental casting alloys, common base metals are titanium (Ti), nickel (Ni), copper (Cu), silver (Ag), cobalt (Co), and zinc (Zn). Base metals often are mistakenly viewed as being "bad" metals. In fact, base metals are *required* in alloys to ensure the strength, flexibility, and wear resistance that is necessary for dental restorations. However, in pure form, base metals have a greater tendency to corrode in the oral environment than noble metals. For this reason, pure base metals are almost never used for dental restorations. One exception is titanium, which is used in nearly pure form for endosseous implants (Chapter 15).

Elements in Dental Alloys

It is beyond the scope of this book to describe the 25 or more elements that are used in dental alloys. However, several of the most common elements are described in more detail here. *Gold* is a noble element that is perhaps the best known of the dental metals (Figure 11-3). Historically, gold played a bigger role than it does today, but it is still a common component of many dental alloys. Gold is used because of its excellent resistance to corrosion, good malleability (ability to be mechanically formed), yellow color, and relatively low melting point (1064° C) for casting. Gold may make an alloy appear yellow, but color is not reliable for identifying gold-containing alloys (see later discussion).

Palladium is a second common noble element component of dental casting alloys (see Figure 11-3). Its corrosion

resistance is excellent, but it has a much higher melting point (1554° C) and is much harder than gold. Thus, palladium is not practical to use in pure form but often is mixed with gold-based alloys to increase their hardness or increase their melting temperature, for example, when ceramics are to be fired onto the alloy substructure of a restoration. Palladium also whitens the color of gold-based alloys. For example, an alloy may have 90% gold and only 10% palladium (by weight), but its color will be white, not yellow. *Platinum* is the third common noble element in dental casting alloys (see Figure 11-3). Platinum has a high melting point (1772° C) and is even harder than palladium. However, platinum is used less in dental alloys because it does not mix as freely with gold as palladium does to form alloys, and it is the most expensive of the three noble metals.

Copper, silver, and zinc are common base metals used in dental casting alloys. Copper is reddish and its addition significantly hardens gold- or palladium-based alloys through a phenomenon called solid-solution hardening. Silver also is used to harden alloys this way. Zinc is a low-melting element (420° C) used to prevent oxidation of the alloy during the casting process; zinc has been used as a hardener for gold-platinum alloys.

Nickel, cobalt, titanium, iron, and indium are other base metals used in dental alloys. These elements may occur in trace amounts to elicit specific properties or may serve as the major element in the alloy. For example, iron is added in trace amounts to enhance the bonding of ceramic to gold-based alloys, or indium may be added to encourage a small grain size. On the other hand, alloys with nickel or cobalt as the most common component are increasingly common because of the low cost of these elements. Alloys of titanium are commonly used as endosseous implants (Chapter 15).

Crystal Structure and Grains of Alloys

Dental alloys have a crystal structure like ice, salt, sugar, or many other solids. For example, when water freezes, microscopic crystals of ice first form in the water then grow slowly in size until the crystals run into one another and all of the water is frozen. There is a period in the freezing process when ice and liquid water coexist. Alloys behave much the same way. When a molten (liquid) alloy freezes after casting, crystals form and grow as the alloy cools. These crystals, or grains as they are called in metallurgy, can be seen clearly under a microscope (Figure 11-4). Each grain consists of a crystal lattice of metal atoms. The boundaries where individual crystals meet are called grain boundaries. The size of the grains is important; a small grain size is generally more desirable in an alloy because it ensures uniform properties of the alloy. Elements called grain refiners often are added to gold-based alloys to reduce the grain size (e.g., iridium or ruthenium). The grain structure of many alloys is far more complex than shown in Figure 11-4 and is highly dependent on the composition of the alloy. Alloys that are predominantly base metals such as nickel generally have larger grain sizes, and grain refiners cannot be used.

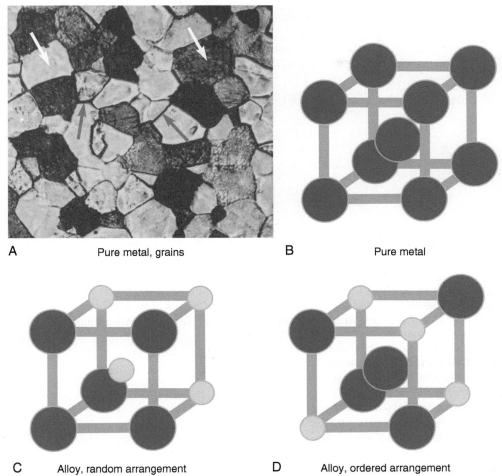

A   Pure metal, grains

B   Pure metal

C   Alloy, random arrangement

D   Alloy, ordered arrangement

FIG 11-4 Grain and crystal structure of alloys. At the level of the light microscope **(A)**, each crystal in an alloy or pure metal is visible as a grain *(white arrows)*. Each grain has different shades because it is oriented differently with respect to incident light. Grains meet and form grain boundaries *(red arrows)*, which are often subject to corrosive attack in the oral environment. Grain size (each grain is about 10 μm across here) is important to alloy performance. At the atomic level, the metal atoms in a pure metal have a specific crystal orientation **(B,** *body-centered cubic shown here).* The different elements in alloys *(denoted by blue or yellow circles)* coexist in crystalline arrays; the ability of elements to coexist depends on their relative sizes and electron configurations. The elements in an alloy may occupy random positions in the crystal lattice **(C)** or be relatively ordered **(D).** The nature of these crystals plays a major role in the electrical, optical, and mechanical properties of alloys. For example, gold-copper alloys with an ordered crystal structure have higher strength and hardness than those with a random crystal structure. Alloys may contain as many as 10 different elements.

The grain structure of an alloy is significantly altered by mechanical forces. For example, if the alloy is rolled into a sheet or drawn into a wire or machined by a cutting instrument, the grains are disrupted. This type of alloy is called a wrought alloy, and the grain structure takes on a fibrous appearance (Figure 11-5). Heating an alloy after casting or mechanical work changes its grain structure. These changes may lead to significant changes in properties of the alloys and clinical problems. For example, if the spring-like qualities of an orthodontic wire rely on a fibrous grain structure, then overheating the alloy and altering the fibrous structure will cause the spring to be weakened. Thus, operations in dentistry that involve heating, such as the application of ceramic or

soldering, must be done with consideration for how the grain structure of the alloy may change.

Other important changes in alloy crystal structure are not visible, even under a microscope. In some dental alloys, how the atoms occupy the crystal lattice of the alloy is exceedingly important. For example, for an alloy of gold and copper, the alloy will be considerably stronger if the copper atoms occupy regularly occurring positions in the crystal lattice (called an ordered crystal structure; see Figure 11-4). The copper atoms can be induced to change lattice positions depending on how the alloy is cast (or reheated) and cooled. Thus, for gold-based alloys with appropriate amounts of copper, heating (to within 100° C of the molten form) and cooling slowly actually may

FIG 11-5 Fibrous grain structure of wrought alloys under the light microscope. If a cast alloy is mechanically worked, it is referred to as a wrought alloy, and its grain structure is altered by breaking up the cast grains (see Figure 11-4, *A*) into a fibrous form seen here. Alloys with a fibrous grain structure are generally stronger and more brittle than their cast counterparts. Fibrous grain structures are common in wires used for orthodontics or in wires for clasps on removable partial dentures. The scale of the figure is approximately 500 µm across.

be used to improve the properties of the alloy. Changes in the order of the atoms in the crystal lattice are invisible to the eye and even invisible in an electron microscope (they must be detected by x-ray diffraction). Not all alloys exhibit ordered-structure hardening. For example, with base-metal alloys, heating and cooling cycles generally deteriorate the

properties of the alloy. Labs use ordered crystal structures to harden some alloys to a clinical advantage.

Important Physical and Mechanical Properties of Alloys

Dental alloys have several properties important to their laboratory and clinical performance. These properties—which include color, melting range, density, modulus strength, and hardness—are discussed in the following paragraphs (Table 11-1).

Color is often used to describe an alloy, and it is often important to patients. Typically, alloys will have yellow or silver hues (the latter often called "white" by metallurgists). Many dental personnel and patients assume that yellow alloys have a high content of gold and white alloys do not. However, the color of an alloy is not a good predictor of its composition or other properties. Yellow and white alloys may contain gold or not; it is impossible to tell from the color. This reality is often confusing for patients; the patient will equate yellow alloys with gold, and white with less expensive ("cheap") content. The dental auxiliary can help resolve confusion for the patient.

> **! ALERT**
>
> The color of an alloy is not a useful predictor of its composition, physical properties, or biocompatibility. Yet it may be important to the patient.

Unlike pure compounds like sugar, alloys do not melt at a single temperature but have a melting range; the melting range reflects to some degree the melting points of the constituents of the alloy. If an alloy has a melting range of

TABLE 11-1	Clinically Important Properties of Alloys	
Property (units)	**Description**	**Clinical importance**
Color	White (silver) to yellow hues	—Has little significance other than personal preference; not predictable for cost or performance
Melting range (°C)	Range of temperatures over which alloy goes from solid to liquid; first melting occurs at the solidus; all liquid occurs at the liquidus	—Soldering (alloy melting range must be higher than melting range of solder) —Application of ceramic (alloy melting range must be higher than ceramic sintering temperature) —Ease of casting (higher ranges are more difficult to cast)
Density (g/cm³)	Mass of alloy per volume of alloy	—Ease of casting (alloys with higher densities are easier to cast) —Cost of purchasing alloy (restorations containing alloys with higher densities are more expensive per restoration)
Modulus (GPa)	Stiffness or flexibility of the alloy	—High moduli (stiff) are important for restorations in which flexure causes failure —Low moduli (flexible) are important for ortho wires and partial denture clasps, in which flexure is needed
Strength (MPa)	Force required to break alloy (usually in tension, by pulling)	—High strength needed to avoid distortion or fracture of restorations, instruments
Hardness (kg/mm²)	Resistance to indentation	—Hardness of restorations to resist scratching (harder is better) —Hardness of restoration for cutting or adjustment (softer is easier) —Ease of polishing (softer is easier) —Wear of opposing teeth (if hardness of restoration is higher than enamel)

950° to 1000° C and the alloy is heated gradually from room temperature, the first sign of liquid formation will be at 950° C. At 975° C, some of the alloy will be liquid, but some will still be solid. Once the temperature reaches 1000° C, all of the alloy will be liquid. When the alloy is cooled again, the reverse process will occur. The temperature at which all of the alloy melts on heating (1000° C in the example) is called the *liquidus,* and the temperature at which all of the alloy freezes on cooling (950° C in the example) is called the *solidus.* The liquidus and solidus of an alloy are important to the casting and soldering of the alloy. An alloy must be heated above the liquidus to be cast. The liquidus also determines the burnout temperatures and which investments are necessary for casting (Chapter 12). The solidus is important to soldering because if the soldering operation heats the alloy above its solidus, then the alloy loses shape, and the soldering procedure is a failure. The solidus is also important for ceramic-bonding alloys, which must be heated to high temperatures to fire the ceramic onto the alloy. The ceramic must sinter and bond to the alloy at a temperature below the solidus ($\leq 50°$ C is needed, Chapter 14).

❗ ALERT

Alloys melt over a range of temperatures versus a single temperature. Melting begins at the solidus temperature and is complete at the liquidus temperature.

By definition, the **density** of an alloy is the mass in grams that occupies a volume of 1 cubic centimeter (g/cm³). Thus, if equivalent sized pieces of several types of alloys are weighed, the alloy with the highest density will weigh the most. The density of an alloy is a function of the densities of the elements that make up the alloy. The densities for dental casting alloys range from 4.5 g/cm³ for the titanium-based alloys to more than 18 g/cm³ for some alloys high in gold and platinum. The density of an alloy is important in the casting of the alloy and its final cost. High-density alloys are easier to cast because gravity can accelerate the molten metal more easily into the casting mold. Furthermore, because alloys are sold by mass, high-density alloys cost more because more mass is present in any given volume of restoration. Of course, the final cost of the alloy also depends on the cost per gram of the alloy; costs of alloys vary considerably and are constantly changing.

The **modulus** of an alloy characterizes its stiffness or resistance to bending. Modulus is important clinically. Some alloys need a high modulus (stiffness) to prevent flexure under load. For example, cast restorations (next section) must be stiff to resist the forces of occlusion. Any flexure might loosen the restoration or cause fracture of a ceramic veneer on the restoration. Other alloys, such as orthodontic wires or partial denture alloys, require a low modulus (flexibility) to allow flexure for the alloy to perform appropriately. Moduli of dental alloys for restorations range from about 90 to 220 GPa (Appendix 11-1).

The **strength** of alloys is important to their clinical success. An alloy must have sufficient strength to resist any permanent

APPENDIX 11-1   Properties of Casting Alloys Clinically Important Properties of Common Types of Dental Casting Alloys

Alloy type	Color	Modulus (GPa)	Strength* (MPa)	Hardness (kg/mm²)
High-Noble Alloys				
Au-Pt (Zn)	Yellow	90	420/470**	175/195
Au-Pd (Ag)	White	100	365/385	255/280
Au-Cu-Ag	Yellow	100	270/400	135/195
Noble Alloys				
Au-Ag-Cu	Yellow	100	325/500	125/215
Pd-Cu	White	120	1145	425
Ag-Pd	White	120	260/320	140/155
Predominately Base-Metal Alloys				
Ni-Cr (Be)	White	180–200	710	340
Ni-Cr (Be-free)	White	200	620	190
Co-Cr	White	220	870	380

*Yield strength, 0.2% offset, tension.
**Lower number indicates soft condition; higher number indicates hardened condition (ordered solution; see Figure 11-4). One number means that no soft/hard transition is possible.

change in shape because many restorations are not successful if they distort. Strength may be cited in tension or compression, but tensile strength (pulling) is used most often. The yield strength of an alloy is the most common strength value used to compare alloys. **Yield strength** is the force per unit area (stress) required to permanently distort an alloy. The units of yield strength are the same as for any strength, megapascals (MPa, Chapter 2). However, an indication of the amount of distortion, called the offset, usually is included. For example, an alloy with yield strength of 750 MPa and 0.2% offset means that a stress of 750 MPa caused a permanent distortion of 0.2% in an alloy. The yield strengths of alloys range from 260 to 1150 MPa (see Appendix 11-1). The yield strength can be increased significantly for some alloys by the proper heat treatment, which changes the order of atoms in the alloy crystal structure.

The **hardness** of an alloy is an indication of how easy the alloy is to indent or polish. The hardness of an alloy is related to its yield strength, so an alloy with high yield strength will have high hardness and will be more difficult to polish. The hardness of alloys generally is measured by indenting the alloy with a diamond tip (very hard) under a certain weight. The deeper the indentation, the larger the area of the indentation will be and the softer the alloy. The units for hardness generally are expressed as kilograms (kg) of force required to form a 1-square-millimeter indentation, or kg/mm². If an alloy is harder than enamel, it may wear the opposing enamel during chewing or other jaw movements. Like yield strength, the hardness of some alloys can be increased significantly by the proper heat treatment to induce ordered crystal structures. The hardness of dental alloys ranges from about 125 to 425 kg/mm² (see Appendix 11-1).

CASTING ALLOYS

Categorizing Casting Alloys

Dental casting alloys (versus wrought alloys) are alloys used clinically in their as-cast form (Figure 11-6). In dentistry, casting alloys are categorized in several ways, but most often on the basis of noble metal content. The *nobility* of an alloy is expressed as a sum of the weight percentages of the noble metals in the alloy. For example, if an alloy contains 60% gold, 10% palladium, 5% platinum, and 25% copper, the nobility

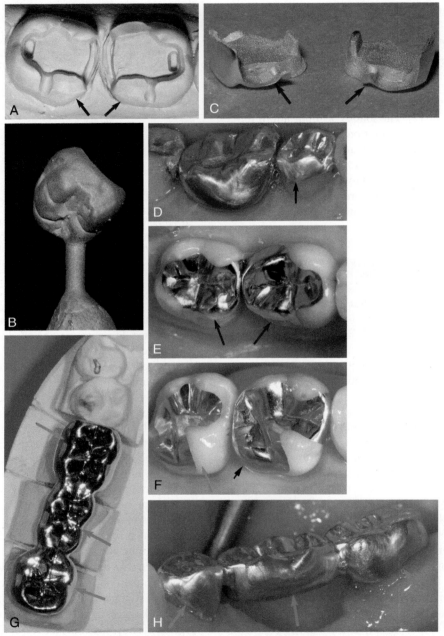

FIG 11-6 Dental restorations that are fabricated entirely from alloys. All-alloy restorations are made by first obtaining a highly accurate model of the surgical preparation of the tooth **(A)**. Through a complex series of steps (see Chapter 12), a casting is made **(B)** that is refined and finished **(C)** to precisely fit the surgical preparation. Cast restorations may cover part or all of a tooth **(D-H)**. Inlay restorations *(blue arrows in* **F**) are intracoronal restorations that do not involve cusp tips and are retained by the internal parts of the tooth. Onlay restorations *(black arrows)* are extracoronal restorations that include at least one cusp. Full crowns *(red arrows)* are extracoronal restorations that involve the entire clinical surface of the tooth. Bridges (or fixed partial dentures) involve several abutment crowns and pontics *(green arrows)* to replace missing teeth. Although ceramic–alloy restorations (see Figure 11-8) are popular today, cast restorations as shown here are more conservative of tooth structure and are generally better able to fit the surgical preparation. (**A, C, E, F,** Courtesy Richard D. Tucker, University of Washington Department of Restorative Dentistry, Seattle, WA; **B,** courtesy Y-W Chen, University of Washington Department of Restorative Dentistry, Seattle, WA; **D, G, H,** courtesy E. R. Schwedhelm, University of Washington Department of Restorative Dentistry, Seattle, WA.)

would be 75% (the sum of gold, palladium, and platinum). Alloys also are described on the basis of their most common metal. For example, an alloy with 75% gold often is described as gold based, or an alloy with 60% nickel may be described as nickel based. The term *based* indicates which metal is the major component in the alloy and should not be confused with the term *base metal*.

Several organizations classify dental casting alloys into broad groups based on nobility. These classifications are intended to simplify selection from the hundreds of alloys that are available to the practitioner and dental laboratory. In addition, these organizations certify that alloys comply with certain requirements set by the organization. Certification verifies not only composition but also physical properties such as hardness or strength. Three major organizations currently classify and certify alloys: the American Dental Association (ADA), the Nordic (Scandinavian) Institute of Dental Materials (NIOM), and the International Standards Organization (ISO). Dentists and dental laboratory technologists use these classifications and certifications when they select casting alloys for prosthodontic restorations. Only the ADA classification system is discussed here.

The ADA currently classifies dental casting alloys into three groups (Table 11-2 and Figure 11-7). High-noble alloys must have a noble metal content of at least 60% by weight and a gold content of at least 40%. Noble alloys must have a noble metal content of at least 25%, but no stipulation exists for gold content. Base-metal alloys have a noble metal content of less than 25%. Thus, the ADA classification includes alloys with reduced gold contents and alloys with little or no noble metal content. The Identalloy Council is a nonprofit group that promotes good communication about the alloys used in dentistry (www.identalloy.org). The group has developed certificates that participating alloy manufacturers use to specify and communicate the type of alloy that a laboratory has used to fabricate a cast restoration (see Figure 11-7). The certificates are approximately consistent with the ADA alloy types discussed in the previous paragraph. The intent is to use the certificates to document the type of alloy used in the patient's health record and to inform the patient of the type of alloy used. Often the dental auxiliary performs these tasks in the dental office. Symbols represent different alloy groups; the dental auxiliary should know these symbols to help ensure good patient and laboratory communication.

TABLE 11-2   American Dental Association Classification of Alloys

Alloy classification	Gold content (wt%)	Noble metal content (wt%)
High-noble	≥40	≥60
Noble	Not required	≥25
Predominantly base metal	Not required	<25

Common Casting Alloys

Hundreds of dental casting alloys are available for use in dentistry from more than a dozen globally based manufacturers. It is beyond the scope of this textbook to introduce all of these alloys. However, an understanding of the properties and compositions of the basic ADA categories of alloys will help the auxiliary to appreciate the wide variety of possibilities for cast restorations in dentistry (see Table 11-3). A basic knowledge of these alloys also will facilitate communication among the auxiliary, dentist, patient, dental laboratory, and insurance companies.

High-noble alloys are expensive because their gold, palladium, or platinum constituents are expensive. There are three common subclasses of high-noble alloys in use today: Au-Pt, Au-Pd, and Au-Cu-Ag alloys (see Table 11-3). These alloys have relatively high densities (above 13 g/cm^3), which make them easy to cast. Copper and silver often are added to the noble elements to increase hardness or strength. If these alloys contain higher amounts of palladium or platinum, then the liquidus of the alloys will be high because palladium and platinum have high melting points (1554° and 1772° C, respectively) relative to gold (1064° C). The high liquidus makes investing and casting more difficult but allows them to serve as alloys for ceramic–alloy restorations (see later discussion under considerations for ceramic alloys). The high-noble metal content of these alloys gives them excellent (low) corrosion properties in the mouth, except for the Au-Pt alloys, which will release zinc if not manipulated correctly by the dental laboratory. Overall, these alloys do not have high moduli and are too flexible for large cast restorations (see Appendix 11-1). The Au-Ag-Cu alloys cannot be used for ceramic–alloy restorations because their melting range is too low.

Noble alloys have at least 25% noble metal content but have no stipulation for gold content. There also are three common subclasses of this alloy type: Au-Ag-Cu, Pd-Cu, and Ag-Pd (see Table 11-3). Noble alloys are the most compositionally diverse of the casting alloys. Gold-based alloys in this class contain about 40% gold but contain higher amounts of copper or silver than the high-noble alloys. Au-based noble alloys are relatively low melting and cannot be used for ceramic–alloy restorations. Palladium-based alloys in this class may contain 77% palladium and almost no gold. The balance in mass of these alloys is commonly made up of copper or gallium. Pd-Cu alloys are extremely strong and hard, but they are difficult to use and have higher corrosion than Au-based alloys. Silver-based alloys (Ag-Pd) in this class usually contain just enough palladium (25%) to classify these alloys as noble by the ADA standard (see Table 11-3). As a group the noble alloys have moderate densities ranging from 10 to 12 g/cm^3, which is significantly less than the high-noble alloys. However, yield strengths and hardness of these alloys are equal to or greater than those of the high-noble alloys. These superior properties are generally attributable to the higher contents of palladium in the alloys. The cost of noble alloys may be less than for high-noble alloys, a fact that has made them popular among dentists. Pd-Cu and Ag-Pd

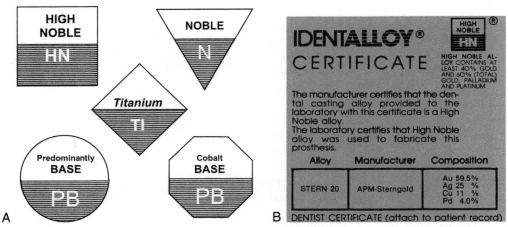

FIG 11-7 The American Dental Association (ADA) classifies alloys into three major groups: high-noble, noble, and predominantly base metal. **A,** Each group has a symbol, which is used on packaging and labeling. The Identalloy Council (www.identalloy.org) promotes full disclosure of alloy composition among manufacturers, laboratories, and dental offices. **B,** Each alloy is issued a sticker that may be scanned into the patient's electronic health record or given to the patient. The Identalloy Council recognizes two additional categories of alloys: the cobalt-based alloys and the titanium-based alloys. Both types are subcategories of predominantly base-metal alloys. Titanium-based alloys are used for endosseous implants (Chapter 15) among other prosthodontic applications. Dental auxiliaries are often asked to communicate with patients, insurance companies, or laboratories about alloys, and knowledge of this system aids accurate communication. The appropriate use of this classification also is important legally and to the patient's health. For example, some patients are allergic to nickel or cobalt and should not receive restorations fabricated from alloys containing these base metals.

TABLE 11-3 Common Casting Alloys and Primary Uses

Alloy type	Uses	Comments
High-noble alloys		
Au-Pt (Zn)	—Full-alloy restorations (without ceramic) —Ceramic–alloy restorations ("porcelain fused-to-metal")	—Some alloys contain small amounts of zinc to harden the alloy. —Alloy has low modulus and tends to corrode.
Au-Pd (Ag)	—Full-alloy restorations —Ceramic–alloy restorations Implant substructures	—Alloys may or may not contain silver. —Most versatile high-noble alloy. —Low corrosion under diverse oral conditions.
Au-Cu-Ag	—Full-alloy restorations (without ceramic)	—Low-melting range alloys. —Cannot be used for ceramic–alloy restorations.
Noble alloys		
Au-Ag-Cu	—Full-alloy restorations (without ceramic)	—Reduced gold alloy. —Cannot be used for ceramic–alloy restorations. —Higher corrosion than Au-Cu-Ag high-noble alloy above.
Pd-Cu	—Full-alloy restorations (without ceramic) —Ceramic–alloy restorations	—Higher modulus than Au-based high-noble alloys. —Corrosion is higher than Au-based alloys. —High strength; moderate hardness. —Difficult to cast and manipulate.
Ag-Pd	—Full-alloy restorations (without ceramic) —Ceramic–alloy restorations	—Ceramics tend to discolor ("green") if precautions are not taken. —Highest corrosion of the noble alloys.
Predominantly base-metal alloys		
Ni-Cr (Be)	—Ceramic–alloy restorations —Partial denture frameworks	—Alloys contain beryllium. —Casting, finishing, and ceramic application challenging. —Among strongest and hardest of the casting alloys. —High modulus, excellent rigidity for restorations. —Highest corrosion among all casting alloys. —Must consider allergy to nickel.

Continued

TABLE 11-3   Common Casting Alloys and Primary Uses—cont'd

Alloy type	Uses	Comments
Predominantly base-metal alloys		
Ni-Cr (Be free)	—Ceramic–alloy restorations —Partial denture frameworks	—Alloys do not contain beryllium. —Casting, finishing, and ceramic application challenging. —Among strongest and hardest of the casting alloys. —High modulus, excellent rigidity for restorations. —Lower corrosion than NiCr (Be). —Must consider allergy to nickel.
Co-Cr	—Ceramic–alloy restorations —Partial denture frameworks —Implant substructures	—Casting, finishing, and ceramic application are challenging. —Strongest and hardest of the casting alloys. —High modulus, excellent rigidity for restorations. —Corrosion intermediate between noble and Ni-Cr alloys. —Allergy to cobalt possible but less common than nickel.

subclasses may be used for crowns or fixed partial dentures with or without ceramic coverings.

The predominantly base-metal alloys may have minor amounts of noble elements, and their primary constituents are nickel or cobalt. Titanium alloys also are in this class but are discussed in Chapter 15 under implants because of their special properties. Of all of the dental casting alloys, these alloys are the most complex and contain six to eight elements including molybdenum, chromium, aluminum, vanadium, iron, carbon, beryllium, manganese, gallium, and silicon in addition to the primary elements. As a group, these alloys have extremely high yield strengths and hardness (see Appendix 11-1) but have relatively low densities. Thus, these alloys are the most difficult to cast and polish of all of the alloys and require special machines and techniques. Base-metal alloys also are the least expensive of all dental casting alloys (see Table 11-3). Combined with their low densities, the cost per restoration is low for these alloys, and this fact has made them popular. However, the use of these alloys, especially those based on nickel and cobalt, remains controversial because of their relatively high corrosion and questionable biocompatibility. Base-metal casting alloys may be used for crowns and fixed partial dentures (with or without ceramic), removable partial dentures, or dental implant substructures.

CERAMIC-BONDING CASTING ALLOYS

Properties Important to Ceramic–Alloy Bonding

Dental casting alloys used for ceramic–alloy restorations (Figure 11-8) are classified identically to the casting alloys already discussed for all-alloy restorations (Figure 11-7, Tables 11-2 and 11-3), but they have special formulations to enhance their bonds to dental ceramics. Properties important to ceramic–alloy bonding are discussed in the next paragraphs.

> **! ALERT**
>
> Ceramic-bonding alloys are formulated to chemically bond the alloy to ceramic via an oxide layer on the alloy surface. Ceramic-bonding alloys are used to make esthetic dental crowns.

The most fundamental property of ceramic-bonding alloys is their ability to durably bond to ceramic. For most alloys, an oxide on the alloy surface mediates this bond (Figure 11-9). The composition and thickness of the metal oxide are crucial to successful long-term bonding of ceramic. For many base-metal alloys (e.g., Ni-Cr and Co-Cr alloys), an oxide layer forms naturally on the surface of the metal and may even be too thick. The oxide films on these alloys must be reduced in thickness before application of the ceramic. However, because of the low reactivity of gold, high-noble and some noble alloys do not form a sufficient oxide layer to ensure reliable ceramic bonding. For these alloys, elements such as iron, gallium, indium, or tin must be added in small quantities to form a surface oxide layer. These trace elements are easily "burned out" of the alloy during casting, so these alloys must not be overheated during casting and should not be recast.

The solidus of ceramic-bonding alloys is critical to the successful fabrication of ceramic–alloy restorations. The ceramic is sintered and fused to the alloy in an oven at temperatures that range from approximately 850° to 1350° C depending on the type of ceramic used (Chapter 14). The alloy substructure must remain intact and undistorted during the firing of the ceramic, or the fit and function of the crown will be compromised. Thus, the solidus of ceramic-bonding alloys must be higher than the sintering temperature of the ceramic. For this reason, elements with high melting points such as platinum and palladium are often more abundant in ceramic-bonding alloys. Not all ceramic-bonding alloys are compatible with all ceramics from the standpoint of melting range. Alloy and ceramic manufacturers specify which ceramics are compatible with a given alloy.

The thermal expansion of ceramic-bonding alloys is another property critical to ceramic–alloy bonding (Chapter 14). Alloys and ceramics expand when heated and contract when cooled. The amount of expansion (or contraction) is called the coefficient of thermal expansion and has units of $(°C)^{-1}$ (Chapter 2). A high coefficient of thermal expansion indicates more expansion on heating and more contraction on cooling. When ceramic is heated with the alloy at a high temperature (e.g., about 1000° C), the ceramic interacts with and bonds to the alloy through the oxide layer. As the ceramic–alloy

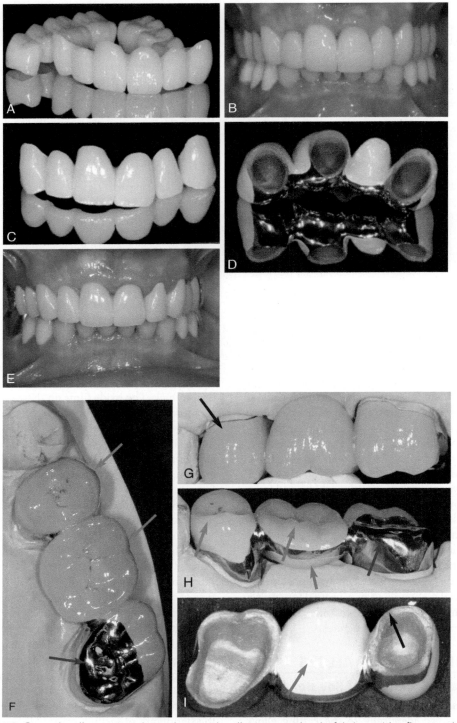

FIG 11-8 Ceramic–alloy restorations. A ceramic–alloy restoration is fabricated by first casting or machining a metal substructure onto which ceramic is fired (see Chapter 14 for details on ceramics). A provisional restoration is worn by the patient while the final restoration is made. In **A,** a provisional (temporary) has been milled from a poly-methylmethacrylate block prior to temporary cementation in the mouth **(B).** Milling of provisionals using a digital impression is a relatively new technique that provides faster, stronger, more accurately fitting temporary restorations. The final restoration is then fabricated and cemented **(C–E).** These restorations have ceramic applied in areas in which esthetics are important but have alloy in other locations **(C, D, F–I).** On the facial margins, the alloy is extremely thin *(black arrows)* to hide the alloy. Clinically, ceramic–alloy restorations may have various configurations for ceramic application. In the posterior **(F–I),** the ceramic may be applied over the entire occlusal surface *(red arrows)* but may be limited to ensure occlusion in alloy *(blue arrows).* On the tissue side of a pontic *(green arrow* in **D, J),** ceramic may be used as well. (**A–E,** Courtesy Y-W Chen, University of Washington Department of Restorative Dentistry, Seattle, WA; **F–I,** courtesy E. R. Schwedhelm, University of Washington Department of Restorative Dentistry, Seattle, WA.)

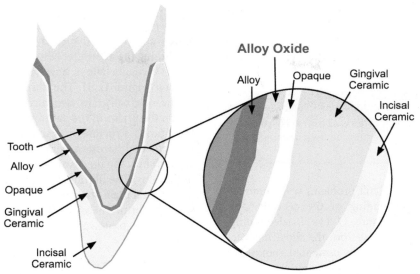

FIG 11-9 Ceramic–alloy bonding. The bonding of ceramic to alloy is nearly always mediated by a thin, adherent alloy oxide that forms on the alloy. The opaquing ceramic (opaque) chemically combines with the alloy oxide, thereby forming covalent bonds that retain the ceramic to the alloy with high affinity. The boundaries between the alloy, oxide, and ceramic layers are not distinct as shown here but form gradients. Any flaw in the alloy oxide will compromise the bond between alloy and ceramic and increase the risk of clinical debonding of the ceramic from the restoration in service. The thickness of the oxide also is an important factor in bonding.

combination is cooled, the contraction of the two materials together must be compatible or the ceramic will crack while cooling to room temperature. In practice, the alloy should contract slightly more than the ceramic to reduce the risk of fracture during cooling or during service. Thus, the coefficient of thermal expansion for the alloy should be about 0.5×10^{-6}/°C greater than that of the ceramic. As with melting ranges, not all ceramic-bonding alloys are compatible with all ceramics in terms of thermal expansion–contraction compatibility. This compatibility issue has become even more complex with the advent of new veneering ceramics. The recommendations of the alloy manufacturer should be followed exactly. Coefficient of thermal expansion is discussed further in Chapter 14.

Problems Encountered with Ceramic–Alloy Bonding

Clinically, ceramic–alloy restorations pose several special problems that do not occur for all-alloy restorations. The color of the oxide on the metal is one such problem. The color of oxides varies from light yellow on high-noble alloys and some noble alloys to dark gray or even black oxides on some base-metal alloys. The color of the oxide must be masked completely by the porcelain, or the restoration will look unnatural (Figures 11-9 and 11-10). Opaquing ceramics are used to mask the oxide color (Chapter 14), but gray and black oxides are much more difficult to mask than the light yellow oxides. For this reason, base-metal alloys are more difficult to use in ceramic–alloy restorations.

During the application of the ceramic, some of the metals in the alloy vaporize and may discolor the ceramic by reacting with the ceramic. Such discoloration is called greening

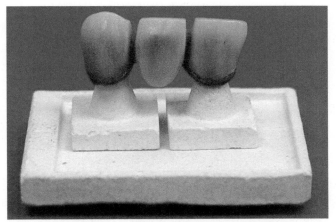

FIG 11-10 Effect of opaquing ceramic–alloy restorations. In this restoration, the opaque layer was purposely omitted. Without the opaque layer, the dark gray metal oxide of the nickel-based alloy shows through the ceramic and discolors the entire restoration. Such a restoration would not be suitable for use in a patient. The ability of the opaquing ceramic to mask the alloy oxide layer depends on the color of the oxide, darker gray hues being harder to mask than light yellow hues found on gold-based alloys. (Courtesy Cindy Oxford, Georgia Regents University, Augusta, GA.)

because the ceramic contaminated in this manner has a slight greenish tinge. Esthetically, the color of the contaminated ceramic is unacceptable. Alloys that contain high amounts of silver and copper are at higher risk for greening problems because these elements are more volatile during ceramic firing. The ceramic oven itself also may be contaminated with copper or silver and subsequently may contaminate ceramics fired in the oven. To a large extent, greening is avoided by selecting an appropriate alloy, firing the restoration at the appropriate temperature, and cleaning the ceramic oven periodically.

> **! ALERT**
>
> Debonding of ceramic from alloy often is a severe clinical challenge and may require replacement of the restoration and re-preparation of the tooth.

Perhaps one of the most difficult problems with ceramic–alloy restorations is the debonding of the ceramic after cementation in the mouth (Figure 11-11). In debonding, some or all of the ceramic fractures from the alloy substructure. Because the crown is permanently cemented, removal of the crown without further damaging the restoration is almost impossible. Even if the crown can be removed successfully, the ceramic is difficult to repair because of many technical issues. Thus, debonding is a challenging clinical problem because it may be esthetically urgent and expensive to correct. The best solution to this problem is to prevent it by the selection of compatible alloy and ceramics and the proper manipulation of these materials during fabrication. When debonding occurs, repair of the restoration is sometimes possible at least temporarily with a composite material bonded to the metal substructure (Chapter 4). However, in general ceramic debonding requires that an entirely new restoration be fabricated. In large fixed partial dentures, the costs in time and money for replacement can be substantial. For this reason, the prevention of ceramic–alloy debonding is particularly important.

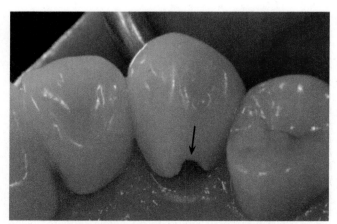

FIG 11-11 Photo of debonding on a ceramic–alloy restoration. On occasion, the ceramic debonds from the alloy, resulting in a clinical defect *(arrow)*. Debonding usually results from inappropriate fabrication processes or poor clinical planning (e.g., parafunction). At the time of permanent cementation, defects are not detectable. The defects cannot easily be repaired intraorally. The need to redo the restoration depends on a variety of clinical factors, including esthetics. (Courtesy Y-W Chen, University of Washington Department of Restorative Dentistry, Seattle, WA.)

WROUGHT ALLOYS

When an alloy is shaped by rolling, drawing, twisting, or machining the alloy after casting, the alloy is called a wrought alloy. Wrought alloys have a grain structure described as fibrous (Figure 11-5). The fibrous structure is what remains of the original grain structure after the mechanical forces act on the grains of the cast form (Figure 11-4). Importantly, the fibrous structure is responsible for the increased yield strength and hardness compared with the cast form of the alloys. Thus, the mechanical work improves some properties of the alloy. The fibrous structure of wrought alloys reverts to the original grain structure if too much heat is applied to the wrought form. Therefore, heat applied to these alloys during soldering or other manipulation degrades important clinical properties.

> **! ALERT**
>
> A wrought alloy is shaped into its final form by mechanical force of some type. These forces change the properties of the alloy to be more advantageous clinically.

Wrought alloys are used in many aspects of dentistry (Figure 11-2). Orthodontic wires are wrought alloys formed by drawing castings of predominantly base-metal alloys, specifically stainless steel, titanium, nickel-titanium (Nitinol), or cobalt-chromium-nickel (Elgiloy) alloys. After the drawing process, the wire has a fibrous grain structure with high strength and other clinically favorable properties. The increased properties of the wrought wire are important to its proper function in orthodontic applications. Endodontic files also are wrought, mechanically formed from wires made of stainless steel or nickel titanium. The ability of the file to bend without being permanently deformed is critical to its function in cleaning the root canal. The fracture resistance of the file during the twisting motions used in endodontic therapy is also critical because files that fracture in the root canal are extremely difficult to retrieve. Wrought wire made from high-noble alloys is used for clasps in removable partial dentures. These wires are called PGP wires, named for the platinum-gold-palladium alloy from which they are formed. These wires must have yield strengths low enough to allow the clasp to be adjusted but must not bend too easily so that they hold their shape and hold the partial denture in place. Clasp wires are soldered to the partial denture framework after the framework is cast. Because excessive heat can degrade the fibrous structure and properties of wrought alloys, the soldering must be done carefully so that the fibrous grain structure of the wire is preserved (Figure 11-12).

SOLDERS

Solders are special alloys used to join other alloys. The alloys to be joined are generally called substrate alloys. In dentistry, solders may be used to join an orthodontic wire to a band in the construction of a space maintainer (Figure 11-12), to join

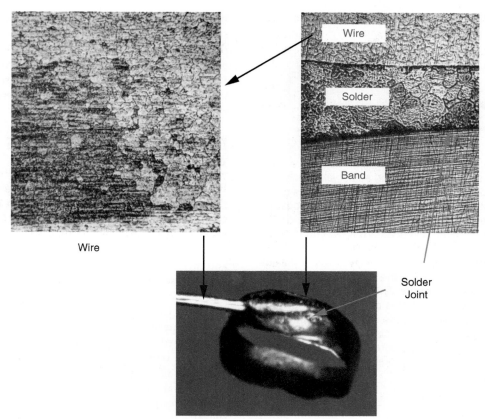

Wire

FIG 11-12 Example of an unacceptable solder joint *(photo)*. The solder was overheated, resulting in a brownish tinge that persists after polishing and pitting in the solder. In the upper right light microscopic image, gaps are evident between the band, the solder, and the wire (which normally has a fibrous form but now has a traditional grain form from the excess heat). The gaps and pits in the solder joint will increase corrosion and deterioration of the appliance intraorally. The upper left light micrograph reveals that the excessive heating has caused the wire to lose its original fibrous form *(top right)* to a traditional grain form *(top left)*. Thus, the advantages of the wrought wire form are lost and the wire will not perform clinically as well.

a clasp wire to a partial denture framework, or to join two units of a fixed partial denture together after each is cast separately (Figure 11-13). Solders also may be used to add a proximal contact to a crown or repair an occlusal defect in a casting. The process of soldering is technically a misnomer because soldering operations are those done below 425° C, and brazing operations are done above 425° C. Because all dental applications are done above 425° C, the processes used in dentistry should be called brazing. However, *soldering* is the term used most commonly.

Solders have several special properties that enable them to function successfully. The solder must melt (have a liquidus) below that of the solidus of the substrate alloy; a 50° C differential is commonly advised. Put simply, if the substrate alloy melts before the solder, then the original cast form will itself melt during the soldering operation. Solders must flow freely against the substrate alloy and must wet the substrate alloy well (Figure 11-14). The property of wetting is the same in principle as impression making or pouring (Chapter 8). The ability to flow and wet the substrate alloy ensures a strong bond between the solder and substrate. Flow and wetting are

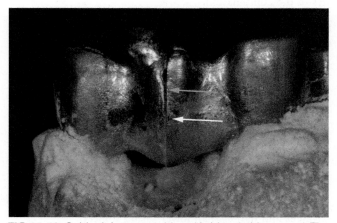

FIG 11-13 Solder joint on a soldered bridge *(white arrow)*. The casting did not fit in the patient at try-in, so the casting was sectioned, seated in the mouth in two pieces, and indexed in the mouth to preserve the appropriate orientation. The indexed pieces were removed and then soldered. The joint was incompletely filled in some areas *(blue arrow)*. (Courtesy Y-W Chen, University of Washington Department of Restorative Dentistry, Seattle, WA.)

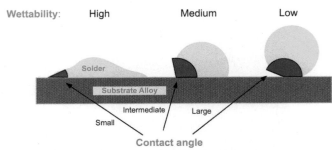

FIG 11-14 Wetting. When solders melt, they must flow freely onto the substrate alloy to ensure good solder–alloy bonding. The ability of the solder to interact with the substrate is called wetting and is illustrated by the figure. If the solder does not wet the substrate alloy well *(right)*, it tends to bead up on the substrate alloy when molten and does not flow onto the substrate alloy. In this case, the contact angle between the solder and its substrate alloy is large and wettability is low. If the solder has a small contact angle on the substrate alloy, it will flow and will have high wettability. The degree of the wettability of a solder is determined by the composition of the solder and substrate alloy, an appropriate soldering temperature, the use of the appropriate flux, and clean surfaces. The concept of wetting also is important to composite–tooth bonding, implant osseointegration, and intra-oral denture retention.

functions of the composition of the solder and compatibility of that composition with the alloy to be soldered. The corrosion of a soldered material is also a concern. Because soldering creates, by definition, a junction between two different alloys, the risk of corrosion in the mouth is higher than if only one metal were present. As with wetting, the composition of the solder and soldered alloys determines the corrosion properties of the combination.

Most dental solders are themselves either gold- or silver-based alloys. These alloys contain special elements such as tin to encourage a lower melting range and better flow. Gold-based solders are used primarily to solder cast prosthetic restorations, whereas silver solders are used more in orthodontic applications. A variety of gold-based solders are available with various melting ranges to meet specific applications. The manufacturers of the cast alloys specify the compatibility of solders with their alloys, and it is common for a manufacturer to offer both a series of dental casting alloys and compatible solders together. The strength, hardness, and corrosion of dental solders also depend on the composition. In general, solders with a higher melting range are stronger and harder than lower fusing solders.

Soldering is an art, requiring immense skill and experience. The increase in the types and compositions of substrate alloys since the late 1990s has made the soldering process even more complex. Furthermore, the increasing use of ceramic–alloy restorations has made soldering more challenging; in these restorations, the solidus of the alloy substructure (substrate alloy), the liquidus of the solder, and the sintering temperature of

the ceramic must all be balanced (Chapter 14). If the alloy substructure is soldered prior to ceramic application (pre-soldering), then the solder cannot melt during firing of the ceramic. If the alloy substructure is soldered after the ceramic is applied (post-soldering), then the heat used during soldering must not damage the color or other properties of the ceramic.

BIOCOMPATIBILITY OF ALLOYS AND SOLDERS

Because dental alloys typically are in long-term contact with the teeth and oral tissues, their effect on those tissues (biocompatibility) is critical. The biocompatibility of dental alloys is related primarily to their corrosion. If an alloy corrodes more, it releases more of its elements into the mouth and increases the risk for unwanted reactions in the oral tissues. These unwanted reactions include unpleasant tastes, burning tongue, irritation, allergy, or other inflammatory reactions. Unfortunately, the connection between the release of elements from alloys and tissue reactions has not been well defined, so public hysteria about the release of metal ions from dental alloys and solders often results. All alloys, regardless of composition, release elements into the oral cavity and oral tissues at some level. Although a wide range of elements can be released from these alloys, little evidence suggests that the released elements cause significant problems for most people. The one exception is for people who are allergic to released metals. Of these, nickel is by far the most common. By current estimates, about 4.2% of the general population is allergic to nickel (Figure 11-15).

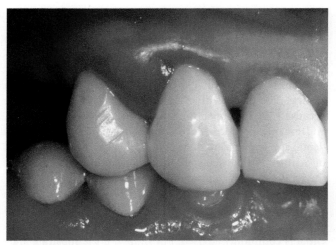

FIG 11-15 Allergy and inflammation in response to a nickel-based alloy. The alloy substructure of the ceramic–alloy crown on tooth number 5 is made from a nickel-based alloy. The gingiva adjacent to this alloy is swollen and red because nickel has corroded from the alloy into the tissue subgingivally, and the patient has had an allergic reaction to the released nickel. (Courtesy M. L. Myers, Georgia Regents University, Augusta, GA.)

In people with other dermatological conditions (e.g., eczema), the frequency of allergy increases to 9.6%. Furthermore, patients with an allergy to cobalt also co-react to nickel 79% of the time. For chromium and palladium, the coreaction rates are 39% and 95%, respectively. Current research focuses on other possible biologic consequences of released elements, particularly nickel.

Although broad-based statements often are not accurate, high-noble alloys corrode less because of their high-noble metal content. On the other hand, predominantly base-metal alloys often corrode significantly more. In this regard, nickel-based alloys have the greatest corrosion rates among casting alloys, and formulations containing beryllium are particularly corrosion prone. Although unwanted reactions are ill defined, alloys that release higher amounts of metals into the mouth pose the biggest risk for unwanted reactions. Thus, some predominantly base-metal alloys pose more biologic risk to the patient than other types of alloys.

QUICK REVIEW

Alloys play many important roles in dentistry. Dental casting alloys are categorized primarily by composition. The American Dental Association system divides alloys into high-noble, noble, and base-metal alloys. High-noble and noble alloys contain specified amounts of the noble elements gold, palladium, and platinum. These alloys are the most resistant to corrosion in the mouth. Ceramic-bonding alloys must form oxides on their surfaces to bond ceramic and must have expansion properties and melting ranges compatible with the ceramic. Wrought alloys are shaped by mechanical forces, and these alloys have superior properties for specialized applications in orthodontics, endodontics, prosthodontics, and implantology. Solders are specialized alloys used to join other alloys together and must have melting ranges lower than the alloys they join. The corrosion of alloys is particularly important because the biocompatibility of alloys depends to a great extent on their corrosion rates and the release of elements into the oral cavity and oral tissues.

SELF-TEST QUESTIONS

Test your knowledge by answering the following questions. For multiple-choice questions, one or more responses may be correct.

1. The noble metals used in dentistry include:
   a. Gold
   b. Platinum
   c. Palladium
   d. Silver
   e. Copper
   f. Titanium
2. Precious metals used in dentistry include:
   a. Gold
   b. Platinum
   c. Palladium
   d. Silver
3. Indicate the function of the components listed in the left-hand column by selecting the correct answer or answers listed in the right-hand column.

a. Gold	1. Increases hardness
b. Copper	2. Increases ductility
c. Silver	3. Produces fine-grained alloys
d. Zinc	4. Reduces corrosion
e. Platinum	5. Increases the melting point
f. Palladium	6. Serves as a scavenger for oxygen during casting
g. Iridium	7. Reduces the melting point
	8. Whitens the alloy
	9. Increases the liquidus

4. The purpose(s) of adding small amounts of iron, tin, and indium to high-noble gold alloys for bonding to ceramic include(s):
   a. To provide corrosion resistance
   b. To cause hardening
   c. To lower the fusing temperature of the ceramic
   d. To form oxides that bond with ceramic
5. Which statements about alloys is/are true?
   a. The strengths of the high-noble gold alloys are comparable to those of predominantly base-metal alloys.
   b. The nickel-chromium alloys contribute to the greening of ceramic.
   c. The main advantages of the nickel alloys are low cost and higher stiffness.
   d. Some patients may be allergic to nickel alloys even when the alloy is covered by ceramic.

Use short statements to answer the following questions.

6. An alloy has 35% by weight of gold, 35% palladium, 10% copper, 10% silver, 5% platinum, and 5% zinc.
   a. What is the percentage of noble metal content?
   b. What is the ADA classification for this alloy?
   c. What is the color of this alloy?
7. A patient complains that his previous dentist made a crown of "cheap" metal because it had a white (silver) color. What is the problem with this patient's statement?
8. An alloy has a liquidus of 1200° C and a solidus of 1100° C.
   a. What temperature must this alloy reach to be cast?
   b. What temperature must this alloy be maintained at or under to solder this alloy or bond ceramic to it?
   c. Could this alloy be appropriate for ceramic bonding?
9. Describe three factors that determine the cost of the alloy needed to cast a crown. Which of these factors is/are fixed and which may vary?
10. Describe the grain structure of a wrought alloy, and compare it to a cast alloy of the same composition. How did the wrought alloy get its grain structure? What can make the wrought structure change? How are wrought forms used in dentistry?

11. What single factor increases the risk the most for a problem with the biologic response to a dental casting alloy? What ADA alloy class generally presents the highest risk for adverse biologic responses?
12. A laboratory made a ceramic–alloy restoration, and on delivery of the restoration to your office, you note that there are cracks in the ceramic. Assuming that the crown was not dropped, what is a possible cause for the cracking? Which properties of alloys are relevant to this problem?

In the following multiple-choice questions, one or more responses may be correct.

13. Alloys categorized by the ADA specification as high noble have:
    a. ≥60 wt% noble metal
    b. ≥60 wt% gold
    c. ≥40 wt% gold
    d. ≥60 wt% gold
14. An alloy has the following composition (in wt%): Au 35, Cu 40, Ag 15, Pd 10. By the ADA standard, this alloy:
    a. Predominantly base metal
    b. Noble
    c. High noble
    d. Precious
15. If the coefficient of thermal expansion of an alloy is $14 \times 10^{-6}/°C$ and that of the ceramic is $10 \times 10^{-6}/°C$, when the ceramic is fired onto the alloy and cooled to room temperature, the ceramic will be in:
    a. Tension
    b. Compression
    c. There will be no net compression or tension in the ceramic
    d. Cannot tell from the information given
16. Yellow alloys are generally:
    a. More expensive per gram than silver (or white) alloys
    b. Harder than silver (or white) alloys
    c. Lower in corrosion than silver (or white) alloys
    d. None of the above
17. ADA specification number 5 states that to be a high-noble alloy, the alloy must contain:
    a. = 40 wt% of Au and = 60 wt% of noble metal
    b. = 25 wt% of noble metal
    c. = 60 wt% of noble metal
    d. None of the above
18. Which ADA class of casting alloys generally has the highest melting range?
    a. High noble
    b. Noble
    c. Predominantly base metal
19. Which elements is/are not noble by the ADA definition?
    a. Au
    b. Pd
    c. Zn
    d. Pt

For the following statements, select true or false.
20. To be successful, a soldering operation must be maintained below the solidus of the substrate alloys.
    a. True
    b. False
21. Grain refiners act in casting alloys by making the grains purer.
    a. True
    b. False
22. Ceramics bond to alloys by interacting with the alloy crystal lattice.
    a. True
    b. False
23. Base-metal alloys are inherently weak and flexible.
    a. True
    b. False
24. Dental solders are alloys.
    a. True
    b. False
25. Wrought alloys cannot be damaged by heat.
    a. True
    b. False

SUGGESTED SUPPLEMENTARY READINGS

Council on Dental Materials, Instruments, and Equipment: Classification system for cast alloys, *J Am Dent Assoc* 109:766, 1984.

Geurtsen W: Biocompatibility of dental casting alloys, *Crit Rev Oral Biol Med* 13:71–84, 2002.

Roberts HW, Berzins DW, Moore BK, Charlton DG, Metal–ceramic alloys in dentistry: a review, *J Prosthodont* 18:188–194, 2009.

Wataha JC: Biocompatibility of dental casting alloys: a review, *J Prosthet Dent* 83:233, 2000.

Wataha JC: Alloys for prosthodontic restorations, *J Prosthet Dent* 87:351, 2002.

Wataha JC, Messer RL: Casting alloys, *Dent Clin North Am* 48:499–512, 2004.

Wataha JC, Shor K: Palladium alloys for biomedical applications, *Exp Rev Med Dev* 4:489–501, 2010.

Wataha JC, Drury JL, Chung WO: Nickel alloys in the oral environment, *Exp Rev Med Dev* 10:519–539, 2013.

Wendt SL: Nonprecious cast-metal alloys in dentistry, *Curr Opin Dent* 1:222, 1991.

Wylie CM, Schelton RM, Fleming GJP, Davenport AJ: Corrosion of nickel-based dental casting alloys, *Dent Mater* 23:714–723, 2007.

evolve Please visit *http://evolve.elsevier.com/Powers/dentalmaterials* for additional practice and study support tools.

12

Casting, Soldering, and Welding

OBJECTIVES

After reading this chapter, the student should be able to:

1. Describe dimensional changes that occur during the casting process, and explain how they are balanced to ensure a clinically acceptable casting.
2. Describe the lost-wax technique and its accuracy in producing a dental casting.
3. Distinguish between casting and milling.
4. Explain the advantages and disadvantages of using wax in the casting process.
5. Define what a sprue is, what it may be made of, and its importance to the casting process.
6. Explain the process of investing and how the properties of the investment regulate the fit of a casting.
7. Explain why the conditions used to burn out the wax pattern influence the fit of a casting.
8. Describe a centrifugal casting machine and how it works.
9. Describe the process for finishing a restoration, and explain why these steps are important to its clinical success.
10. Compare solders with casting alloys in terms of composition and properties.
11. Describe the soldering process and critical techniques that must be followed to ensure a good soldered joint.
12. Distinguish soldering from welding.

In dentistry, casting is a process by which a detailed wax pattern of a dental restoration is converted into alloy or ceramic. The casting process allows the dentist and dental laboratory to custom-make precision restorations for missing or damaged teeth. Casting is complex and takes place largely in commercial dental laboratories. However, dental auxiliaries must understand the casting process to communicate effectively with the dentist, patients, insurance companies, and dental laboratory. This chapter provides an overview of casting at an introductory level. Milling of restorations, in which a block of alloy or ceramic is cut back to a final restorative shape by a precision machine (usually computer-directed), is growing in use, particularly for ceramic restorations. Regardless of the method used to form the restoration, its fit and retention intraorally are the primary considerations for clinical success.

> **! ALERT**
>
> Casting uses the lost-wax technique to fabricate precision restorations for teeth.

Casting is used to fabricate inlays, onlays, crowns, ceramic–alloy crowns, some all-ceramic crowns, partial dentures, implant restorations and frameworks, and occasionally a complete denture. Thus, the casting process plays a large role in dentistry. In dentistry, casting often uses a technique called the lost-wax technique. Figure 12-1 shows a diagrammatic summary of the steps involved in the lost-wax technique: making the wax pattern, spruing the pattern, investing, burnout, casting, removal of investment (devesting), and finishing.

In many cases, such as with a ceramic–alloy crown, the casting is not the final restoration but is modified to obtain the final restoration through ceramic application, machining, or soldering. Castable or pressable ceramics have been developed that also use the lost-wax technique to form either the final restoration or a substructure onto which other ceramics are applied.

If done correctly, casting is exceedingly accurate, which is truly remarkable because each step in the process influences the final size of the casting (see Figure 12-1). The accuracy of a cast restoration can be as good as 0.05%. This accuracy translates into a tolerance of less than 20 µm for most dental restorations. To achieve this degree of accuracy, each step in the casting process must be done carefully. An error in any step will result in a final restoration that is clinically unacceptable. In general, the casting should be slightly oversized to optimize clinical fit and space for the luting cement. The remainder of this chapter discusses each step of the casting process in the order presented in Figure 12-1.

Milling is an alternative to casting for fabricating restorations (Figure 12-2). Milling starts with an alloy or ceramic material (sometimes itself cast) and precisely carves it back to the shape of the restoration. Improvements in computer-aided machining (CAM) technology and digital imaging have made milling increasingly popular; current techniques even allow for chair-side fabrication of some restorations such as inlays or onlays. Although milling can be used for alloys or ceramics, its most common current use is with ceramic materials. The focus of this chapter will therefore be casting.

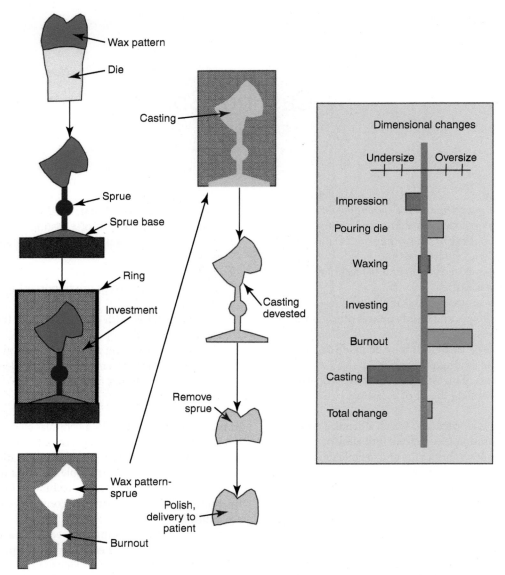

FIG 12-1 Sequence of steps for dental casting using the lost-wax technique. The wax pattern is formed on the die of the prepared tooth. A sprue (generally made of wax or plastic) is added and the wax pattern is transferred to a sprue base. A ring is added and the ring is filled with casting investment, embedding the wax pattern and sprue. The sprue base is removed, and the ring is placed into a hot oven that burns away the wax pattern and sprue. Molten alloy is cast into the space formerly occupied by the wax pattern and the investment is broken away (devested). The sprue is removed and the crown is polished and ready for try-in in the patient. Each step in the casting process has an effect on the overall final dimension of the casting: some steps tend to make the casting too small, whereas others tend to make it too big. At the end of process, most castings are slightly oversized to allow for discrepancies in the casting surface and space for cement.

WAXING AND SPRUING

Waxing

A wax pattern is a detailed model of the final dental restoration, including all anatomy, contours, occlusal function, and proximal contacts. Wax is used because it is easy to manipulate, inexpensive, and well suited to making custom restorations. Wax also is easy to completely eliminate (via **burnout**) after investing. Wax patterns are formed most often on a working die of the tooth or arch. These dies retain detailed information about the teeth to be restored and the oral structures around them. When the wax pattern is formed on a die versus the tooth itself, the waxing technique is described as indirect (Figure 12-3). In past times, the wax pattern of small restorations was formed directly on the tooth. This "direct technique" was used for relatively simple restorations such as small two-surface inlay restorations. The direct technique is technically demanding and uses special waxes that do not distort at mouth temperature. The direct technique is seldom used today; use of the indirect technique is nearly ubiquitous.

Although wax is a convenient material for making a pattern of the dental restoration, it also has a tendency to flow,

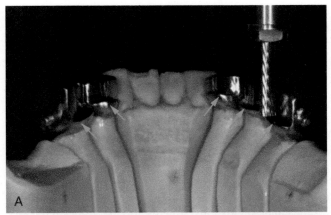

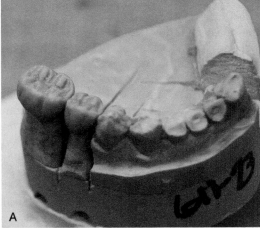

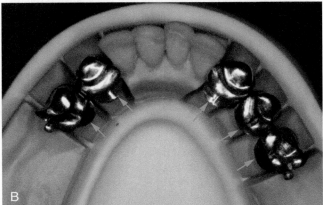

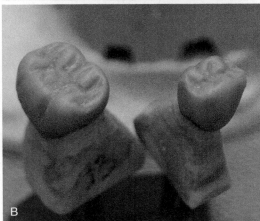

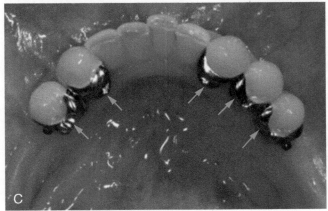

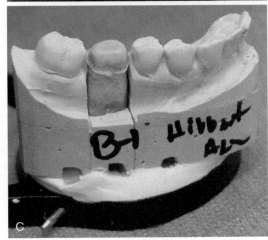

FIG 12-2 Milling of metallic restorations. One alternative to casting dental restorations is milling. In the case shown **(A)** cast crown substructures are milled *(blue arrows)* to provide a precision fit of a partial denture framework that must engage all the crowns simultaneously. Milling is used because casting all the crowns to this coordinated level of precision would be difficult. **(B)** The milled crown substructures are shown from the occlusal. **(C)** Ceramic has been fired onto the crowns, which are cemented in the patient's mouth, ready for the partial denture framework. Milling is far more common today in fabrication of all-ceramic restorations (see Chapter 14). (Courtesy Y-W Chen, University of Washington Department of Restorative Dentistry, Seattle, WA.)

FIG 12-3 Wax patterns. Wax replicas of teeth to be restored with castings are fabricated on stone dies **(A),** themselves fabricated from impressions of the prepared tooth. The dies are removable **(B)** so that all aspects of the patterns can be evaluated and adjusted. When a ceramic–alloy restoration is constructed, the wax pattern is not to full contour but is "cut back" to a thickness that will support the ceramic and allow adequate ceramic thickness for an esthetic result **(C).** In this latter case, the casting is referred to as an alloy substructure. For ceramics that are cast or pressed, this process is similar. (Courtesy M. Owens, C. S. Bemis, and D. E. Owens CDT, Georgia Regents University, Augusta, GA. Photography by R. Messer, Georgia Regents University, Augusta, GA.)

release stress, and expand or contract with changes in temperature. The waxing process itself does not oversize or undersize the dimensions of a restoration (see Figure 12-1), but distortion of the wax pattern is a serious risk. Even when supported by the die, a wax pattern may distort significantly if the ambient temperature changes or time (days) passes. However, when the wax pattern is removed from the die, distortion may occur in only 1 to 2 minutes. Thus, the shortest time possible should elapse between the time the pattern is removed from the die and the time it is invested. For this reason, the wax pattern is generally sprued while it is still on the die.

Spruing

A sprue forms a channel in the investment through which the molten alloy or ceramic travels to form the restoration. Sprues often are wax but also may be plastic or even metal. If metal, the sprue must be removed before casting because the metal will not burn out. The decision of where to place one or more sprues onto a wax pattern is complex and depends on the type of restoration, the type of casting material, and the experience of the technician. In the simplest case, a single sprue is placed on one of the cusps of the wax pattern (Figures 12-1 and 12-4). In more complex cases, multiple sprues may be placed.

> **! ALERT**
>
> A sprue forms the channel through which molten alloy or ceramic travels to form the restoration in the space formerly occupied by the wax pattern.

The other end of the sprue is attached to a base made of rubber (Figures 12-1 and 12-4). The sprue is attached at the apex of the cone of the sprue base. The cone ultimately forms a depression in the investment to help guide the molten alloy into the sprue hole. Sprue diameter and length vary considerably depending on the type of restoration but should be selected to ensure that the cast material solidifies last in the sprue. This strategy allows the sprue to continue to "feed" the casting as it solidifies and shrinks. To prevent premature freezing in the sprue channel, sprues are generally as big in diameter and as short as possible; a reservoir is often added in the sprue itself to increase the sprue mass. The wax pattern is ready to be invested after it is sprued and the sprue is attached to the sprue base (Figure 12-4).

INVESTING AND BURNOUT

Investments

During investing, the wax pattern and sprue are embedded in investment, a stone-like material that withstands the high temperatures and forces of burnout and casting. Investments are composed of a binder, which holds the investment together, and a refractory, which helps them to resist the heat of burnout and casting. The refractory in most dental investments is a form of silica (SiO_2). Both the binder and the refractory material contribute to expansion of the investment, which is necessary to compensate for shrinkage of the alloy

during casting and produce a casting that fits the tooth (Figure 12-1).

Investments that use gypsum as a binder are described as "gypsum bonded." Gypsum-bonded investments are used to cast alloys for inlays, onlays, full-alloy crowns, and some Ni-based partial denture frameworks. Gypsum alone (without silica) cannot be used for investing because it lacks sufficient resistance to heat. Even with the silica refractory added, the melting temperature of an alloy cannot exceed 1200° C, and the burnout temperature cannot exceed 700° C or the gypsum will decompose and degrade the casting. If higher melting alloys are needed, then phosphate-bonded investments are used.

Phosphate-bonded investments also use a silica refractory but use a monoammonium phosphate-magnesia binder. The binder is the product of the reaction of ammonium hydrogen phosphate with magnesium oxide. During burnout, the binder undergoes additional chemical reactions that increase its resistance to damage at high temperatures. Phosphate-bonded investments are much stronger than gypsum investments and are used for ceramic–alloy restorations, all-ceramic restorations, implant substructures, and partial denture frameworks in which casting alloys with high melting ranges are used. If ceramics are to be pressed, there are still other types of investments available to withstand the higher burnout and casting temperatures.

Investing

Investing the wax pattern captures all details of the wax pattern into the investment and, once the wax is burned away, provides a defined space into which the molten alloy or ceramic is cast. To retain the investment as it sets, a casting ring is placed onto the sprue base (Figure 12-4). The casting ring also supports the investment during the casting process. The ring is commonly lined with a ceramic-paper liner to help the investment to expand during setting and burnout. The liner is moistened before the investment is added to prevent it from absorbing water from the investment. Before investing, the wax pattern may be treated with a surfactant that aids flow of the water-based (hydrophilic) investment material over the water-hating (hydrophobic) wax pattern. The surfactant generally is sprayed onto the pattern with a fine atomizer.

After these preparatory steps, the investment is mixed. Most manufacturers provide the powder bulk quantities, but it also comes in premeasured packets (Figure 12-4) so the operator needs to measure only the water. However, the water *must* be measured. The investment generally is mixed in a power-driven vacuum mixer. The water is added to the bowl; then the powder is sprinkled into the water to eliminate air in the powder. The lid is applied to the bowl, and a vacuum is attached to remove air from the container so that it will not be incorporated during mixing. The entire apparatus is applied to the power mixer for the exact number of seconds specified by the manufacturer. Once mixed, the investment is poured slowly into the casting ring, taking extreme care to flow the investment around the wax pattern without forming bubbles or voids (see Figure 12-4). A vibrator often is used to

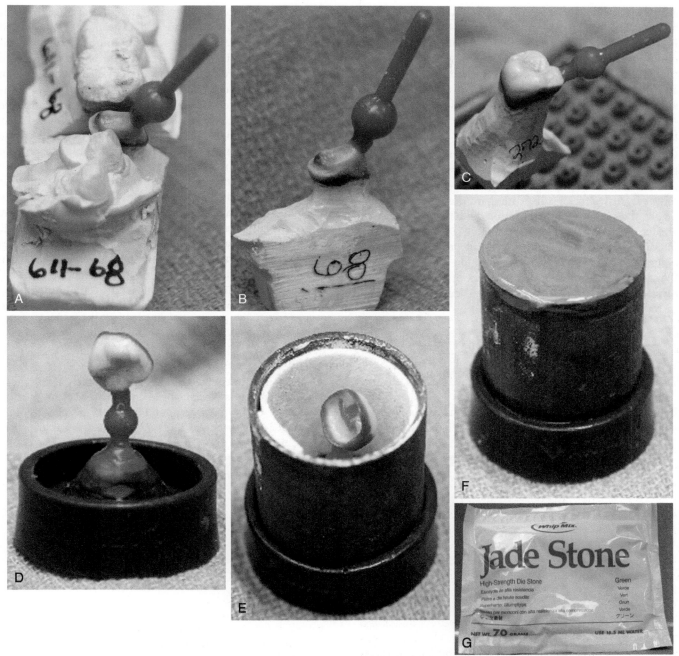

FIG 12-4 Sequence of steps for investing. Whether the wax pattern is a cut-back **(A** and **B)** or to full contour **(C),** a sprue is attached with wax onto a cuspal area that is least involved with the occlusal function of the tooth. The sprue is then attached to a rubber sprue base with wax **(D);** then a steel ring is placed onto the sprue base **(E).** A surfactant may be sprayed onto the wax pattern to improve the wettability of the pattern by the investment at this step. A ceramic liner is generally placed inside the ring to allow for investment expansion (see Figure 12-1). Finally, the investment is mixed under vacuum at a precise water–powder ratio **(F** and **G)** and carefully poured into the ring, embedding the wax pattern and sprue. Bubbles in the investment must be avoided during the pour. The investment must set for approximately 45 minutes before it is placed into the burnout oven in preparation for casting. (Courtesy M. Owens, C. S. Bemis, and D. E. Owens CDT, Georgia Regents University, Augusta, GA. Photography by R. Messer, Georgia Regents University, Augusta, GA.)

aid in the flow of the investment material and to eliminate bubbles. The investment is added until the casting ring is full. Because the wax pattern is dimensionally unstable once removed from the working die, the time taken to invest should be minimized but certainly should be less than 10 minutes. The invested wax pattern is allowed to set for at least 45 minutes but should not be allowed to desiccate.

Expansion of the Investment

Once the molten casting material freezes in the investment, the alloy shrinks as it cools from the solid state at a high temperature to room temperature (Figure 12-1). The shrinkage ranges from 1% to 2.5% depending on the type of alloy; the higher the melting temperature of the alloy (liquidus), the greater the shrinkage. Although 1% to 2.5% shrinkage seems minor, it is too large to ignore in a casting process that must be accurate to 20 μm. Without compensation for this shrinkage, the casting will be too small and will not fit the tooth. Casting investments are designed to expand to compensate for the casting material shrinkage.

> **! ALERT**
>
> Investments must expand to compensate for shrinkage of the casting material, or the casting will not fit the tooth.

Both hygroscopic and thermal mechanisms cause an investment to expand. Expansion of the binder from added water (from the addition of the water after the original water is added for mixing but before the investment sets) is called hygroscopic expansion, which is common with gypsum-bonded investments but also relevant to phosphate-bonded investments. Extra water allows the crystals of the gypsum or ammonium phosphate-magnesia binder to grow in a manner than promotes expansion. In an older procedure, the unset investment is submerged into a water bath immediately after it is poured into the casting ring, referred to as the "immersion technique." The immersion technique is seldom used today.

Investment expansion in response to temperature is referred to as thermal expansion. The silica refractory expands when heated because the crystals of the silica assume different lattice arrangements with greater volumes. The amount of thermal expansion may be regulated by the types of silica refractories used and the temperature used during burnout of the ring. All types of investments use thermal expansion to some extent. The total expansion of the investment is thus a sum of the hygroscopic and thermal expansions, but today's investments rely primarily on thermal expansion to compensate for casting shrinkage of the alloy (Figure 12-1).

Burnout

Once the investment has set (after approximately 45 minutes), the casting ring is placed, sprue end down, into an oven to burn out the wax pattern and sprue (Figures 12-1 and 12-5). It is important to understand that the wax does not

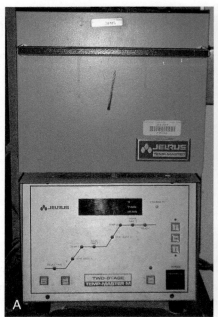 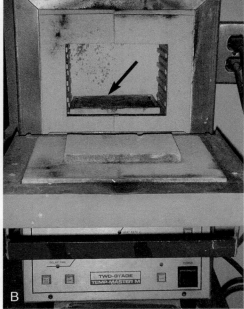

FIG 12-5 Burnout oven. The invested wax pattern (without the sprue base) is placed into an oven **(A)** to burn out the wax prior to casting. The oven maintains a temperature compatible with the investment used (600° to 900° C for alloys, higher for ceramics); this particular oven allows the operator to program several temperature–time combinations. The muffle (heated area) of the oven is in the upper half. When the oven door is opened **(B)**, the casting ring is placed into the central area of the muffle *(arrow)* to ensure even heating. Once the wax has burned out, the ring is ready to be cast with molten alloy or pressed with ceramic; the ring must not cool to any extent before casting or pressing.

simply melt but combusts to allow complete removal. After burnout, a space remains that was occupied by the wax pattern and sprue. The sprue thus forms a channel through which the molten casting material can flow to the space formerly occupied by the wax pattern. Burnout temperatures also cause thermal expansion of the investment (see the previous discussion). Finally, burnout provides temperature compatibility between the hot, molten casting material and the investment. If the molten casting material were cast into the investment at room temperature, the rapid change in temperature would likely crack the investment. This phenomenon is similar to the effect of pouring boiling water into a glass just removed from the freezer. The relatively cold investment also would cause the casting material to solidify prematurely before the restoration space was completely filled. A rule of thumb is that the melting temperature (liquidus) of an alloy should not be more than 500° C higher than the burnout temperature. Ceramics do not melt, per se, but must be fluid enough (hot enough) to press into all facets of the investment.

The temperature in the burnout oven is commonly 500° to 600° C, but it varies depending on the type of investment, the temperature of the casting material, and the amount of expansion needed. The length of burnout time depends on the size of the ring, the burnout temperature, the number of casting rings in the oven, and whether the oven was hot at the beginning of the burnout. Generally, at least 1 hour at full temperature is needed to completely eliminate wax from the ring and provide the necessary investment expansion. However, burnout times of up to 4 hours can be used, particularly for alloys with lower melting ranges. Once the casting ring and investment are heated, the ring should be cast before it cools to any degree; any delay of more than 20 to 30 seconds will severely compromise the fit and quality of the cast restoration. The thermal expansion of the investment is not reversible, and if the ring cools before it is cast, either the investment will crack or the casting will be distorted.

CASTING

Casting

Successful casting requires the coordination of the burnout of the ring, the melting of the casting alloy, and the manipulation of the casting machine. Most casting of alloys is done in a centrifugal casting machine (Figures 12-6 and 12-7). Centrifugal casting machines operate on the principle of centrifugal force, in which the molten material is accelerated outward by rapid spinning. This principle is similar to that used to spin the water out of wet clothing in the final cycle of a washing machine. The casting machine is driven with a spring or electric motor. Casting or pressing of ceramics often uses pressure instead of centrifugal force; discussion of these techniques is beyond the scope of this chapter. Subsequent discussion will focus casting alloys.

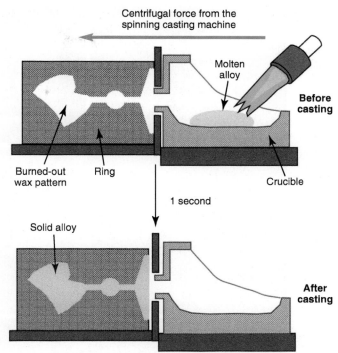

FIG 12-6 Schematic diagram of the alloy casting process. After burnout of the wax from the ring, the ring is moved from the burnout oven to the cradle in the casting machine *(left)*. At this point, the alloy has been melted with the torch in the crucible *(right)*, which remains in place to maintain the molten state. As soon as possible, the casting arm is released and the spinning force of the casting arm generates centrifugal force *(red arrow above)* that drives the molten alloy toward the ring. The molten metal is accelerated at high speeds (>600 km per hour!) into the ring in under a second. The torch is removed and the molten alloy freezes rapidly (1 to 2 seconds) to the solid state. The casting is then ready to devest. The process for pressing ceramics is similar in principle but uses different techniques and materials.

> **! ALERT**
>
> Casting takes less than 1 second, but the solidification of the casting material must occur in a specific pattern to avoid an unacceptable restoration.

The casting alloy is heated in a crucible made of heat-resistant ceramic (see Figures 12-6 and 12-7). A flux is usually added to minimize the formation of oxides that impair the heating and casting of the alloy and decrease the final quality of the casting. The type of flux used depends on the temperature of casting, the type of heat source used, the type of casting alloy, and the type of investment. When the alloy is completely molten, the casting ring is removed from the oven and is placed behind the crucible and the crucible–ring assembly is spun rapidly. Spinning accelerates the alloy into the casting ring and into the space previously occupied by the sprue and wax pattern. The process of casting takes less than 1 second.

Casting alloys may be heated by blowtorch or electric current. The most common method for heating low-temperature alloys (<1200° C) is by blowtorch. The blowtorch may

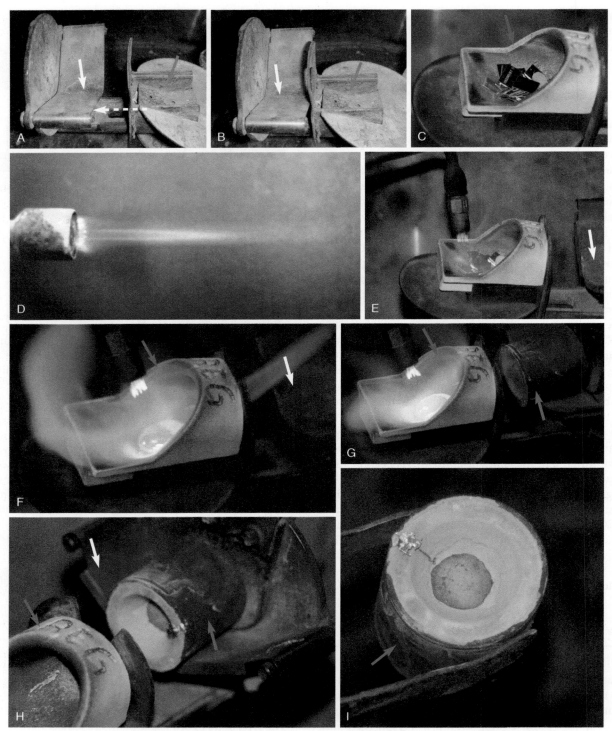

FIG 12-7 Casting alloys. The arm of the casting machine has a cradle to support the ring *(white arrows)* and a support to secure the crucible *(red arrows* in **A** and **B**). The crucible support slides *(white dashed arrow* in **A**) to place the crucible in close proximity to the ring **(B).** The alloy is added to the crucible itself *(green arrows)* **(C),** and the torch is adjusted to provide a large brushlike inner cone *(orange arrow* in **D**), indicating a reducing flame. The torch is applied **(E)** to gradually heat the alloy to its molten state **(F).** While the flame is maintained on the molten alloy, the ring *(blue arrows)* is added to the cradle **(G).** The casting arm is released, accelerating the molten metal into the ring **(H).** In only a few seconds, the alloy solidifies in the ring **(I)** and the casting is ready to be devested. Note that excess alloy is always used to ensure adequate mass to cast the restoration and acceleration force for casting. (Courtesy M. Owens, C. S. Bemis, and D. E. Owens CDT, Georgia Regents University, Augusta, GA. Photography by R. Messer, Georgia Regents University, Augusta, GA.)

operate on a combination of natural gas and compressed air or natural gas and oxygen (see Figure 12-6). The latter combination is hotter and is used for alloys that melt between 1100° and 1300° C. An electric current is used for higher temperatures, using a process called induction casting (also used for pressing ceramics). Regardless of the method used, the proper heating of the alloy is critical to a successful casting. If heated too little, the alloy will be too viscous to flow into all of the finest details of the casting ring. If heated too much, the alloy may be damaged by the oxidation of elements, or the investment may crack from thermal shock. When a blowtorch is used, the adjustment of the flame is critical to ensure the appropriate heating environment and rate.

After casting, the casting ring either is allowed to cool slowly on top of a bench or is submerged immediately in cold water. For some gold-based alloys, bench cooling produces a harder, stronger state of the alloy, and rapid cooling in water (also called quenching) produces a softer condition. For these alloys, the best type of cooling thus depends on the type of metal and whether the operator wants the casting in a hardened or softened condition. However, many types of alloys do not obey this principle. In either case, the casting is removed from the investment (devested) and rinsed with water. Investment that clings to the casting is removed with a toothbrush and water.

Pickling

Many times, a freshly cast alloy restoration will be covered with dark surface oxides. These oxides are easily removed from gold-based alloys by **pickling** the casting with an acidic solution. The casting is grasped with special insulated tongs and submerged for 5 to 10 seconds in a hot solution of phosphoric acid, potassium dichromate, and urea (Prevox). Protection from the acid, which can cause severe burns and blindness, is imperative. High-gold alloys are pickled in this manner, but acidic treatment of predominantly base-metal alloys will significantly corrode and damage them.

> **! ALERT**
>
> Pickling removes surface oxides on the casting alloy that formed during the casting process and makes polishing easier. Pickling is not used for ceramics.

FINISHING

After casting, devesting, and pickling (if applicable), a casting is ready to be finished and polished. The first finishing step is to remove the sprue from the restoration (Figure 12-8). The sprue is removed with a thin carborundum disk on a handpiece. Care must be taken not to scar the restoration with the disk in this step. Carborundum stones or green stones are then used to recontour the restoration if necessary. After the recontouring, the goal is to make the external surface of the restoration as smooth as possible. A variety of techniques are available, but all use a series of polishing steps to polish the surface with progressively finer abrasives (see Figure 12-8). Procedures and materials are distinctly different for ceramics

and alloys; polishing and finishing materials should also be used exclusively on one or the other of these types of restorations. For alloys, rubber wheels with impregnated abrasive generally are used first, and several stages of rubber wheel polishing may be used. Then tripoli and rouge polishing compounds may be applied (separately) on felt wheels or cloth wheels. Throughout the polishing procedure, the margins of the casting must be protected; even the slightest contact of abrasives with the margin of the restoration will irreparably damage it. The operator also must protect the proximal contact areas and occlusal contact areas. Overpolishing in any of these areas results in a restoration that will fail clinically and must be recast. Once polished, an alloy or ceramic restoration should have a high luster and be perfectly smooth (see Figure 12-8). Ceramic restorations may be glazed as a final step in the finishing process.

Supplementary Steps for Alloy-Based Restorations

Although inlays and full-coverage crowns are ready for cementation after the finishing and polishing, other types of restorations require additional steps before delivery to the patient. For example, ceramic–alloy crowns go through many steps to apply the ceramic (Chapter 14). Partial dentures generally need to have acrylic teeth bonded to them in specific areas and may need to have some clasps soldered onto the metal framework (Chapter 13). Implant restorations may need ceramic application. Finally, some castings require soldering or welding with other components to make them complete for use in the mouth (Figures 12-9 and 12-10, next sections). In all cases, the clinical success of these supplemental steps relies heavily on the quality of the initial casting.

SOLDERING

Solders are alloys used to join other alloys; joined alloys are referred to as **substrate alloys**. Dental solders join orthodontic wires to bands in the construction of a space maintainer, a clasp wire to a partial denture framework, two units of a fixed partial denture, or components of an implant substructure. Solders also may be used to restore a missing proximal contact or repair an occlusal defect on a crown. Technically, soldering operations occur below 425° C; brazing occurs above 425° C. Because all dental operations occur above 425° C, dental procedures mentioned earlier should be considered brazing but are nearly ubiquitously referred to as soldering.

> **! ALERT**
>
> Solders are alloys used to join other alloys for orthodontic, prosthetic, or implant restorations.

Most dental solders are either gold- or silver-based alloys that contain special elements such as tin or phosphorus to lower the melting range and increase flowability when molten. These elements are rarely present in dental casting alloys. Gold-based solders are used primarily to solder cast

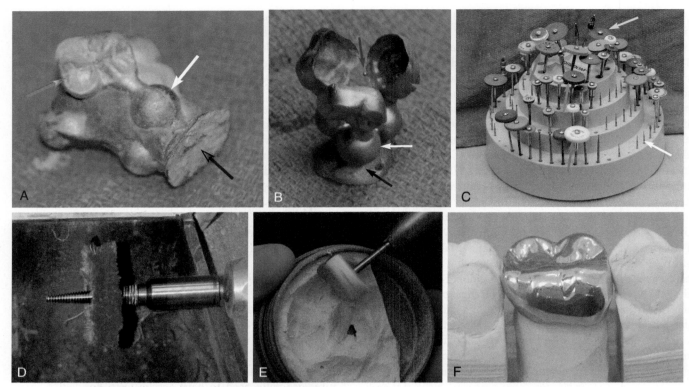

FIG 12-8 Finishing and polishing the casting. When the casting is removed from the investment, it is covered with residual investment and oxides **(A).** Note that in these photos, several crowns have been cast at the same time, a common practice in commercial labs. The residual investment is removed, the oxides are removed **(B),** and the castings (*red arrows* in **A** and **B**) are visible. The casting button (*black arrows* in **A** and **B**) and sprue (*white arrows* in **A** and **B**) will then be removed. The casting is inspected closely for voids or positives (*blue arrow* in **B**) that may or may not make it unacceptable for clinical use. If the casting is complete, it is polished using a variety of instruments. **C,** Carborundum disks (*yellow arrow*), rubber wheels with impregnated abrasives (*orange arrow*), burs (*white arrow*), and felt wheels (*green arrow*) are used. Polishing agents also may be applied on a rag wheel with a high-speed lathe **(D)** or handpiece **(E),** resulting in the finished restoration ready to cement **(F).** (**A–D,** Courtesy M. Owens, C. S. Bemis, and D. E. Owens CDT, Georgia Regents University Augusta, GA. Photography by R. Messer, Georgia Regents University, Augusta, GA. **E,** Courtesy Rich Lee, Department of Restorative Dentistry, University of Washington School of Dentistry, Seattle, WA.)

restorations such as bridges, whereas silver solders are used more for orthodontic applications. The manufacturers of the cast alloys generally specify the compatibility of solders with their alloys, and it is common for a manufacturer to offer a series of dental casting alloys and compatible solders together. The strength, hardness, and corrosion of dental solders also depend on the solder composition. Ideally, solders should have low corrosion, a low melting range, and high hardness and strength. Unfortunately, solders with a higher melting range, which are more difficult to use, are stronger and harder than lower fusing solders.

Solders have special properties that enable them to function successfully. The solder must melt (have a liquidus) below that of the solidus of the alloys to be soldered (substrate alloys). Put simply, if the substrate alloys melt at a lower temperature than the solder, then soldering will destroy the substrates. Solders must flow freely against the alloys to be soldered and must wet the alloys well (Figure 11-14). The ability to wet and flow onto the soldered alloy ensures a strong bond between the solder and substrate. Wetting and flow are functions of the composition of the solder and compatibility of that composition with the alloys to be soldered. The corrosion of a soldered material is also a concern. Because soldering creates, by definition, a junction between two or more different alloys, the risk of corrosion in the mouth is higher than if only one alloy were present. As with wetting, the composition of the solder and substrate alloys determines the corrosion properties of the combination.

Flux is nearly always used during the soldering process. Flux cleans the substrates and dissolves any surface oxides. For an alloy to be soldered successfully, its surface oxide must be eliminated to allow wetting and flowing of the solder on the substrate alloy surface. Fluxes come in pastes, liquids, or powders, but all serve the same purpose. A flux must be compatible with the alloy being soldered. Gold-based alloys generally use a borax-containing flux, whereas stainless steel or other

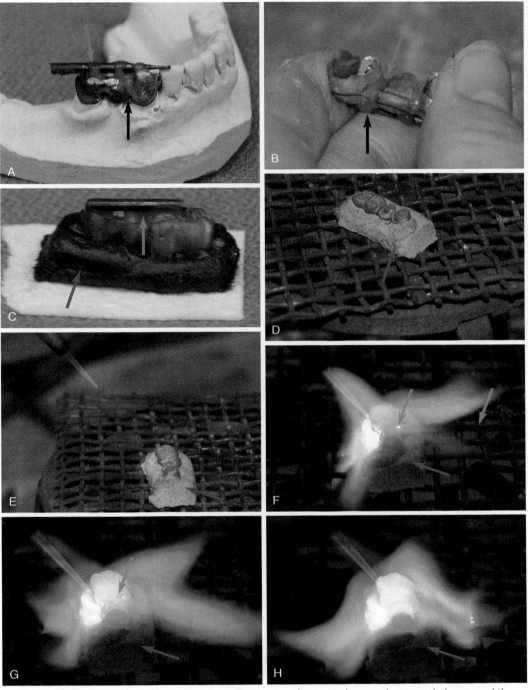

FIG 12-9 Soldering alloys. Sometimes, an alloy restoration must be cast in several pieces and then soldered together before cementation. In general, the pieces of the restoration are juxtaposed in the mouth and temporarily held together ("indexed") with sticky wax or a resin material. In these images, the juxtaposed pieces are shown on a master cast **(A)**. The final desired shape of the solder joints are then waxed **(B)**, followed by investment of the restoration into soldering investments (*blue arrows* in **C**). Once the investment has set, the wax and index are removed and the investment is placed onto a soldering stand **(D)**; flux paste is generally added at this point. A small reducing flame is gradually applied to the investment and restoration **(E)**, and then solder (*red arrows* in **F, G**) is added while maintaining the reducing atmosphere of the flame. Heating continues until the ball of solder (*red arrow* in **G**) flows into the solder joint **(H)**. At this point the temperature of the castings is about 50 to 100° C below the melting point of the alloy, so the heat must be removed to prevent damage to the castings. It is significant to note that with all-ceramic restorations, soldering is not possible. (Courtesy M. Owens, C. S. Bemis, and D. E. Owens CDT, Georgia Regents University, Augusta, GA. Photography by R. Messer, Georgia Regents University, Augusta, GA.)

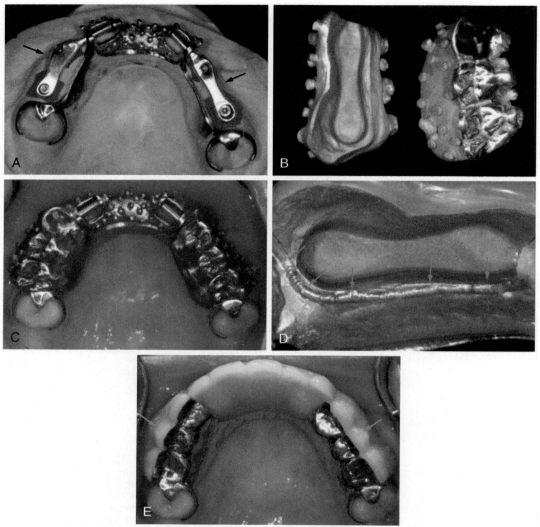

FIG 12-10 Welding. In this patient, the "bite" (vertical dimension) had collapsed over the years, leaving inadequate interarch room for the maxillary partial denture framework and acrylic posterior teeth (**A,** areas marked by black arrows). To solve this problem, alloy teeth (stronger and thinner than the acrylic option) were cast **(B):** at the left is the tissue side of the casting; at right are the occlusal surfaces. **(C)** The cast pieces are positioned in the mouth onto the framework and indexed (red material), which holds them in precise position relative to the framework. **(D)** A laser welding machine is used to seal the cast teeth to the framework *(red arrows)*. In this case, soldering such a long joint would be nearly impossible. The laser welding allows control of the heat applied to and location of the welded area. **(E)** The welded partial denture is seated in the mouth. Note that acrylic has been bonded to the anterior areas and buccals of the posteriors *(blue arrows)*. (Courtesy Y-W Chen, University of Washington Department of Restorative Dentistry, Seattle, WA.)

base metals require a potassium fluoride-containing flux. The type of flux required depends on the metallurgy and chemistry of the substrate alloy and its oxide layer.

Soldering begins with cleaning and positioning of the substrate alloys. Typically, the pieces to be joined are held in place using a gypsum product called soldering investment (see Figure 12-9). A flux is added to the substrate; then the alloys are heated slowly until the melting range of the solder is reached. At this point, the solder is added, and if all conditions are correct, it will flow onto the surface of the substrate alloys. Heating is accomplished using a blowtorch (most common), a burnout oven, or a laser.

Technically, soldering is art requiring immense skill and experience. The increase in the types and compositions of substrate alloys since the late 1990s has only made the soldering process more complex. Furthermore, the increasing use of ceramic–alloy restorations poses significant challenges; the solidus of the substrate, liquidus of the solder, and sintering temperature of the ceramic must all be balanced. If the metal substructure is soldered prior to ceramic application (presoldering), then the solder cannot melt during firing of the ceramic. If the metal substructure is soldered after the ceramic is applied (postsoldering), then the heat used during soldering must not damage the color or other properties of the ceramic.

WELDING

Welding is distinct from soldering; welded components do not generally use a second alloy (solder) to join components. Rather, the components are pre-positioned (or indexed, as in soldering); then a high-energy source is focused on the area to be joined. Lasers are commonly employed for this purpose and are often positioned and guided through a microscope. The high energy melts the alloys locally such that they fuse with one another (Figure 12-10) without distorting the bulk of the joined components. As welding does not involve another alloy, the risk of electrochemical corrosion is minimized. However, the fusion of the components in the joint often forms a hybrid alloy due to vaporization of components or changes induced from high temperature. Because of this, the risk of corrosion of welded joints is somewhat higher than the component alloys joined.

> **! ALERT**
>
> Welding joins components by locally fusing them through the application of focused high energy, often from a laser.

Welding does not require flames and is far more precise than soldering. It also is possible to weld alloys that are exceptionally difficult to solder (titanium alloys, for example). However, the equipment for welding is expensive and relatively complex to use. Furthermore, the ability to weld an alloy is greatly dependent on the type of alloy. In recent years, welding has increased in popularity along with the growth of titanium alloy use and implantology.

> **↻ QUICK REVIEW**
>
> Casting is a process by which a wax pattern of a dental restoration is converted into alloy or ceramic. The casting process is extremely accurate but requires strict attention to detail. The lost-wax technique is used to fabricate most cast restorations in dentistry; machining is increasing as an alternative method. Casting occurs in several steps. First, a sprue is added to the finished wax pattern that forms a channel through which the molten casting material will flow. Next, the pattern and sprue are invested in a casting ring, and the wax and sprue are burned out in an oven. The investment thus contains a space in the exact shape of the original wax pattern. Next, the alloy or ceramic is melted and accelerated into the casting ring by centrifugal force or application of high pressure. After the casting solidifies, the investment is removed, and alloy castings may be pickled to remove any surface oxides formed during casting. The sprue is then removed, and the casting is polished, taking care to preserve the occlusal and proximal contact areas. In some alloy restorations such as ceramic–alloy crowns, the casting is processed further before delivery to the patient. In still others, solders are used to join or repair cast components of the restoration. Welding also joins component alloys but does not require a second alloy. Ceramics are not soldered or welded.

> **? SELF-TEST QUESTIONS**

In the following multiple-choice questions, one or more responses may be correct.

1. Once the wax pattern has been created, which procedures will give acceptable results?
   a. Store at room temperature for 24 hours to allow any distortion to occur before investing.
   b. Store in a refrigerator but warm to room temperature before investing.
   c. Store in a refrigerator and invest when cold.
   d. Invest immediately.
2. Which statements about gypsum-bonded investments is/are true?
   a. The binder is calcium sulfate hemihydrate, and the refractory is a form of silica.
   b. The investment powder must be mixed with a special liquid supplied by the manufacturer.
   c. The components of the investment must be proportioned accurately to obtain a suitable casting.
   d. The investment may be mixed mechanically under a vacuum to reduce porosity in the set investment.
3. Why is the investment heated before casting?
   a. To increase the hygroscopic expansion of the investment
   b. To expand the investment
   c. To eliminate the wax pattern from the investment

4. Which of the following describe(s) phosphate-bonded investments?
   a. The powder contains only ammonium phosphate and magnesium oxide.
   b. Phosphate investments are weaker than gypsum investments.
   c. Phosphate-bonded investments are used with high-fusing gold- and palladium-based alloys and base-metal alloys.
5. Precautions to consider when pickling include
   a. Avoid contact between the casting and metal tweezers in pickling acid.
   b. Protect eyes, skin, and clothing from pickling acids.
   c. After pickling, carefully rinse acid from the casting with water.

Use short statements to answer the following questions.

6. Two technicians make all-alloy crowns. Technician A adds the sprue to the wax pattern when it is on the working die, whereas technician B adds the sprue to the pattern after it is removed from the working die. Which technician is most likely to have a well-fitting casting and why?
7. A sprue is designed for a wax pattern that is too long and narrow. What consequence is this design likely to have on the success of the casting process?
8. By mistake, a technician invests a wax pattern in pure gypsum rather than a gypsum-bonded investment. What are the consequences?

9. An invested ring is submerged in water immediately after investing. The ring then is heated to 600° C during burnout. What can you predict about the fit of the crown?

10. A technician burns out a ring for casting but does not have time to cast the ring at the end of the day. So the technician removes the ring from the burnout oven and reheats the ring again the next day before proceeding with the casting. When the technician breaks the investment away, the technician notices large fins (thin metal extensions from the casting) on the casting. What caused the fins? What can you predict about the fit of the casting?

11. A dentist receives a crown from a dental lab. On trying it in the patient, the dentist notes that the crown is missing a distal contact. Assuming that the position of the teeth has not changed, what were the possible causes of this problem related to the casting process? How can this problem be remedied?

12. The dentist tries in a crown and makes occlusal and proximal adjustments. The auxiliary repolishes the crown, and on reinsertion, the casting has no proximal contacts. What were the possible causes? What can be done about this problem?

13. The dentist tries in a casting in the mouth and notes that the cast seats incompletely. Assuming that the proximal contacts are not preventing seating, what are the possible sources of this problem related to the casting process?

For the following questions, select the one best answer.

14. Wax is the only material from which a casting sprue can be made.
    a. True
    b. False

15. When should the investing of a wax pattern be done?
    a. Within 24 hours of finishing the wax up
    b. Within 48 hours of finishing the wax up
    c. Only after the wax is warmed to body temperature
    d. As soon as possible after the wax up is completed

16. The two most common types of investments for casting are which of the following?
    a. Gypsum bonded and silica bonded
    b. Gypsum bonded and phosphate bonded
    c. Silica bonded and calcium bonded
    d. Phosphate bonded and calcium bonded

17. Pickling is the process of preserving the casting after it cools to room temperature.
    a. True
    b. False

18. The primary shrinkage that must be accommodated for in the casting process comes from which of the following materials?
    a. Wax
    b. Investment
    c. Casting alloy
    d. Gypsum

19. To be sure that the casting alloy has a sufficiently low viscosity for casting, slightly overheating the alloy when casting is always better.
    a. True
    b. False

20. The pathway for the molten casting alloy to reach the invested wax pattern is formed by the:
    a. Crucible
    b. Casting ring
    c. Ceramic liner
    d. Sprue

21. All-ceramic restorations can be fabricated using the lost-wax technique.
    a. True
    b. False

22. Welding generally uses a secondary alloy to join substrate alloys.
    a. True
    b. False

23. Soldering can be accomplished with a flame, an oven, or a laser.
    a. True
    b. False

24. All-ceramic restorations can be soldered and welded.
    a. True
    b. False

25. All alloys can be soldered.
    a. True
    b. False

SUGGESTED SUPPLEMENTARY READING

Mackert JR: An expert system for analysis of casting failures, *Int J Prosthodont* 1:268, 1988.

evolve   Please visit *http://evolve.elsevier.com/Powers/dentalmaterials* for additional practice and study support tools.

13

Polymers in Prosthodontics

OBJECTIVES

After reading this chapter, the student should be able to:

1. Describe a polymerization reaction and how the properties of monomers compare with those of polymers.
2. Explain why by-products or residual monomer from a polymerization reaction may be a clinical liability in dentistry.
3. Explain how free-radical polymerization is initiated for dental polymers.
4. Describe what polymer cross-linking is, how it is created, and its importance to the clinical performance of dental polymers.
5. Describe how copolymers are formed, give several examples of copolymers in dentistry, and explain why they are important clinically.
6. Describe how a complete denture is made and how the processing methods affect the physical properties of the denture.
7. Describe the properties of poly(methyl methacrylate) that are most important to the clinical performance of a dental prosthesis.
8. Correlate the recommendations for the care of dentures with the properties of poly(methyl methacrylate).
9. Explain how soft liners are formed on a denture, why they are used, what types are available, and how long each type can be expected to last in service.
10. Explain how acrylic polymers are bonded to alloys to form combination prostheses.
11. Describe the nature of polymers used in denture teeth and how the properties of the polymer network are controlled to ensure the best clinical service; explain why ceramic denture teeth are rarely used today.
12. Aside from denture construction, describe other uses of polymers in prosthodontics, and explain how the properties of polymers are exploited to facilitate these uses.

> **! ALERT**
>
> Polymers play important roles in many areas of dentistry, and their roles are increasing.

Polymers are nearly ubiquitous in dentistry and widely used in prosthodontics, primarily for removable prostheses such as complete or partial dentures (Figure 13-1). However, polymers also are used for denture teeth, impression trays, temporary crowns, and maxillofacial prostheses. Prosthodontic polymers have specific compositions and physical and chemical properties to ensure appropriate clinical performance, but the properties of these polymers overlap to some extent with those used for direct esthetic restorative materials (Chapter 4), mouth protectors (Chapter 3), impression materials (Chapter 8), and cements (Chapter 7). This chapter focuses on the properties and manipulation techniques that are most critical to polymers used in fixed, removable, and maxillofacial prosthodontics.

Some prosthodontic polymers may not be manipulated in the dental office. For example, many of the fabrication steps of a removable complete or partial denture occur in a dental laboratory. Yet all members of the dental team need a basic knowledge of these materials. This knowledge ensures effective communication among dental office staff, patients, the dentist, and the laboratory personnel—resulting in optimal patient care. Furthermore, the dental auxiliary may be asked to manipulate other polymers for temporary crowns, impression trays, orthodontic appliances, preventive restorations, or cements. Thus, knowledge of prosthodontic polymers is paramount.

POLYMERIZATION

Polymerization chemically links small organic compounds called monomers into long chains of repeating monomer ("mer") subunits (Figure 13-2). A single polymer chain commonly contains 10,000 to 100,000 linked monomer subunits. Because polymerized chains have molecular weights thousands of times greater than their parent monomers, the physical and chemical properties of polymers are always distinct from monomers. For example, methyl methacrylate, a common monomer used to make complete dentures, is a liquid that boils at about 100° C. Yet poly(methyl methacrylate) (PMMA) polymers (composed of methyl methacrylate monomer) never boil but are rigid solids that decompose before they even melt! The simplest polymers consist of many long chains that behave much like long strands of spaghetti. In the simplest case, each polymer strand is not chemically linked to the other, but the strands entangle to create a polymer network that gives the polymer its particular physical properties (see Figure 13-2).

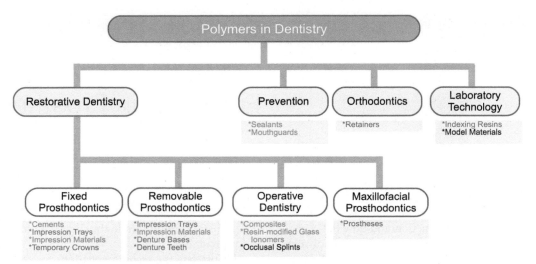

FIG 13-1 The role of polymers in dentistry continues to expand. Polymers are used for diverse applications including fixed, removable, and maxillofacial prosthodontics; orthodontics; preventive dentistry; operative dentistry; and laboratory technology. Applications in blue text are discussed in this chapter; those in orange text are discussed in other chapters.

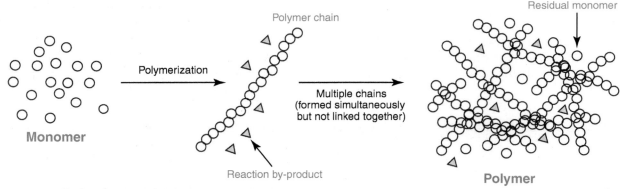

FIG 13-2 Polymerization is a chemical reaction that links a starting compound, a monomer, into long chains of repeating monomer units, a polymer chain. The polymer chains formed by polymerization entangle with one another but in the simplest case are not themselves linked together. These entangled chains form the polymer. Depending on the type of reaction, polymerization may produce by-products that are initially trapped in the polymer. Furthermore, not all monomer reacts, leaving residual monomer trapped in the polymer. Both residual monomer and reaction by-products may have negative clinical consequences because they may leach out of the polymer into the oral cavity over time, potentially affecting oral tissues and changing the clinical properties of the polymer itself.

> **! ALERT**
>
> Polymerization is the process of chemically linking many small monomers together to form a large polymer that has advantageous clinical properties quite different from those of the monomer.

The chemical nature of a monomer greatly influences the properties of its resulting polymer. Each monomer has at least one chemical group that participates in the polymerization reaction but may have other chemical groups that influence the polymer to be flexible, rigid, or water absorbing. For a number of complex reasons, not all monomers may be able to participate in the polymerization reaction, and any unreacted residual monomer in the polymer may have significant clinical consequences. For example, residual monomer may cause allergic reactions or chemical "burns." The extent to which all monomer is converted to polymer is the degree of conversion. Polymers with high degrees of conversion have low levels of residual monomer; a high degree of conversion is generally desirable clinically.

The chemical reactions during polymerization may produce by-products such as water, hydrogen gas, or alcohols (see Figure 13-2). Because these by-products are at least temporarily trapped in the polymer network, they are important to the physical nature of the polymer. For example, some impression material polymers form volatile alcohol by-products shrink as the alcohol evaporates from the polymer network over a period of hours. Shrinkage may or may not be important to the performance of a dental prosthesis. The nature of the polymerization reaction also regulates dimensional changes during polymerization. If a monomer expands as it links to other monomers, then the polymer may not shrink as much as a monomer that loses mass by formation of a by-product. Most prosthodontic polymers used in dentistry shrink significantly as polymerization proceeds, and shrinkage generally has negative clinical consequences.

All chains in a polymer network are not of identical length. As polymerization proceeds, monomer is consumed by thousands of growing chains, each adding monomer units independently of the other. Each polymer chain will grow until monomer is no longer accessible, but the number of monomer units will be somewhat different for each chain. Thus, in a polymer network, the chains will have a distribution of sizes. The extent to which monomer is converted into polymer is called the degree of polymerization (to be distinguished from the degree of conversion, discussed previously). Polymers with a high degree of polymerization have fewer polymer chains that are longer (on average); those with a lower degree of polymerization have more polymer chains, but each is shorter. The degree of polymerization influences the physical properties of a polymer because shorter strands interact differently from longer strands in the polymer network. As a rule of thumb, high degrees of polymerization lead to more rigid, less soluble polymer networks, which is desirable in clinical applications.

Methyl Methacrylate, Acrylic Polymers (PMMA), and Free-Radical Polymerization

In prosthodontics, acrylic polymers are a major class of polymers used for complete dentures, portions of removable partial dentures, maxillofacial prostheses, temporary crowns, custom impression trays, and denture teeth. Acrylic polymers also are used in orthodontic appliances and in several laboratory procedures in casting and soldering (for example, indexing resins). Acrylic polymers are formed through free-radical polymerization. Free-radical polymerization uses monomers that have a carbon–carbon double bond as their reactive group. The most common acrylic monomer is methyl methacrylate, but hydroxyethyl methacrylate and butyl methacrylate also are common in dentistry. Methyl methacrylate is a sweet-smelling liquid that boils at 100° C. The odor of methyl methacrylate is present in many dental laboratories, but chronic inhalation should be avoided because of potential toxicity to the liver. Methyl methacrylate also is highly flammable and allergenic. The careers of dentists and dental auxiliaries have ended when they developed a severe allergy to this chemical.

Addition polymerization of methyl methacrylate to form poly(methyl methacrylate) (PMMA, acrylic) begins when a free radical (a highly reactive molecule with a free electron) is formed. Free radicals can be formed in a number of ways (Figure 13-3). The free radical attacks the carbon double bond of the monomer and initiates a series of reactions of monomer additions. For this reason, free radicals are commonly referred to as initiators. The free-radical reaction rapidly adds methyl methacrylate molecules in this manner (thousands per second!), one after the other. In this fashion, the polymer chain grows until no more monomer is available. When accessible monomer is depleted, the last free radical "terminates" via one of several complex reactions, and polymerization is complete. Some monomer cannot be added to the polymer chains and becomes trapped in the polymer as residual monomer.

Acrylic free-radical polymerization is distinctive because it produces no reaction by-products. Because no by-product is formed, this type of polymerization is called addition polymerization; monomer units are added to the growing

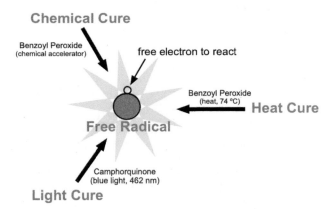

FIG 13-3 Free radicals *(center)* are highly reactive chemicals that initiate polymerization of acrylic polymers (poly[methyl methacrylate]). The reactivity of these chemicals stems from a free electron that is formed in three basic ways in dentistry. Benzoyl peroxide is used in denture base polymers to generate free radicals by either heating (so-called heat cure) or by adding a chemical accelerator (so-called chemical cure) to form the radical. Both types of these strategies are used in dentistry, particularly in the construction of removable complete and partial dentures. A third strategy is to irradiate a chemical such as camphorquinone with blue light (so-called light cure). Light causes the camphorquinone to decompose to form the initiating free radical. Light cure strategies are used in some prosthodontic polymers but are most common in polymers used for direct restorative materials (see Chapter 4) or preventive materials (see Chapter 3).

polymer. Addition polymerization reactions are used to form other dental polymers in impression materials (Chapter 8), restorative composites (Chapter 4), and cements (Chapter 7). Addition polymerization is preferred clinically because, without reaction by-products, there is no risk of leaching of the by-product intraorally, which can increase shrinkage of the polymer or toxic reactions to the patient. In spite of the absence of reaction products, acrylics have significant polymerization reaction shrinkage, approaching 6 vol%. This degree of polymerization shrinkage poses significant problems for the fit of dental prostheses and temporary crowns (see later sections). The free-radical polymerization reaction also is highly exothermic, which means that heat is generated during polymerization. Heat generation is so great that it can boil unreacted methyl methacrylate, creating porosity in the final polymer. In the laboratory, steps must be taken to avoid this porosity. Heat generated during the fabrication of temporary crowns may burn adjacent tissues or even damage the pulp of the tooth!

Cross-Linking, Copolymers, Plasticizers, and Fillers

In PMMA (acrylic) polymers, each polymer strand is chemically unbonded to the other (see Figure 13-2). However, the physical and chemical properties of the polymer can be markedly changed if the polymer strands are linked together. Such linkages are called cross-links (Figure 13-4). The cross-links are created by adding a cross-linking agent to the monomer before polymerization occurs. The degree of cross-linking may be controlled by the amount of cross-linking agent added

to the monomer. Cross-linked acrylic polymers are more rigid, more temperature resistant, and less soluble than their uncross-linked counterparts. In dentistry, cross-linking improves wear resistance and susceptibility to organic solvents in foods containing ethanol (e.g., wine). Cross-linked acrylics also are easier to grind and polish. Cross-linked polymers are used in acrylic denture teeth and direct esthetic restorative materials (Chapter 4). They also have been used occasionally in some dentures to increase fracture resistance in patients prone to denture failure because of heavy biting forces or occupational activities (e.g., contact sports).

> **! ALERT**
>
> Cross-linking during polymerization changes the properties of polymers by chemically linking polymer chains together. Linked chains are more rigid, providing more stability for a dental prosthesis during use, and are resistant to dietary "solvents" such as wine.

The acrylics discussed so far are homopolymers—that is, the polymer strands contain only one type of monomer. However, it is possible to use more than one type of monomer in a free-radical polymerization reaction (Figure 13-5, *lower diagram*). Polymers that have two or more types of monomers in their polymer network are called copolymers. When polymerization proceeds, the two monomers are randomly incorporated into the polymer strands. There also are methods to control the order of monomer addition (such as block polymer formation), but these strategies are beyond the scope of this discussion.

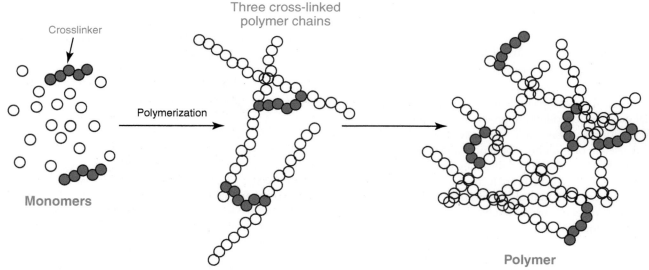

FIG 13-4 Several polymers in dentistry use a phenomenon called cross-linking in the polymerization process. In this case, a cross-linking agent is added to the monomer. The cross-linker is a small molecule and is difunctional, meaning that each end of the molecule can be polymerized into a different polymer chain. The net effect is a web of polymer chains that are all linked together. Cross-linking has profound effects on the melting temperature, strength, and flexibility of polymers. In prosthodontics it is used in denture teeth to increase resistance of the teeth to degradation from solvents in foods such as alcohol and to increase the rigidity of the teeth to provide a more solid biting sense for the patient. Cross-linking is common in polymers for composite restorations (see Chapter 4).

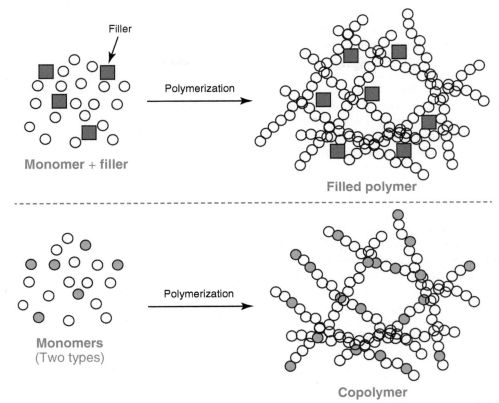

FIG 13-5 *(Upper diagram)* Prosthodontic polymers are commonly filled with a solid phase that does not participate in the polymerization reaction but changes the properties of the polymer. For example, fillers are used in denture acrylic polymers to add opacity, color, strength, wear resistance, and decreased water sorption. The filler may or may not be chemically linked to the polymer chains. *(Lower diagram)* Some dental polymers use two or more different monomers to form a copolymer. The occurrence of the two monomers is generally random in the polymer chains. Copolymers are used to optimize polymer properties. A common application is in polymers for mouthguards, denture bases with altered properties, or composite materials.

> **! ALERT**
>
> Copolymers contain two or more different monomers, which creates different polymer properties to optimize the clinical success of dental prostheses. Copolymers are used in dentures, mouth protectors, and restorative composites.

Copolymers are fabricated to modify the physical and chemical properties of the polymer network. For example, in **denture bases**, copolymerization of the monomers methyl methacrylate and butyl methacrylate results in a copolymer that is more fracture resistant. Addition of comonomers such as octyl methacrylate makes the copolymer soft and flexible, and these copolymers are used for denture soft liners. Addition of hydroxyethyl methacrylate increases the wettability of the polymer by water and improves complete denture retention in a patient with xerostomia (dry mouth). Copolymers also are common in direct esthetic restorative materials (Chapter 4) or mouth protector materials (Chapter 3). For example, a vinyl acetate-ethylene copolymer is used for mouth protectors to maximize energy absorption and prevent the energy of facial trauma from being transferred to the oral structures.

On occasion, chemicals called **plasticizers** are added to a polymer that do not participate in the polymerization reaction and do not become part of the polymer strands, yet are trapped in the polymer network. These chemicals are used to modify the physical properties of the polymer. For example, liquid oils such as dibutyl phthalate will cause a PMMA to become rubbery. Plasticizers dissolve into the polymer network and modify the interactions between the polymer strands. Plasticizers are most often used in polymer networks that are not cross-linked. Often, the polymer will expand when plasticized as the chemical dissolves into the network. Plasticizers are used in dentistry to soften polymers for denture soft liners. However, because plasticizers are not chemically linked to the polymer network, they leach out of the polymer over time, and their effect on the polymer network is lost. For this reason, denture soft liners harden with time, requiring periodic replacement. The effect of the released plasticizer on oral tissues must also be considered.

> **! ALERT**
>
> Plasticizers are liquids that are not part of the polymer chains but soften the polymer and make it more flexible. Fillers are particles that are often bonded to the polymer network to increase strength, reduce water sorption, or change the color or transparency of the polymer.

Fillers are solid particles added to polymers to change their optical or physical properties (Figure 13-5, *upper diagram*).

Denture polymers are sometimes filled with small particles of butadiene-styrene rubber (itself a copolymer) to increase the resistance of the PMMA to fracture. Because filled denture bases have impact strengths of twice that of unfilled bases, these modified polymers are used in patients who have a history of denture base fracture. Inorganic fillers such as glass particles are added to PMMA to give the polymer color or change its handling properties during fabrication. For example, impression tray materials are filled to give the setting polymer a heavy dough-like consistency. The shape and thickness of the tray are then controllable as the material is formed onto a working cast to make the impression tray. Without the filler, the setting polymer would be too runny and sticky. Filler also improves the working consistency of elastomeric dental impression materials (Chapter 8), and it is used to modify the esthetic and wear properties of direct restorative materials (Chapter 4).

Fillers may be chemically linked into the polymer network. This strategy is used to maximize the ability of the filler to strengthen the polymer network, and these polymers have better wear resistance. The advantage of chemically linked fillers is that they cannot easily be dislodged from the polymer network by oral forces such as chewing. This strategy also minimizes polymerization shrinkage. Chemicals called coupling agents are used to link the filler to the polymer. Chemically linked fillers are used in light-activated impression tray materials and denture repair materials.

COMPLETE DENTURES

Complete dentures and partial dentures use filled PMMA (acrylic), uncross-linked homopolymers for the denture base, chemically bonded to denture teeth made of filled, cross-linked acrylic homopolymers. In this section, we first describe the process of complete denture fabrication and the options available for processing the denture. We then discuss the physical and chemical properties of acrylic polymers that influence clinical performance of the denture and how inappropriate care of the denture by the patient or the dental auxiliary may adversely affect dentures. Knowledge of this process enhances the ability of the auxiliary to aid chairside as well as in the laboratory and in communication to the patient.

> **! ALERT**
>
> Complete dentures are constructed of acrylic polymers using chemical- or heat-cured polymerization techniques. This process is the basis for the construction of many dental prostheses and is therefore considered in-depth here.

Fabrication of Complete Dentures: An Overview

Complete dentures are fabricated in a rather complex series of steps over several appointments with the patient (Figures 13-6 and 13-7). Initially, a preliminary alginate impression is made, and preliminary working models are poured in dental stone. From these preliminary models, a custom impression tray is fabricated from a filled PMMA polymer (custom impression trays, often light-cured), and this tray is used to obtain the final impression using an elastomeric material in

a second appointment. The final impression is poured in dental stone to obtain the master cast on which the denture will be constructed. Record bases are then made from unfilled PMMA, and a wax rim is added. This record base–wax rim combination serves as a trial denture that is used to determine jaw relations and tooth position for the final denture. The master casts are mounted on an articulator to capture the patient's upper and lower jaw relationship, and the acrylic denture teeth are selected (Figure 13-8) and set into the wax rim. The esthetic and functional positions of the teeth are verified by inserting the record bases–wax rims into the patient's mouth, and the teeth are moved as necessary to finalize esthetics, speech, and occlusion.

Once the final position of the teeth is determined clinically, the record base–wax rim is sealed onto the master cast with wax, and each denture (with the acrylic teeth in place) is invested with gypsum in a metal flask (see Figures 13-6 and 13-7). After the investment has set, the flask is opened, and the wax is softened using boiling water, referred to as "boil out." The record base, now loose, is removed and discarded. The denture teeth remain, locked into the gypsum investment. The mixed but unpolymerized denture acrylic is then "packed" into the space formerly occupied by the record bases and wax. The flask is reassembled, and any excess base material is removed (referred to as "trial packing"). Polymerization is initiated either chemically or by heat (see Figures 13-3 and 13-9). After polymerization is complete, the flask is opened, and the denture is removed from the master cast and polished (Figure 13-10). The denture is adjusted and delivered at a final appointment with the patient.

> **! ALERT**
>
> Dentures are fabricated in a dental laboratory, but many important steps in this process are completed by the dental team with the patient present. Understanding this process improves the ability of office staff to assist the dentist, explain the procedure to the patient, and improve patient outcomes.

Manipulation of Poly(Methyl Methacrylate) in Complete Denture Construction

Most dentures are made using a PMMA homopolymer that is filled but not cross-linked (see Figures 13-2 and 13-4). PMMA materials are usually powder–liquid systems, and both the powder and liquid contain multiple components (see Figure 13-9). The polymerization of the material may be initiated either by chemicals or more commonly by heat. For custom trays or record bases, the light-activated materials are often used. In heat-cured systems, the powder contains small spheres of prepolymerized PMMA, a benzoyl peroxide initiator (see Figure 13-3), ceramic oxide to add translucency, inorganic pigments for color, and small colored fibers to mimic blood vessels. The liquid contains methyl methacrylate monomer and traces of an inhibitor (hydroquinone) to prevent inappropriate polymerization by room light (the monomer also is stored in dark-colored bottles to prevent light exposure). When the powder and liquid are mixed, the monomer dissolves into the prepolymerized PMMA spheres, and

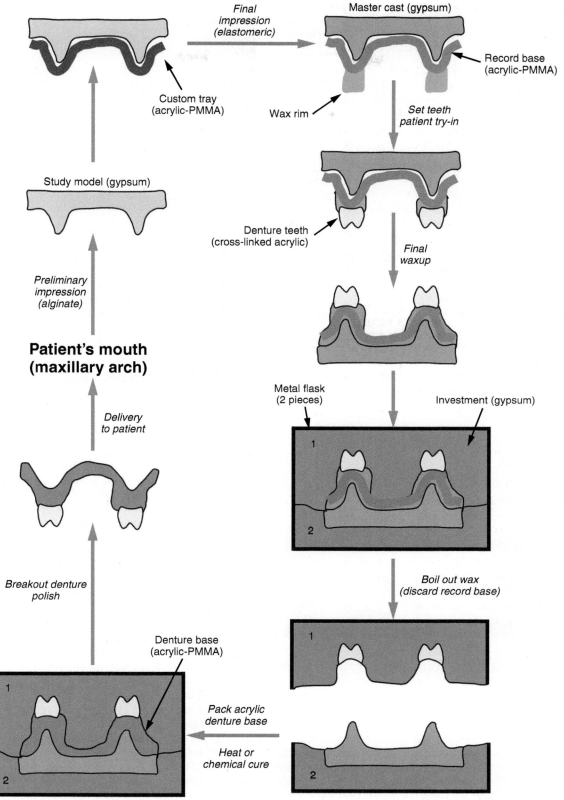

FIG 13-6 Construction of a complete denture diagrammatically showing key steps. A complete explanation is in the legend to Figure 13-7.

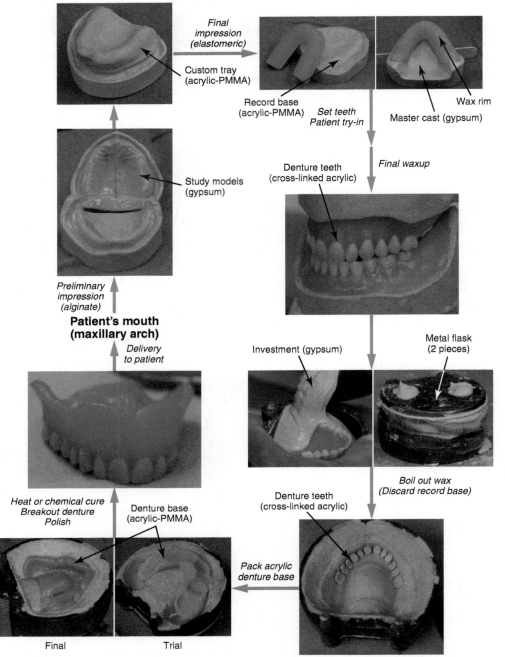

FIG 13-7 Construction of a complete denture begins by taking a preliminary alginate impression of the patient's residual edentulous ridges in the mouth. *(Note that construction of a maxillary denture is shown here.)* From the preliminary impression, a study model is poured in gypsum, and a custom tray (made from acrylic polymers or light-cured dimethacrylate polymers) is prepared. In a second appointment, a final impression is taken, and the master cast (separate from the study model) is poured in gypsum. A record base (made of acrylic polymer) is constructed on the master cast, and wax rims are added. Plastic denture teeth (made of cross-linked acrylic polymer) are added in the wax, and their position is checked by inserting the record base/tooth provisional restoration into the patient's mouth. When all teeth are satisfactorily positioned, the record base is waxed onto the master cast, and the master cast and waxup are invested with gypsum in a metal flask. The flask is then boiled in water and the flask separated. The wax and record base are removed, but the teeth and master cast remain locked in the investment. Denture resin material is then packed into the space formerly occupied by the record base and wax, and the flask is reassembled and heated to cure the polymer completely. After curing, the flask is disassembled, and the denture is removed (called "breakout"), polished, and delivered to the patient for final adjustments. (Photos courtesy M. Adams, D. Idels, and J. Nalley, Georgia Regents University, Augusta, GA. Photography by R. Messer, Georgia Regents University, Augusta, GA.)

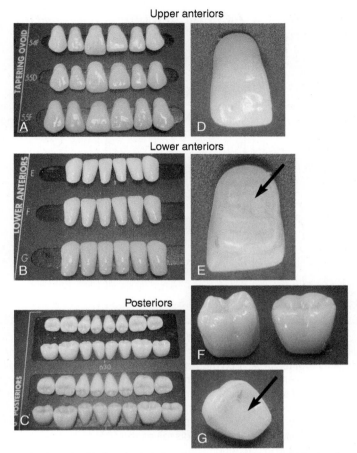

FIG 13-8 Polymer denture teeth for dental prostheses. **A–C,** Upper anterior, lower anterior, and posterior teeth are available in different shapes (moulds) and sizes. Teeth are selected to fit the patient's edentulous arch and for esthetics. In addition, different shades are available. Anterior teeth have highly characterized facial surfaces for a lifelike appearance **(D).** Occlusal surfaces of teeth are highly cross-linked to decrease wear. Anterior and posterior teeth have a surface (*black arrows* in **E** and **G**) that is not cross-linked to promote bonding to the acrylic base. Posterior teeth are available with different types of cusps **(F)** to allow different types of occlusions to be designed.

the mixture progresses through a series of consistencies. In heat-cured systems, these changes in consistency do not result from polymerization; rather, they occur because the monomer dissolves and swells the prepolymerized particles. Initially, the mixture is grainy or sandy, but then it rapidly becomes sticky and stringy. Within a few minutes, the mixture becomes doughy, and it is in this stage that the material is "packed" into the denture flask (see Figures 13-6, 13-7, and 13-9). If too much time expires, then the mixture becomes rubbery, which is inappropriate for packing. During packing, the dough is molded into the flask, and then the flask is compressed to remove excess (see Figures 13-6 and 13-7). Several compression sequences are necessary to completely remove the excess material. Polymerization of heat-cured materials occurs only when the mixture is heated in a water bath to 74° C for a minimum of 8 hours (see Figure 13-9).

For chemical-cured materials, the process of packing the denture flask is similar, but timing is more critical. Chemical-cured materials contain all of the components of the heat-cured materials but also contain an accelerator in the liquid (see Figure 13-9). When the accelerator is combined with the benzoyl peroxide in the powder, free radicals are produced, and polymerization begins (see Figures 13-3 and 13-9). The polymerization reaction is therefore superimposed on the dissolution and swelling of the prepolymerized particles that occur in heat-cured materials. Thus, a similar evolution of consistencies (sandy, stringy, doughy, rubbery) occurs, but these stages have shorter lifetimes because the polymerization is occurring at the same time. For the same reason, denture packing must be done in a shorter time.

Other ingredients may enhance the properties of the denture base material to better serve the special needs of some patients. Some materials contain a cross-linking agent, which increases the rigidity of the material and strengthens it (see Figure 13-4). These reinforced polymers would be used for individuals inclined to drop the denture. In other denture base materials, small particles of rubber are added to the powder to increase the impact strength of the denture. The rubber particles contain a chemical group that links the particles into the polymer network. Rubber-reinforced materials might be

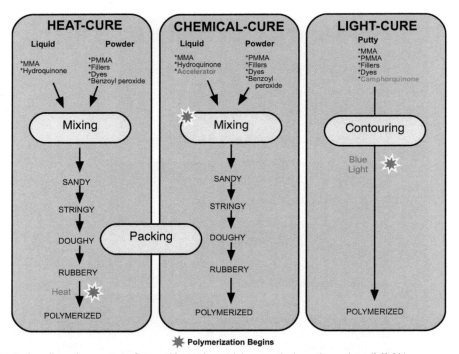

FIG 13-9 Acrylic polymers are formed by polymerizing methyl methacrylate (MMA) monomer into poly(methyl methacrylate) (PMMA). Polymerization of MMA is achieved either by heat (heat cure), the addition of amine accelerators (chemical cure), or blue light (light cure). In the first two cases, the material is a powder–liquid system, and the components of both heat- and chemical-cure systems are shown. Both systems contain benzoyl peroxide, which is the source of the free radicals that initiate polymerization (see Figure 13-3). The powder and liquid are mixed and proceed through a series of consistency changes as the MMA dissolves the PMMA beads in the powder. Packing of the denture is only possible in the doughy consistency. Thus, the laboratory technician has a limited time in which to complete the packing. The heat-cured polymerization process does not begin until the material is heated, but polymerization begins immediately on mixing in the chemical-cure system. In light-cure systems, the premixed material is supplied as a thick paste, which is manipulated to the desired shape before blue light is used to initiate polymerization. Packing of light-cure systems can take place any time prior to curing.

used in patients with severe clenching habits or those in sports such as football. Because denture base materials are inherently radiolucent, pieces of a fractured prosthesis that might be aspirated during an accident would not be visible radiographically unless heavy metal salts were added to provide radiopacity.

Properties of Acrylic (PMMA) Polymers

Acrylic polymers used for complete and partial dentures are relatively low in strength and modulus, brittle, and soft (Table 13-1; also see properties of other materials in Chapter 2). Biting forces tend to cause a denture base to flex. If flexure is excessive, the retention and function of the denture will be compromised as the patient bites. Excess flexure during biting also increases fatigue-mediated fracture (see later discussion). Therefore, denture base materials should have a high modulus to minimize flexure under occlusal loads (see Table 13-1).

The impact strength of a polymer predicts its resistance to fracture if placed under high, short-term stress such as during dropping. Traditional PMMA denture bases have mediocre impact strengths. However, the addition of butadiene-styrene

rubber fillers to PMMA improves the impact strength significantly. Because these fillers also decrease the modulus of the base, rubber-modified denture bases are only used in patients who have a high risk of dropping the denture or experiencing facial blows or excessive occlusal forces.

Denture acrylic polymers are fairly resistant to fatigue-mediated fractures. Fatigue strength is defined as the number of cycles of low stress that a material can experience without failure (fracture). Fatigue strength is particularly important to denture performance because low stresses are applied to the denture as the patient chews. Most acrylic polymers can withstand more than 1.5 million cycles of low stress (17 MPa) application, which provides an excellent service life for most patients.

Denture acrylic polymers have high water sorption (see Table 13-1). Water sorption is critical to performance of the denture because it causes denture expansion of as much as 2%. Although expansion seems like a liability to the clinical fit of the denture, sorption-mediated expansion compensates to some degree for the polymerization shrinkage that occurs during fabrication of the denture, particularly those that are heat cured. It is important to note that hours to days are

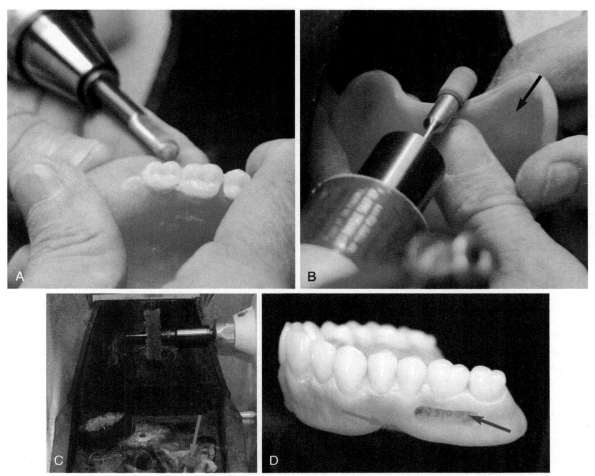

FIG 13-10 Denture finishing and polishing. A high-speed lathe with a special acrylic-cutting bur is used to shape the outside of the denture **(A)** and the periphery **(B).** The tissue side of the denture *(arrow* in **B)** is not adjusted before try-in. After shaping, rag wheels **(C)** coated with polishing compounds *(red arrow)* are used to put a final finish on the denture. The patient's name *(blue arrow* in **D)** is generally embedded into the denture, sometimes on the tissue side. Clinically the denture is inserted and checked for proper extensions, particularly in areas of the frenae *(green arrow).* Further adjustments are normally needed after initial insertion. **(A–C,** Courtesy M. Adams, D. Idels, and J. Nalley, Georgia Regents University, Augusta, GA. Photography by R. Messer, Georgia Regents University, Augusta, GA. **D,** Courtesy Richard Lee, Sr., University of Washington Department of Restorative Dentistry, Seattle, WA.)

TABLE 13-1   Selected Properties of Acrylic Polymers and Clinical Relevance

Property	Description	Clinical relevance
Elastic modulus	Stiffness	High modulus is desirable to prevent flexure of denture or other prosthesis. Acrylic polymers have relatively low elastic moduli.[†] Higher moduli are clinically desirable.
Impact strength	Resistance to fracture upon high-energy impact (dropping)	Important to resist fracture when dropping or blow to facial area. Acrylic polymers have moderate impact strength. Cross-linking increases by two-fold. Higher impact strengths are clinically desirable.
Fatigue strength	Number of repeat stresses to fracture at low loads (chewing)	Important to resist fracture under long-term intraoral forces (chewing, clenching). Acrylic polymers have moderate fatigue strength. Cross-linking can increases fatigue strength. Higher fatigue strengths are clinically desirable.
Water sorption	Mass of water that absorbs into the polymer after sufficient time to reach equilibrium (oral use)	Important because acrylic polymers expand after contact with oral fluids, affecting fit of prostheses such as dentures. Acrylic polymers have high water sorption. Lower sorption is clinically desirable.

Continued

TABLE 13-1	Selected Properties of Acrylic Polymers and Clinical Relevance—cont'd	
Property	Description	Clinical relevance
Water solubility	Mass released into water over time (oral leaching)	Important because mass release compromises the integrity of the prosthesis. Acrylics have low solubility but release residual monomer that may cause allergic reactions in some individuals, particularly in the first 1 to 2 weeks of service. Lower solubility is clinically desirable.
Thermal conductivity	Ability to transmit heat or cold (intraoral foods)	Important to allow patient to sense food temperatures. Acrylic polymers have low thermal conductivity. A higher conductivity would be clinically desirable.
Polymer shrinkage	Shrinkage that occurs during polymerization (processing)	Important because shrinkage alters the fit of the denture or other appliance or, if restricted, leads to residual stresses. Acrylics are moderate to high in polymer shrinkage. Lower shrinkage is clinically desirable.
Heat distortion temperature	Temperature above which residual stresses may be released and lead to distortion (cleaning or very hot foods)	Important because exposure of a prosthesis to hot water can cause distortion compromising fit and function. A high distortion temperature is clinically desirable.

†Among various materials used in dentistry (alloys, ceramics, polymers, waxes).

necessary for the full water sorption to occur. The water sorption of some copolymers, such as those containing hydroxyethyl methacrylate, is greater than that of traditional PMMA.

The water solubility of acrylic polymers is related to but distinct from their water sorption. In general, the water solubility of acrylic polymers is low, and most mass release from these polymers is from residual (unreacted) methyl methacrylate monomer (see Table 13-1). Residual monomer acts as a plasticizer in the denture base. As the monomer is released (leached) from the denture, the modulus of the denture increases somewhat. Released monomer also may trigger allergic reactions in individuals hypersensitive to methacrylates. Residual monomer levels are highest in chemical-cured acrylic polymers because heat-cured polymers tend to release monomer in the hot water bath during processing. Free monomer levels in chemical-cured polymers can be reduced to acceptable levels if the denture is soaked in water for several days before delivery to the patient.

During processing, all acrylic polymers develop residual stresses. Residual stress results from polymerization shrinkage that is constrained by the master cast (see Figure 13-6). Because the gypsum master cast is rigid, the full shrinkage of polymerization cannot occur, and the polymer network is strained as a result. As polymerization proceeds and the polymer increases in rigidity, these strains are "frozen" into the polymer network. Residual stresses are not a problem unless the polymer is heated, which makes the denture more flexible and promotes the release of residual stresses (without the support of the master cast) (see Table 13-1). In this situation, the denture becomes distorted. Distortion from the release of residual stresses may be sufficient to destroy the fit of a denture! Because of residual stresses, the clinical fit of heat-cured dentures is somewhat inferior to that of those cured chemically. In heat-cured polymers, the rigid polymer network essentially forms at the elevated temperature of the processing water bath. When the denture is cooled to room temperature, additional shrinkage because of cooling (related to the coefficient of thermal expansion; see Chapter 2) tends to occur. This residual

stress is released when the denture is removed from the master cast, leading to an undersized denture. Chemical-cured dentures do not suffer from these types of residual stresses and therefore are closer to the ideal size. The bottom line is that patients and dental auxiliaries should not place a denture in hot water. A well-intentioned auxiliary can destroy the fit of a denture by washing or soaking it in hot water!

> **! ALERT**
>
> Denture base materials should have a high modulus, high fatigue strength, high impact strength, moderate water sorption, and good wettability to function optimally in the mouth.

Dentures are retained via a close approximation of the tissue-bearing surface of the denture with the oral tissues. A close approximation between denture and tissue forms "suction" when forces try to separate the denture from the tissue. However, for this suction to form effectively, the saliva must form a "gasket" in the small space between denture and tissue. The contact angle of water on the polymer surface plays a major role in the retention of the denture. This property is also known as wettability (see Chapter 2). Water and saliva form low contact angles with acrylic polymers, ensuring good wettability of the polymer surface, a thin gasket-like layer of saliva on the denture, and favorable retention of the denture. The surface tension and viscosity of the saliva itself also play a significant role in denture retention. Increased salivary viscosity, which occurs when the mouth is dry, does not allow good wetting and increases the thickness of the salivary gasket, leading to impaired retention of the denture. Denture adhesives, such as pastes and powders, should not be needed for denture retention if the denture is well constructed and well fitting. In patients with a chronically dry mouth, the use of a hydroxyethyl/methyl methacrylate co-polymer will improve the wetting of the saliva on the denture.

Acrylic polymers conduct thermal energy poorly, and low thermal conductivity limits the patient's ability to sense changes in oral temperature (see Table 13-1). Although this property rarely affects the performance of the denture, low thermal conductivity may contribute to patient dissatisfaction with eating.

Care of Dentures

Complete or partial dentures should be removed each night and cleaned to ensure the health of the supporting oral tissues. Inappropriate care of the denture during cleaning or extraoral storage can severely compromise the fit and performance of the denture. When removed from the mouth, dentures must remain wet and are best stored in water. Because acrylic polymers have high water sorption, desiccation results in a significant loss of water and shrinkage of the polymer. If cycles of hydration and desiccation continue, the denture will gradually distort as it expands and contracts and its clinical fit will deteriorate.

Acrylic polymers should be cleaned with a soft brush and mild abrasives, as more aggressive cleaning will scratch the soft polymer (Figure 13-11). A soft toothbrush and low-abrasivity toothpaste are suitable for cleaning. Stain-removing toothpastes and whitening toothpastes should be avoided. Particular care should be taken to avoid excessive scrubbing of the tissue-bearing surface of the denture, because even minor wear will compromise the fit and retention of the denture. Disinfection of the acrylic polymer also is important to destroy organisms such as *Candida albicans* (yeast) that tend to accumulate and grow in pores and recesses on the polymer surface. For complete dentures without a metal component, overnight immersion in Clorox (hypochlorite, 5%) and Calgon (a liquid soap, 1 to 2 g per 300 mL) will normally disinfect a denture. However, the use of hypochlorite is contraindicated in appliances that contain alloys as part of the prosthesis, because hypochlorite will corrode the alloy. Electronic ultrasonic cleaners are sold for denture cleaning, but studies indicate that they do not clean the polymer surface any more effectively than the simpler, less expensive measures. However, for patients with physical or mental limitations, ultrasonic cleaners may be an effective alternative.

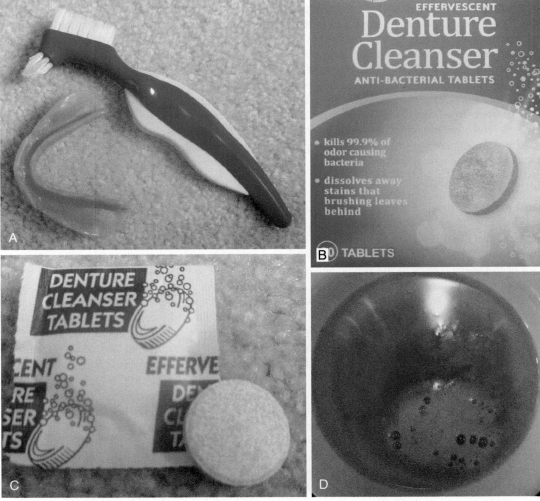

FIG 13-11 Materials for care of complete dentures. A soft-bristled brush **(A)** with either a traditional brush form or a more pointed brush for the tissue side of the denture *(shown here)*. Abrasive pastes should be avoided. Often an effervescent denture cleanser **(B)** is used, consisting of tablets **(C)** that are placed into water **(D)** with the denture. Both the chemical and the bubbling action help to clean the denture and to disinfect it to some extent. Partial dentures with alloy may not be appropriate for these or other cleaning solutions.

Dentures should not be exposed to alcohol or acetone, as these or other solvents will dissolve and swell the polymer network and irreversibly damage the denture surface. This problem is especially important for PMMA polymers that are not cross-linked and therefore cannot resist swelling. For patients who drink alcohol frequently, the use of cross-linked polymers is recommended to help resist solvent-induced swelling and damage. Denture acrylic polymers should never be cleaned or otherwise placed in hot (greater than 35° C [95° F]) water. Hot water increases the risk that residual stresses in the polymer network will be released, leading to significant distortion of the denture.

Manipulation of the denture outside of the mouth increases the risk of dropping the denture. Although acrylic polymers have good impact strengths, fracture from impact is commonplace. Given the expense and complexity of denture fabrication, fracture of the denture base is a significant clinical problem. Care should be taken to manipulate the denture over a sink filled with water to prevent high impact if the denture is dropped. For patients at higher risk of dropping dentures (e.g., those with physical or mental limitations), dentures can be fabricated from butadiene-styrene rubber-reinforced polymers (see the previous discussion). These rubber-reinforced polymers have significantly higher impact strengths and may reduce the risk of fracture.

Repair of Dentures

Given the expense of denture prostheses, repair of a fractured denture is a significant service to the patient. Fortunately, the fracture of a denture most often results in two pieces that can be repositioned accurately. The tendency to fracture "cleanly" is a consequence of the brittle nature of the acrylic polymer. Typically, dentures fracture across the midline where the thickness of the denture is least, near notches built to accommodate the frenular attachments of the tongue in the mandibular arch and upper lip in the maxillary arch. Repair may be done in the office or the denture may be sent to the laboratory, but it is almost always a "one-day" service because the patient is without the prosthesis during the repair.

The development of light-activated polymers has revolutionized denture repair. These materials are close in composition to the polymers for direct restorative materials (Chapter 4) but are shaded to match the tissue color of the acrylic polymers. Repair materials are highly cross-linked to add strength and rigidity (see Figure 13-4). The light-activated material is provided in light-proof packages to avoid premature polymerization (see Figure 13-9).

The procedure for repair of a fractured denture involves assembling the broken pieces and securing their relationship with sticky wax, pouring a stone model on the inside of the denture, opening up the fracture line with a bur, coating the ground surface with a bonding agent, placing the repair material into the opened space, carving the surface, and then placing the model and denture on a turntable in an oven with high-intensity blue light. Polymerization requires 5 to 10 minutes of exposure, and the entire repair can be done in less than 1 hour. Repair with the light-cured materials is noted for its simplicity, high bond strength to acrylics, and no measurable heat release during processing.

DENTURE SOFT LINERS

Denture soft liners are materials that coat the tissue-bearing surface of a complete or partial denture. As their name implies, these materials are soft or rubbery and are less likely to traumatize the oral soft tissues than the harder acrylic polymer. Soft liners are used for patients with severe undercuts of the edentulous ridges or for those patients whose ridges are continually sore. They also are useful as a tissue treatment after oral surgery and in obturators for congenital or acquired defects of the palate, such as cleft palate or postsurgery for oral-facial cancer. Despite divergent opinions about the usefulness of soft liners, some patients tolerate dentures significantly better when a soft liner is used (Figure 13-12).

Soft liners are classified as long-term (months) or short-term (days) materials. Long-term materials are commonly methacrylate- or silicone-based polymers. Methacrylate-based materials often consist of poly(methyl/ethyl methacrylate) copolymers with plasticizers. Plasticizers are not generally chemically bonded to the polymer network (see the previous discussion in this chapter). Methacrylate-based liners are cured either by heat or chemically at room temperature, depending on their formulation. Heat-cured formulations are processed in a laboratory, whereas chemical-cure materials may be processed either in the laboratory or at chairside. If the soft liner is processed at chairside, care must be taken to avoid burning the patient's tissues, since heat is released during the exothermic polymerization reaction. The hardness of the long-term acrylic materials increases slowly as the plasticizer is leached out by exposure to oral fluids.

Silicone-based polymers also are used as long-term soft liners. As these materials polymerize, they produce acetic acid or other by-products. Silicone soft liners are either heat cured or chemical cured, but they are processed in a laboratory regardless of the initiation mechanism. Unlike methacrylate-based liners, silicone liners do not harden as time passes because they contain no plasticizer. Rather, the soft nature of the liner is from the flexible nature of the polymer network itself. Yet because of their flexible nature, silicone liners are difficult to finish at the periphery, and this makes irritation or yeast infection more likely. The bond strength of silicone liners to acrylic denture base material is not high, but it is adequate to retain the soft liner in service in most cases. Clinically, silicone liners may support the growth of *Candida albicans* (yeast), and with some patients, hard, raised spots occur on the surface of the liner as the result of yeast infection. *Candida* infection is more likely with formulations that have a low contact angle with water (good wettability) because wetting more easily permits penetration of oral fluids into the polymer.

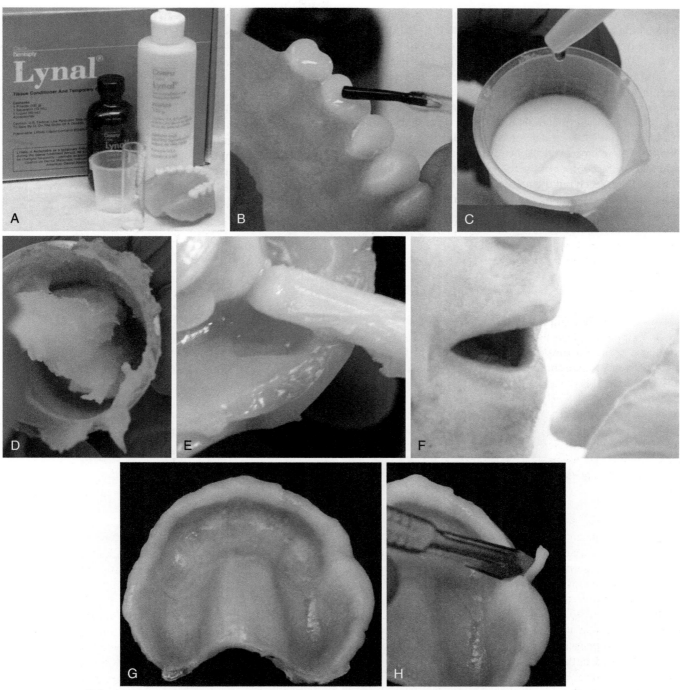

FIG 13-12 Denture soft lining materials are used to help patients tolerate denture prosthetics when the tissue is inflamed or otherwise sore. Temporary lining materials **(A)** do not undergo polymerization. They are prepolymerized particles that swell, soften, and stick to the denture (except when a separating agent **(B)** is added) when a plasticizer is added **(C** and **D)**. The mixed material is applied to the tissue side of the denture **(E)**; then it is inserted into the patient's mouth **(F)** until it gels. The material thinly coats the entire tissue-bearing surface of the denture **(G)**. Excess is easily trimmed **(H)** prior to insertion. The soft liner hardens over a period of days as the plasticizer leaches out of the polymer. The liner is then replaced. (Courtesy Richard Lee, Sr., and Bradley Jonnes, University of Washington Department of Restorative Dentistry, Seattle, WA.)

Short-term materials are used in clinical situations in which the edentulous tissues are inflamed or swollen, are easily irritated or damaged, or are likely to change contours significantly over a period of days. Short-term liners are often used after oral surgery or if the patient has a significant oral infection. Short-term lining materials consist of a polyethylene methacrylate powder and liquid plasticizers. When these materials are mixed, there is no polymerization reaction.

Rather, the plasticizers penetrate and soften the prepolymerized acrylic polymer, providing adhesion to the denture base and a soft texture that serves the purpose of the liner. Short-term materials, also known as "treatment" materials, are always applied at chairside, and the liner is replaced frequently (every 3 days or sooner). Heat generation during mixing is not a problem because there is no polymerization reaction. Treatment materials flow under static load but are elastic (do not flow) under intermittent loads produced by chewing. As irritated and swollen tissues heal, the liner flows and follows the contour of the tissues. They become harder as the oral fluids leach out the plasticizers. When the tissue contours are more stable, a longer-term liner may be used before a new denture is constructed.

ACRYLIC POLYMERS COMBINED WITH ALLOYS

Acrylic polymers often are combined with alloys to fabricate permanent or temporary oral prostheses. Permanent alloy–acrylic restorations include removable partial dentures. Removable partial dentures consist of an alloy framework, which rests on and is retained by the remaining teeth. The alloys used are rigid (high modulus), low-density alloys such as cobalt–chromium alloys (Chapter 11). Because acrylic polymers do not bond to alloys without special treatments, the acrylic is locked mechanically into retentive areas in the alloy framework (Figure 13-13), and the acrylic also retains

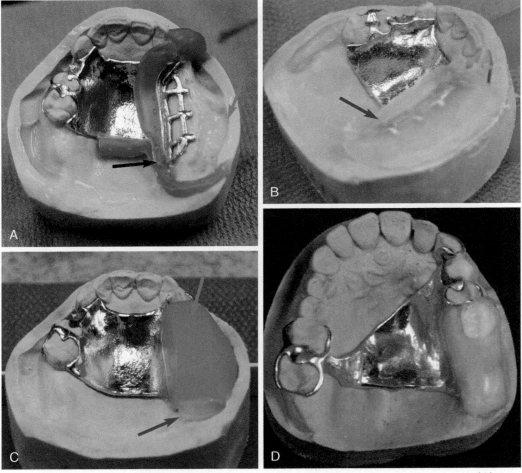

FIG 13-13 Partial denture fabrication. A partial denture contains a rigid metal framework **(A)** that uses the existing teeth to support occlusal function in edentulous areas. Once the framework is cast and its fit verified in the mouth, acrylic and teeth are added to the edentulous areas **(A–D)**. Beading wax is added to define the boundaries of the acrylic *(black arrow)*; the land area of the cast *(red arrow)* is used as well. A temporary acrylic record base is added *(blue arrows)*, and a wax rim *(green arrow)* is added. From this point, the teeth are added into occlusion with the opposing arch, and the denture waxed to the master cast **(D)**.

(Continued)

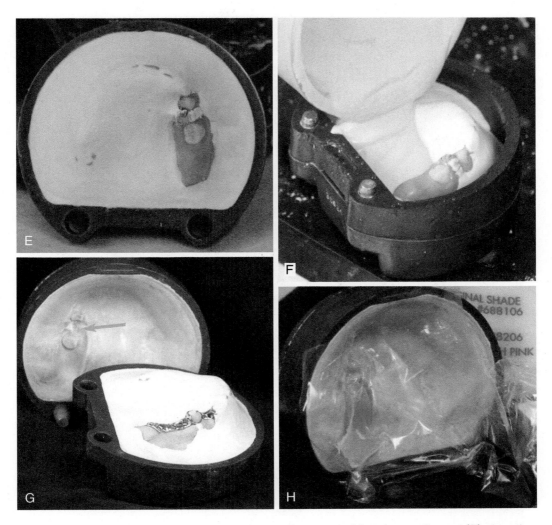

FIG 13-13, CONT'D A gypsum investment is used to cover all but the acrylic area **(E)**; then the appliance is invested with yellow stone in a flask **(F)**. Once the flask is separated, the teeth remain in the upper investment (*orange arrow* in **G**), and the appliance is packed with acrylic **(H)** and processed as for a complete denture. **(A–C,** Courtesy M. Adams, D. Idels, and J. Nalley, Georgia Regents University, Augusta, GA. Photography by R. Messer, Georgia Regents University, Augusta, GA. **D–H,** Courtesy Richard Lee, Sr., University of Washington Department of Restorative Dentistry, Seattle, WA.)

the artificial teeth. The processing of partial dentures is similar to that described for a complete acrylic denture, except that the alloy is retained in the investment mold along with the artificial teeth, and the acrylic is packed into the space that results from the loss of the baseplate wax and record base. The acrylic bonds chemically to the denture teeth and mechanically to the alloy framework. Removable partial dentures use uncross-linked PMMA polymers identical to those used to fabricate complete dentures.

Acrylic polymers also are used in conjunction with stainless steel or other types of wires to construct temporary partial dentures or orthodontic appliances (Figure 13-14). These appliances are made by a hand-painting procedure that use chemical-cured, unfilled, uncross-linked PMMA. The acrylic liquid is painted on the desired areas, and then the acrylic powder is added to the same areas; the procedure is repeated until the proper thickness is attained. This technique is commonly referred to as the "salt and pepper" technique. The cast that contains the wire framework and the acrylic is placed in a pressure cooker, and 0.14 MPa of air pressure is applied during polymerization. The pressure minimizes the porosity in the acrylic and eliminates the need to invest or flask the appliance. Light-cured dimethacrylate polymers also are used to fabricate orthodontic appliances.

POLYMER DENTURE TEETH

Although ceramic materials were first used for teeth in removable complete and partial dentures, ceramic denture teeth are rare today. Denture teeth made of acrylic and modified acrylic polymers have replaced ceramic teeth because acrylic teeth do not wear natural opposing teeth, chemically bond to the acrylic denture base, and better absorb occlusal forces to preserve edentulous ridges (see Figure 13-8).

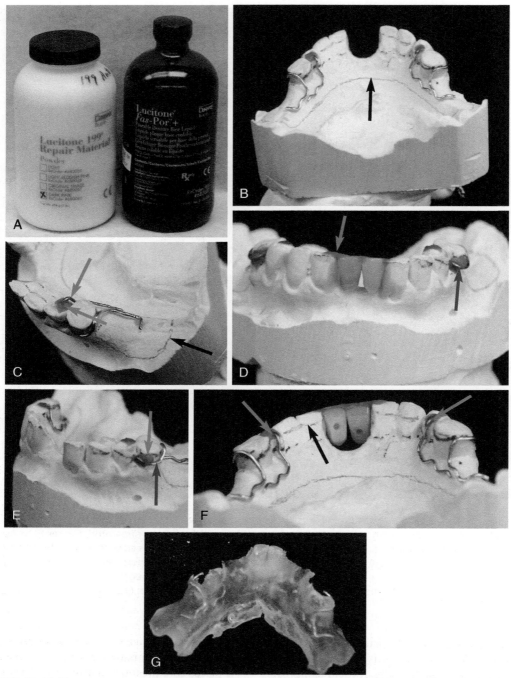

FIG 13-14 Temporary partial denture fabrication using PMMA polymer **(A),** orthodontic wire, and denture teeth **(B–F).** The extent of the appliance is marked with a red line *(black arrows).* Orthodontic wires are bent and adapted to provide rests for the appliance *(green arrows)* and clasps *(blue arrows).* Wire and denture teeth are temporarily secured to the cast using sticky wax *(red arrows).* Finally, the resin is added to the cast to embed the wires and bond to the teeth **(G).** The rough resin appliance is a chemical-cure, uncross-linked PMMA that is trimmed and polished before insertion. (Courtesy Richard Lee, Sr., University of Washington Department of Restorative Dentistry, Seattle, WA.)

Polymer teeth also are substantially easier to modify and equilibrate during denture design and adjustment. In general, the properties (including esthetics) of polymer teeth are sufficiently favorable that the use of ceramic teeth is discouraged, except in special clinical circumstances.

> **! ALERT**
>
> Acrylic denture teeth have largely replaced ceramic denture teeth in partial and complete dentures. Acrylic teeth preserve opposing natural teeth and edentulous ridges.

Acrylic denture teeth are fabricated from the same materials as a denture base (see Figure 13-8), and the physical properties of these polymers are similar to those of the denture base polymers (see Table 13-1). The principal difference in the composition of polymer teeth is that different pigments are used to produce the various tooth shades. To produce teeth with appropriate esthetics, plastic teeth are made in layers of different colors, translucencies, and thicknesses so that the tooth is lighter at the incisal or occlusal portion. Color and translucency can be modified by regulating the fillers in the polymer.

However, there also are differences in the polymer network itself in polymer denture teeth. Polymers in the gingival, or body, portion of the plastic teeth have minimal cross-linking to ensure that the denture base can bond to the denture base material when it is applied in the packing step of processing (see Figure 13-7). With minimal cross-linking, the monomer in the uncured denture base can slightly swell the polymer of the denture tooth and promote penetration of the monomer and chemical bonding. On the other hand, the coronal portion of the tooth is constructed of a cross-linked polymer to provide resistance to crazing when the teeth are exposed to solvents such as alcohol during eating. Cross-linking also provides better wear resistance and a more solid feel when the patient chews.

Polymer denture teeth will wear substantially over their surface life, but this wear is considered an advantage because it spares trauma to the edentulous ridge, thereby helping to preserve ridge integrity. Furthermore, when polymer teeth are worn heavily, the patient is encouraged to replace the denture, which accommodates for changes in the ridge and ensures better occlusal function and ridge longevity.

OTHER USES OF POLYMERS IN PROSTHODONTICS

Polymers play many roles in prosthodontics beyond those for denture construction (see Figure 13-1). These additional roles include maxillofacial prostheses, temporary crowns and bridges, and custom impression trays.

Maxillofacial Prostheses

Trauma or diseases such as cancer may cause extensive loss of oral-facial tissues. The restoration of facial esthetics as a result of an accident or disease is generally treated by a prosthodontist. The replacement of a lost ear, nose, eye, or intraoral tissue such as the palate requires the construction of a maxillofacial prosthesis. Because the tissues being replaced are often soft, flexible polymers play a central role. For example, plasticized acrylic polymers or silicone elastomers have been used to construct these appliances (Figure 13-15). The clinical replacement of facial structures is complex and demanding of the materials used. Facial tissues may be rigid (bone), semirigid (cartilage), or soft (skin), or the structure may move (muscle). These tissues also are subjected to a significant temperature range in service, and they must be esthetic. The materials in maxillofacial prostheses ideally accommodate all of these demands.

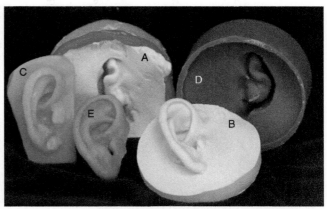

FIG 13-15 Fabrication of an ear prosthesis using silicone polymers. An alginate impression of the patient's ear is made **(A)** and poured in gypsum **(B)**. Wax is used to customize the replacement prosthesis, changing any attribute of the ear that is desired or replacing anatomic features destroyed by disease or trauma **(C)**. A silicone mold of the waxup is made **(D)**, which allows a silicone-based prosthesis to be poured **(E)**. From this point, the prosthesis is colorized and tailored to the patient. (Courtesy Richard Lee, Sr., and Calvin Cowen, University of Washington Department of Restorative Dentistry, Seattle, WA.)

> **! ALERT**
>
> Maxillofacial polymers are made from a variety of different polymer types designed to be flexible and esthetic.

Maxillofacial materials should remain soft over a broad range of temperatures. They also should resist staining from body oils and should be color stable, easily cleaned, and compatible with adhesives to attach the appliance to soft tissue. Because the edges of the appliance are generally thin, the materials must have high resistance to tearing. In addition, the materials should be colored readily to match skin tones and should accept cosmetics. No currently available polymer or combination of polymers fulfills all of these requirements; however, silicone elastomers currently have the best overall properties.

The social, psychological, and nutritional consequences of the loss of facial tissues cannot be underestimated. Because maxillofacial materials are not used in large quantities, there has been little economic incentive to develop new materials with better properties since the 1980s. Clinicians at all levels should recognize that the successful development and application of these materials are extremely important for patients who require such service.

Temporary Restorations

The fabrication of a crown or fixed partial denture (bridge) is a laboratory-based procedure, and several weeks (and sometimes months) may lapse between the preparation of the teeth and the cementation of the permanent restoration; thus, a temporary restoration must be provided. Uncross-linked acrylic polymers are commonly used to make temporary crowns; their composition and manipulation are essentially

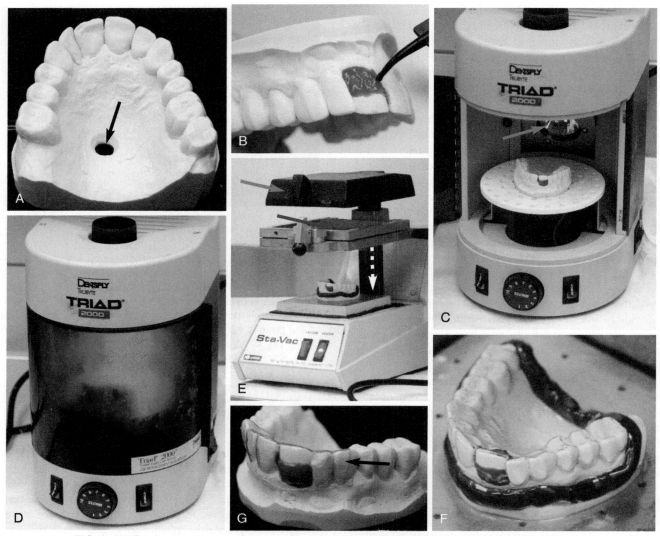

FIG 13-16 Fabrication of a matrix for a temporary crown. A model of the original tooth is captured in alginate and poured in stone **(A).** A hole is added to the palate to facilitate suction for subsequent steps *(black arrow).* A light-cured polymer blockout material *(blue* in **B)** is added to provide some space for the temporary material; it is cured in a light oven **(C, D),** which uses an intense quartz-tungsten-halogen light *(green arrow)* to cure the blockout material. The cast is placed onto a suction machine **(E),** and a sheet of heat-softenable polymer material is placed into the machine *(blue arrow)* and heated until soft by a heating element *(red arrow).* Once the polymer is soft, the platform with the polymer sheet is rapidly moved down *(white dashed arrow)* onto the cast and a suction is applied. The polymer adapts to the cast and cools **(F);** then it is trimmed back to cover the tooth of interest and several teeth mesial and distal *(border of trim at arrow* in **G).** (Courtesy Richard Lee, Sr., University of Washington Department of Restorative Dentistry, Seattle, WA.)

the same as for chemical-cured denture bases (see Figures 13-9, 13-16, and 13-17). The powder and liquid are mixed to a creamy consistency, and the temporary restoration is formed using a cellulose acetate crown former, a vacuum-formed plastic, an elastomeric impression, or an alginate impression of the area before tooth preparation. A separating medium is used to provide a release from the tooth structure. Once in the mouth, the material reaches a rubbery condition in a few minutes, and the temporary restoration is removed and placed in warm water (~57° C) to harden. The temporary restoration is trimmed before cementation with temporary cement.

Many clinicians use resin composites to make temporary crowns or bridges. These materials are supplied as an auto-mixing system with a cartridge and gun that mix two components together as the material is injected into the crown former or impression. These materials may be light cured, chemical cured, or dual cured (see Figure 13-9) and form a highly cross-linked polymer network (see Figure 13-4). Resin composite temporary crowns wear better than their acrylic counterparts and are stronger and more easily trimmed, particularly at the margins of the restoration. They also have a better shade availability and better polishability; however, they are more expensive.

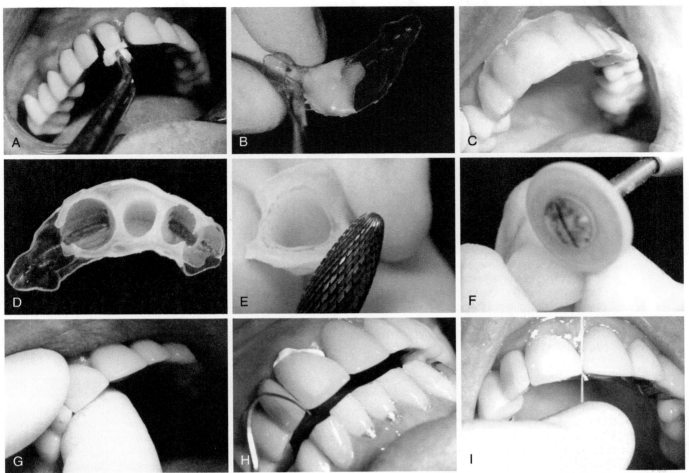

FIG 13-17 Temporary crown fabrication. The tooth is prepared for a crown **(A)** and cleaned. The temporary crown polymer material is mixed and added to the matrix **(B;** see Figure 13-16) and is then immediately seated in the mouth over the preparation **(C)**. After setting, the matrix and polymer are removed **(D)** and the crown is shaped **(E)** and polished **(F)** before trying into the mouth **(G)**. Temporary cement is applied **(H),** and excess cement is removed before dismissing the patient **(I)**. (Courtesy Dr. Xavier Lepe. Photography by Richard Lee, Sr., University of Washington Department of Restorative Dentistry, Seattle, WA.)

Impression Trays

Custom impression trays provide a rigid, closely fitting impression tray and are essential for the appropriate construction of both removable and fixed prostheses (Figure 13-18). These trays are usually constructed on a gypsum study model obtained from an alginate impression during the diagnostic appointment. Custom impression trays may be made from either chemical-cured acrylic polymers or light-cured polymers.

Highly filled powder–liquid acrylics used to make custom impression trays are still common today. The gypsum study model with or without a wax spacer, or stop, is placed in cold water; absorbed water prevents the acrylic from sticking to the model. The recommended amount of liquid and powder is placed in a disposable cup and thoroughly mixed for 1 minute or until the gloss on the surface disappears and the mix develops a slight firmness. A patty is prepared and adapted by gloved hands to the model. After a proper thickness is obtained, the excess is trimmed away with a knife. The excess

then may be used to form a handle. Acrylic materials for custom impression trays are generally highly filled to give the setting polymer a stiffer consistency during manipulation. The acrylic tray material is allowed to polymerize for 6 to 10 minutes, and then the model and tray are placed in warm water to speed up polymerization. The tray is trimmed with acrylic finishing instruments. Retention holes may be drilled into the tray, or the inner surface of the tray may be painted with an adhesive to retain the final impression material.

More recently, custom trays are made from a light-cured material. The tray material is supplied as a sheet, which is adapted carefully over the gypsum study model. The excess material is trimmed away with a sharp knife, and a handle is formed. The tray material then is polymerized on the model by placing it in an "oven" containing a high-intensity blue light (see Figure 13-16). Polymerization takes 4 to 8 minutes, depending on whether the sheet is colorless, translucent, or blue. Because the material has low polymerization shrinkage,

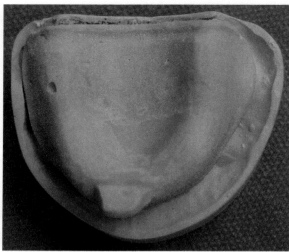
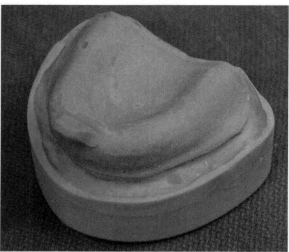

FIG 13-18 Custom impression trays used in denture construction commonly are made from highly filled poly(methyl methacrylate) polymers. Light-cured dimethacrylate polymer materials also are increasingly used. These trays are designed to provide a rigid base that closely approximates the surface of the master cast. Impression material for the final impression is added and adheres to the tray via adhesives that are painted onto the tray. (Courtesy M. Adams, D. Idels, and J. Nalley, Georgia Regents University, Augusta, GA. Photography by R. Messer, Georgia Regents University, Augusta, GA.)

QUICK REVIEW

Polymerization is the process of chemically linking thousands of small organic molecules called monomers into large polymer networks. Polymers are used extensively in many areas of dentistry but are central to prosthodontics. The polymerization process may be modified by using copolymers, cross-linkers, or plasticizers to produce polymer networks with the diverse properties that are necessary for prosthodontic applications. Removable dentures and denture teeth are made of acrylic polymers, which form through a mechanism called free-radical addition polymerization. Acrylic polymers may be combined with alloys to form other types of prostheses. Polymerization of acrylic polymers may be initiated ("cured") by heat, chemicals, or light, and all three initiation mechanisms are used in dentistry today. Most dentures are formed by heat curing. Processing of acrylic dentures is complex and primarily done in the laboratory, but the dental auxiliaries must understand this process to ensure

good communication and the best patient care. Acrylic polymers may be modified by the addition of rubber compounds or other comonomers to provide dentures with greater resistance to fracture or better wettability by saliva. The appropriate care of acrylic prostheses by patients and dental auxiliaries will ensure a better fitting and longer-lasting denture; avoiding overheating of the denture is one prime example of proper care. Polymers also serve as soft liners for dentures or as the primary components of maxillofacial prostheses that are necessary after cancer- or trauma-induced damage to the facial architecture. Polymers for these applications may be based on acrylic, silicone, or other chemistries. Light-cured polymers are supplanting acrylic polymers for several prosthodontic applications, including custom impression trays, denture record bases, temporary crowns and bridges, and some components of maxillofacial prostheses.

SELF-TEST QUESTIONS

Test your knowledge by answering the following questions. For multiple-choice questions, one or more responses may be correct.

1. Which statement(s) is/are true of methyl methacrylate?
    a. It is used as a monomer.
    b. It has a high vapor pressure at room temperature.
    c. It is polymerized by a free-radical polymerization mechanism.
    d. After polymerization, it is commonly called acrylic.
    e. It forms a cross-linked polymer.
    f. It forms a homopolymer.

2. Which of these statements applies to the polymerization of methyl methacrylate?
    a. Can be initiated by heating
    b. Can be initiated at room temperature
    c. Is exothermic

    d. Can be initiated by blue light
    e. Is initiated by free radicals

3. Which statement(s) is/are true of cross-linked polymers?
    a. They have a network structure.
    b. They are formed when monomers with two reactive groups are polymerized.
    c. They do not swell as much as uncross-linked polymers.
    d. They are generally soluble.
    e. They are less susceptible to degradation by solvents such as alcohol.
    f. They are routinely used in denture bases.

4. Which statement(s) is/are true for copolymers or modified acrylic polymers?
   a. Acrylic polymers that are plasticized often become harder with time in the mouth.
   b. Rubber-modified acrylic polymers have lower impact strength than poly(methyl methacrylate).
   c. Addition of hydroxyethyl methacrylate as a co-monomer will make the copolymer more wettable and improve intraoral retention of a complete denture.
5. Indicate whether the following components are found in the liquid or the powder of a heat-cured acrylic denture base material.
   a. Polymer
   b. Amine accelerator
   c. Monomer
   d. Inorganic pigments
   e. Inhibitor
   f. Poly(methyl methacrylate)
   g. Methyl methacrylate
   h. Peroxide initiator
   i. Dyed fiber
   j. Cross-linking agent
   k. Titanium dioxide
   l. Light-active initiator
6. Indicate the function of the components in acrylic denture base materials listed in the left-hand column by selecting the correct answer listed in the right-hand column.
   a. Methyl methacrylate
   b. Poly(methyl methacrylate)
   c. Titanium dioxide
   d. Organic peroxide
   e. Hydroquinone
   f. Organic amine
   g. Inorganic pigments
   h. Bismuth or uranyl salts
   i. Accelerator
   j. Initiator
   k. Inhibitor to provide shelf life
   l. Monomer
   m. Polymer
   n. Adds color
   o. Controls translucency
   p. Provides radiopacity
7. Compared with acrylic denture base polymers, which statement(s) is/are true of a butadiene/styrene–reinforced acrylic polymer?
   a. It has lower modulus.
   b. It is less color stable to light.
   c. It has lower impact strength.
   d. It is polymerized by a condensation mechanism.
8. Denture patients should be instructed to do which of the following?
   a. Clean all surfaces of the denture with an abrasive dentifrice to remove debris.
   b. Avoid placing the denture in hot water.
   c. Keep their dentures in water when not in the mouth.
   d. Use dental adhesives to improve denture retention.
   e. Clean the denture daily.
   f. Soak the denture in concentrated bleach every week.

Use short statements to answer the following questions.
9. To speed up the processing of dough-molded acrylic denture base, polymerization was done in a 100° C water bath. Although polymerization was complete at 1 hour rather than the usual 8 hours, porosity was observed when the denture was polished. What was the cause of the porosity?
10. A patient complained that her complete acrylic dentures fit too tightly in the morning after the dentures sat on the nightstand overnight. What could cause this problem, or was it the patient's imagination?
11. A patient wishing to have clean dentures cleaned them with a nonabrasive dentifrice in very hot (95° C) water. After the cleaning, the dentures did not fit well, and the occlusion was no longer correct. What was the cause of this problem?
12. A patient consistently cleaned all surfaces of his dentures with a highly abrasive dentifrice, and after a period of time found the dentures fit poorly and lost some of their retention. What caused this problem?
13. Inadequate cooling of dentures during polishing makes the acrylic in the denture very hot. Give two reasons that these temperatures are harmful to dentures.
14. What clinical problem can be created by residual monomer in a processed complete denture? How can the dentist ensure that the levels of residual monomer are minimized?
15. Surface cracking (crazing) of acrylic dentures can result from contact with organic solvents such as alcohol. What strategies may be taken to minimize such crazing?
16. Why should patients be instructed to avoid the use of hot water when cleaning their dentures?
17. Why should patients use nonabrasive dentifrices and a soft brush to clean the tissue-bearing surface of a denture?
18. Why can a hypochlorite type of denture cleaner be used periodically on a complete denture with no exposed Ni- or Co-base alloy but should not be used on a removable partial denture or metal-based denture that consists of part acrylic polymer and part Ni- or Co-alloy?
19. Why should the dentures be stored in a moist or wet environment when they are not in the mouth?
20. How are polymer acrylic denture teeth retained in the denture?

an accurate and stable tray can be produced in a short time. However, the light-cured materials are substantially more expensive than their acrylic counterparts.

SUGGESTED SUPPLEMENTARY READINGS

Bunch J, Johnson GH, Brudvik JS: Evaluation of hard direct reline resins, *J Prosthet Dent* 57:512, 1987.

Craig RG: Denture materials and acrylic base materials, *Curr Opin Dent* 1(2):235, 1991.

Dootz ER, Koran A, Craig RG: Comparison of the physical properties of eleven soft denture liners, *J Prosthet Dent* 67:707, 1992.

Dootz ER, Koran A, Craig RG: Physical property comparison of 11 soft denture lining materials as a function of accelerated aging, *J Prosthet Dent* 69:114, 1993.

Johnson GH, Taylor TD, Heid DW: Clinical evaluation of a nystatin pastille for treatment of denture-related oral candidiasis, *J Prosthet Dent* 61:699, 1989.

Kawano F, Dootz ER, Koran A, Craig RG: Comparison of bond strength of six soft denture liners to denture base resin, *J Prosthet Dent* 68:368, 1992.

Kawano F, Dootz ER, Koran A, Craig RG: Bond strength of four processed soft denture liners as influenced by artificial aging, *Int J Prosth* 10:178, 1997.

Murata H, et al: Dynamic viscoelastic properties and the age changes of long-term soft denture liners, *Biomaterials* 21:1422, 2000.

Nikawa H, et al: Growth and/or acid production of *Candida albicans* on soft lining materials in vitro, *J Oral Rehabil* 21:585, 1994.

Smith LT, Powers JM, Ladd D: Mechanical properties of new denture resins polymerized by heat, light, and microwave energy, *Int J Prosthodont* 5:315, 1992.

14

Dental Ceramics

OBJECTIVES

After reading this chapter, the student should be able to:

1. Describe the major types of ceramics used in dentistry today and how they differ in composition, physical properties, optical properties, and clinical applications.
2. For the properties of ceramics:
   - Explain which physical properties are most important to the clinical success of all-ceramic and ceramic–alloy restorations and why these properties are important.
   - Explain the differences between transparency, translucency, and opacity and how these terms apply to dental ceramics.
   - Explain how the color of dental ceramics is described and assessed.

3. Describe the sequence of steps in fabrication of ceramic–alloy restorations.
4. Describe the nature of the bond between alloy and ceramic and what factors may contribute to failure of this bond. Explain why failure of this bond is a major clinical problem.
5. Describe the process of sintering, and explain why it is important in ceramic dental restorations.
6. Describe several fabrication processes for all-ceramic crowns and how these processes differ from the fabrication of ceramic–alloy restorations.
7. Explain what veneers and ceramic inlays are and when they are used to restore teeth. Explain the advantages and disadvantages of ceramic versus composite inlays.

Ceramic materials are fundamentally distinct from alloys or polymers because they contain strong, directional, ionic bonds between metals and oxygen that impart strength but will not tolerate distortion. In dentistry, it is the esthetic qualities of ceramics that drive their use; the interaction of light with ceramics mimics tooth structure better than any other material. The first use of ceramics in dentistry was for denture teeth; however, ceramic denture teeth are rarely used today because of their tendency to wear natural teeth and damage edentulous ridges (Chapter 13). But since about 1950, ceramics have been used in esthetic restorations for teeth. Because ceramics are brittle, the first ceramic-containing dental restorations required that a ceramic veneer (covering) be supported by an alloy substructure. These ceramic–alloy restorations are still used in today's dental practice. Yet new, stronger ceramics are now available to restore teeth with all-ceramic restorations, and this method of restoration has become commonplace. Other roles for ceramics in dentistry include implant abutments and implants, also covered in Chapter 15.

CERAMICS IN DENTISTRY

Basic Ideas about Ceramics

At the atomic level, ceramics are composed of metal–oxygen ionic bonds (see Figure 14-1). Silicon (Si), zirconium (Zr), and aluminum (Al) are common metallic elements that occur in ceramics in combination with oxygen. Ionic bonds, unlike the metallic bonds of alloys or covalent bonds of polymers, result from the complete transfer of electrons from the metal to oxygen. Ionic bonds are strong and they are directional—that is, they do not tolerate bending. This intolerance to distortion makes ceramics brittle. A second distinguishing feature of ceramics is that the metal–oxygen ionic bonds occur in vast crystalline arrays (see Figure 14-1). Metals also occur in crystalline arrays, but bonds are not ionic and are not as directional because electrons are shared (Chapter 11). Polymers also may be crystalline in nature, but the unit of the crystal is the polymer molecule, itself composed of covalent bonds (Chapter 13).

> **! ALERT**
>
> Ceramics differ from alloys and polymers in that they are composed of arrays of metal and oxygen atoms bonded together with rigid ionic bonds that are resistant to and will not tolerate distortion. These ionic bonds give ceramics their physical and esthetic properties.

Ceramic crystalline arrays are not flawless, however. The continuity of the array may be interrupted by the presence of metal ions of sodium (Na) or potassium (K) that cannot bond in a manner consistent with the parent metal in the array (Figure 14-2). These interrupting ions are called fluxes and have several profound effects on ceramic properties, including reduced strength, lower fusing temperature, and more transparency (see the following section on properties).

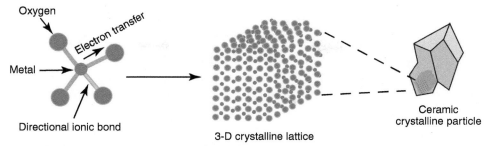

FIG 14-1 Ceramics are composed of arrays of metal atoms and oxygen held together by ionic bonds. These ionic bonds result from the transfer of electrons from the metal to oxygen, and they are strong and highly directional (i.e., the bonds do not tolerate distortion). The metals and oxygen form arrays in a three-dimensional crystalline lattice that makes up the ceramic particle. Because of the directionality of the ionic bonds, ceramics are brittle and will fracture if distorted even slightly.

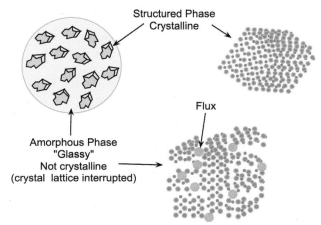

FIG 14-2 Most dental ceramics contain areas (phases) that are amorphous in structure (glassy) and areas that are crystalline. The amorphous areas have disruptions in the metal-oxygen crystal arrays; these areas tend to be transparent. In amorphous areas, metal ions called fluxes (like sodium or potassium) interrupt the array formed by the parent metal and oxygen. Crystalline areas have a more ideal crystal structure; these areas are opaque. The overall strength and optical properties, as well as the clinical use of a ceramic, depend on the relative abundance of the amorphous and glassy phases.

When the crystalline array is disrupted sufficiently, it is described as amorphous or glassy. The latter term is used because amorphous ceramics are transparent (like window glass, which is an amorphous ceramic). The ratio between crystalline and amorphous areas in a ceramic fundamentally determines how the ceramic will behave clinically in the mouth and is the topic of the next section.

The terms *ceramic* and porcelain are often used interchangeably, but incorrectly. Ceramic refers to any material composed of the arrays of metallic oxygen bonds described previously. Porcelain, on the other hand, is a type of ceramic that results when feldspar (K_2O-Al_2O_3-SiO_2), silica (SiO_2), and alumina (Al_2O_3) are fired together with fluxes such as sodium carbonate (Na_2CO_3) or potassium carbonate (K_2CO_3). During the firing, large areas of amorphous ceramic are formed, with small islands of a crystalline phase called leucite ($K[AlSi_2O_6]$). Porcelains are often referred to as feldspathic ceramics in

dentistry, and they are the most esthetic but weakest of the ceramics (see the section on properties). Feldspathic ceramics are still common in dental restorations today, particularly as esthetic veneers on either alloy or ceramic cores.

> **! ALERT**
>
> Feldspathic ceramics (porcelains) are glassy ceramics that form from the combination of feldspar, silica, and alumina; feldspathic ceramics are the oldest of the dental ceramics and are very esthetic but relatively weak.

Types and Uses of Ceramics in Dentistry Today

Dental ceramics may be roughly classified into four types: traditional feldspathic (or glassy), glass dominated, crystalline dominated, and crystalline (Figures 14-3 and 14-4). Each of these is discussed briefly in the text that follows, and all are a consequence of the ratio of amorphous to crystalline phases and how the phases interact with one another.

Feldspathic or glassy ceramics are porcelains that are composed primarily of an amorphous phase (often called a *matrix*) with embedded leucite crystals (see Figures 14-3 and 14-4). Leucite makes the porcelain more opaque, stronger, and higher fusing and creates expansion upon heating (see the properties section). Feldspathic ceramics also contain small amounts of metal oxides for coloring and fluorescence to optimize their esthetics. Feldspathic ceramics were used at one time for all-ceramic (so-called porcelain jacket) crowns, but because of their low strength, porcelain jacket crowns had high failure rates. Today, these ceramics remain among the most esthetic of the dental ceramics and are primarily used as veneers over alloys or ceramic substructures that impart strength to the restoration and support the weaker veneer (Table 14-1). Feldspathic ceramics also are used for veneers that are bonded directly to tooth structure, particularly in the upper anterior region. In this case, strength is imparted by the bond of the ceramic to tooth enamel.

Glass-dominated ceramics contain increased amounts of crystalline phase relative to the glassy ceramics; crystals may be leucite or fluoroapatite (see Figures 14-3 and 14-4). The increased crystalline phase gives the ceramic higher strength but sufficient translucency to serve in esthetic

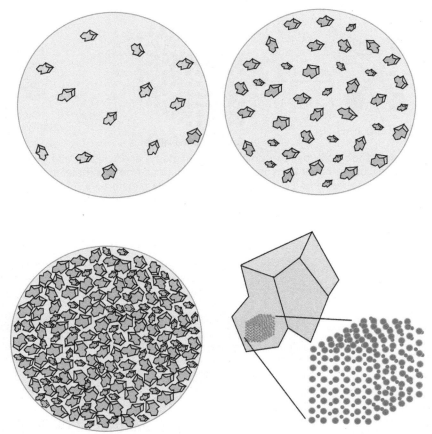

FIG 14-3 Ceramics in dentistry can be roughly divided into four categories. Feldspathic or glassy ceramics *(upper left)* are the oldest ceramic in dentistry. They consist of mostly amorphous glass with islands of a crystalline phase, often leucite. Glass-dominated ceramics *(upper right)* have mostly a glassy phase but have an increased abundance of crystalline phase that may be leucite or other compounds. Crystalline-dominated ceramics *(lower left)* have mostly a crystalline phase, which may be composed of several types of crystals but have a glassy phase that surrounds the crystals. Finally, crystalline ceramics *(lower right)* have no glassy phase; these ceramics are the newest and strongest of the ceramics used in dentistry.

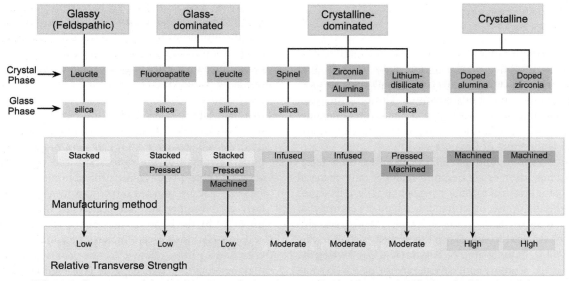

FIG 14-4 Summary of the major types of ceramics used in dentistry today; listing the identity of the crystalline phase, glass phase, common methods of manufacture, and relative transverse strength.

TABLE 14-1 Possible Uses of Ceramics in Dental Restorations*

Ceramic	Anterior veneer	Anterior crown		Inlay, onlay	Anterior bridge	Posterior crown		Posterior bridge
Glassy								
All-ceramic**	**	full***	veneer		veneer	veneer		veneer
Alloy–ceramic	na	veneer			veneer	veneer		veneer
Glass-dominated								
All-ceramic		full	veneer		veneer	full	veneer	veneer
Alloy–ceramic	na	veneer			veneer	veneer		veneer
Crystalline-dominated (all-ceramic only)								
Spinel-infused		core						
Alumina or alumina-zirconia infused		core			core	core		core
Lithium disilicate		core		full	core	full	core	
Crystalline (all-ceramic only)								
Doped-alumina		core		full	core	core		core
Doped zirconia		core		full	core	core or full		core or full

*According to manufacturer's literature; evidence incomplete on long-term survival in many cases.
**Green = indicated; yellow = caution needed; red = ill-advised.
***Full = full-contour restoration; veneer = veneer layer over core; core = substructure of restoration.

applications. The increased strength allows these ceramics to occasionally be used for anterior all-ceramic crowns that are not under excessive occlusal force (see Table 14-1). But except as veneering ceramics, these materials cannot be used for posterior crowns or bridges. They are, however, excellent choices for alloy-veneering ceramics or ceramic cores.

> **! ALERT**
>
> Amorphous ceramic phases are weaker and more soluble than crystalline phases. A pure amorphous phase is transparent, like window glass.

Crystalline-dominated ceramics are composed, as their name implies, mostly (about 70 vol %) of a crystalline phase (see Figure 14-3). The spaces between the crystals are occupied by an amorphous silica glass, and the two phases synergize to increase the strength of the ceramics substantially (see the properties section). The crystalline phase is generally spinel ($MgAl_2O_4$), zirconia (ZrO_2), alumina (Al_2O_3), or lithium disilicate (see Figure 14-4). Crystalline-dominated ceramics are much more opaque and therefore are far less suitable in esthetic roles such as veneers or veneers on alloys (see Table 14-1). One exception is the lithium disilicate ceramics, for which newer forms have been developed to provide sufficient esthetic qualities for some posterior and some anterior restorations. In contrast, crystalline-dominated ceramics often serve as cores for anterior or posterior all-ceramic crowns, onto which veneering porcelain (either glassy or glass-dominated) is added. They may be used with caution for inlays, onlays, or crowns

when occlusal forces are minimal. Of the crystalline-dominated ceramics, the spinel-based ceramics have the lowest strengths, whereas the zirconia-alumina–based ceramics have the highest strengths.

The crystalline ceramics are the newest and strongest of the ceramics used in dentistry (see Figure 14-3). These ceramics are formed from either alumina or zirconia that has been seeded, or "doped," with other ions such as magnesium or yttrium to optimize them for use in dental applications (see Figure 14-4). Crystalline ceramics have no glassy phase and are opaque. They cannot serve as esthetic veneers on alloys or teeth. However, as high-strength cores, they are plausible for use in nearly any other dental restoration, including posterior crowns and bridges (see Table 14-1). If esthetic considerations are not paramount, doped zirconia may be used for full-contour posterior restorations (so-called monolithic restorations).

Fabrication Techniques

One consequence of the strong ionic bonds in ceramics is that these materials melt only at relatively high temperatures. For this reason, ceramic restorations are not generally cast like alloy restorations in Chapter 12 (although castable ceramics do exist). Other techniques are used to form the final dental restoration including stacking, infusing, pressing, or machining. Each of these techniques is discussed briefly in the following text.

In stacking, the parent ceramic is ground into particles that are manipulated into an approximation of the final form in a "green" state (weak state). The green state is achieved through a process called condensation (Figure 14-5). A viscous slurry

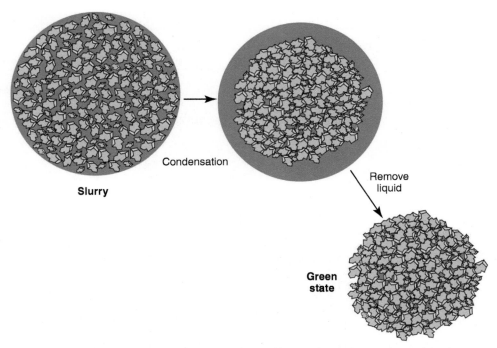

FIG 14-5 Ceramic condensation. During ceramic stacking, a slurry of ceramic particles in water or glycerin-water is applied to an alloy or high-strength ceramic substructure and then vibrated to condense the particles together onto the substructure, expelling the liquid. The liquid is removed by absorption, and the particles interlock with one another to form a green state in which the approximate final form of the restoration may be carved or otherwise shaped.

of the porcelain particles in water or water-glycerol is applied to a substructure, using vibration to pack the particles and expel the liquid to the surface. The liquid is removed by a sorbent tissue. By alternatively vibrating the liquid to the surface and then removing it, the particles become packed quite tightly into the green state. In the green state, the ceramic can be carved and shaped into approximate final form. Superior condensation leads to less shrinkage during sintering (see next paragraph). Stacking is used to apply ceramics to alloys or high-strength ceramic substructures or to fabricate laminate veneers. Stacking is used primarily for glassy and glass-dominated ceramics (see Figure 14-4).

After forming the green state, the ceramic is fired in a specialized oven in a process called sintering (Figure 14-6). During sintering, the particles only melt and fuse at their surfaces. After a short time (minutes), the particles are cooled to room temperature, and the fired ceramic is formed. To reduce the "dead" air spaces in the ceramic, a vacuum is often applied. Changes in the ratio of crystalline to amorphous phases also may occur when firing. During sintering, significant shrinkage (up to 10% linearly) occurs, and this shrinkage must be accounted for in the fabrication of a restoration. Occlusal and proximal contacts, heights of contour, and embrasures are all affected; for this reason, the green state form is often made a bit larger than final desired contours. The sintering temperature is often referred to as the fusing temperature of the ceramic.

❗ ALERT

Today's dental ceramic restorations may be fabricated by traditional stacking and sintering or by infusion, pressing, or machining.

Infusion is a fabrication method by which a porous sintered form is infiltrated with a silica glass (Figure 14-7). In the initial step, a ceramic slurry is stacked onto a refractory model of a tooth preparation, sintered to provide an intermediate strength, and trimmed to near-final form. Trimming of this intermediate form is far easier and faster than trimming the final ceramic. Next, a silica glass is added and the restoration is sintered again. During the second sintering, the silica melts and flows into all the capillary spaces of the initial structure. The infused ceramic has markedly higher strengths. Infusion is used on a subset of crystalline-dominated ceramics (see Figure 14-4).

Pressing techniques are used to force a viscous mass of molten ceramic into a mold to get the desired final form (Figure 14-8). This process is similar to casting alloys (Chapter 12), except that the ceramic, unlike the alloy, is too viscous to accelerate into the mold, and high pressure is used to move the ceramic. In addition, special investments (called refractories) are needed to survive the high temperatures of the molten ceramic; the goal is to avoid chemical reactions between the ceramic and the investment, which itself is a

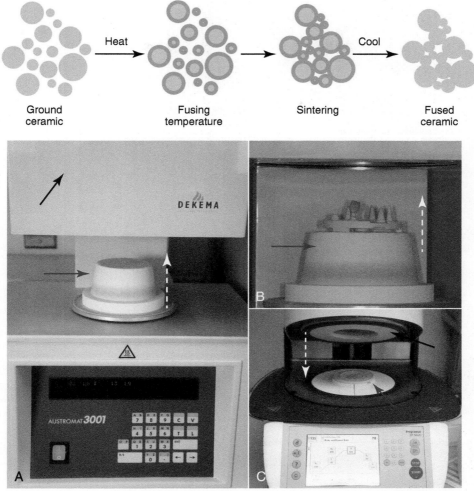

FIG 14-6 *(Top)* Ceramic particles are fused together in a process called sintering. After the green state is formed (see Figure 14-5), particles are heated to a temperature at which only the surfaces of the particles melt (brighter orange color). The particles then fuse together at their surfaces (or sinter). During cooling, the spaces between the particles may be minimized by applying a vacuum. In general, ceramics shrink significantly from the green state to the fused state. *(Bottom)* Ceramic firing ovens used to sinter dental ceramic restorations. The oven muffle *(black arrows)* contains the heating elements. Restorations are placed on a platform *(blue arrows)* that is then introduced into the muffle by raising **(A** and **B)** or lowering **(C)** the muffle *(white dashed arrows)*. Depending on the ceramic, a vacuum also may be applied to the muffle during firing to limit porosity in the ceramic. The oven has controls to regulate the temperature of the muffle, time of firing, and degree and time of vacuum. When the firing cycle is completed, the vacuum is released, and the platform is lowered **(A** and **B)** or raised **(C)** slowly. Firing does not melt the ceramic but causes the ceramic particles to sinter. (Courtesy Kavita Shor, University of Washington Department of Restorative Dentistry, Seattle, WA.)

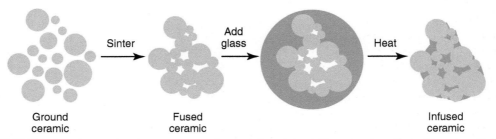

FIG 14-7 Infused ceramics. In some ceramics, a sintered crystalline structure (fused) is secondarily surrounded by a lower fusing (melting) glass to strengthen the ceramic. The amorphous glass, which is often silica, infiltrates throughout the ceramic to form an infused ceramic. The infused ceramic is capable of withstanding higher forces without fracture in many clinical applications.

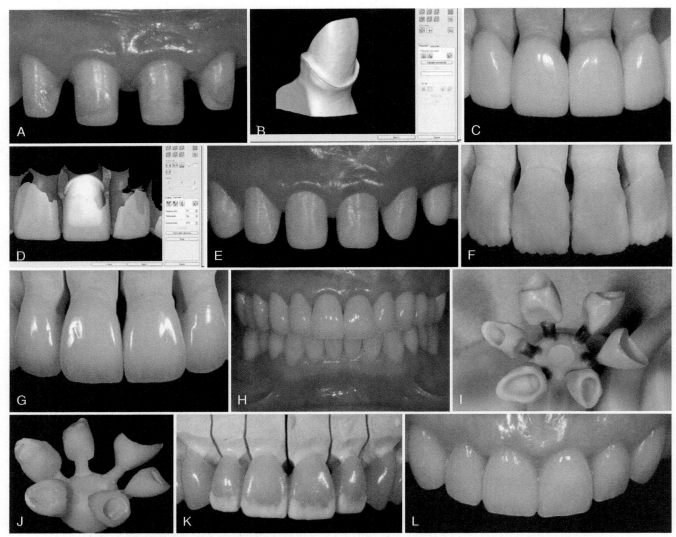

FIG 14-8 Milling **(A–H)** and pressing **(I–L)** of ceramics are increasingly common ways to fabricate all-ceramic dental prostheses. Milling is closely linked with digital scanning techniques. The tooth preparations **(A)** are scanned, resulting in a digital image **(B)** of each preparation. Waxups of the full-contour restorations **(C)** are prepared and scanned **(D)**. The computer calculates the volumetric difference between the preparation and full contour and then directs a milling machine to fabricate copings for the restorations (here in a crystalline ceramic-zirconia). The copings are shown seated on the preparations in **E.** Stacking is used to veneer the copings with glassy or glass-dominated ceramic **(F)**, which is then fired **(G)** and cemented onto the preparations **(H)**. (Courtesy Y-W Chen, University of Washington Department of Restorative Dentistry, Seattle, WA.) In pressing, the full-contour waxups are made and then sprued onto a button **(I)**. A pressing machine is used to "cast" the ceramics in crystalline-dominated ceramic—here lithium disilicate—**(J)** then the sprues are removed and the restorations are seated on the working cast. For anterior cases in which esthetics is paramount, areas are cut back and veneered in a glassy or glass-dominated ceramic **(K)**. After firing and polishing, the restorations are cemented into the mouth **(L)**. (Courtesy Jae-Seon Kim, University of Washington School of Dentistry, Seattle, WA.)

ceramic. Pressing has an advantage that, to some extent, the pressure can compensate for shrinkage of the ceramic and create a final form that is closer to the desired size. Pressing is often employed today for making all-ceramic cores from glass-dominated or crystalline-dominated ceramics (see Figure 14-4).

Newer ceramics are machined into final form; no condensation or sintering or melting is needed (Figure 14-8). The replica of the tooth preparation is scanned into a computer, and then a highly sophisticated program drives fine machining tools to mill a ceramic block to the final form, usually in several minutes. In the most advanced techniques, the shape of the tooth preparation is captured digitally (so-called digital impression), and these data are sent to the lab for milling. Computer-aided design–computer-aided manufacturing (CAD-CAM) fabrication has several advantages over other ceramic fabrication techniques. First, because there is no heat and no condensation, shrinkage associated with stacked ceramics is not an issue (although some shrinkage is associated with ceramics milled in a green state). Second, the properties of the restoration are more predictable because manufacturing of the starting ceramic block can be tightly controlled, without the influence of a sintering or casting process to alter properties. CAD-CAM techniques are used for fabrication of high-strength ceramic cores from glass-dominated, crystalline-dominated, or crystalline ceramics (see Figure 14-4).

PROPERTIES OF CERAMICS

Physical Properties

As a group, ceramics exhibit extremely high compressive strengths and moduli but relatively low tensile strengths and elongation (Table 14-2; see Chapter 2). Thus, from a clinical perspective ceramics are inherently stiff, brittle materials relative to alloys or polymers; their brittleness has limited their use in restorative dentistry over the years. The concern that a ceramic will fracture in service remains a problem for ceramic–alloy and all-ceramic restorations alike, although the newest crystalline ceramics (see Figure 14-3) are beginning to challenge this notion. Two physical properties in particular are used to assess the clinical performance of today's dental ceramics: flexural strength and hardness, both described in the following paragraphs.

Flexural strength (also referred to as transverse strength) is the ability of a suspended ceramic bar to resist fracture when loaded from above (Figure 14-9). Flexural strength is influenced by compressive and tensile strength but is used in place of these other strengths because it is the best predictor of clinical performance. Based on empiric evidence, a high flexural strength suggests that a ceramic will better resist fracture in clinical service. Flexural strengths of glassy dental ceramics range from 70 to 90 MPa, depending on the type of ceramic. However, crystalline-dominated or crystalline ceramics have remarkably high flexural strengths (see Table 14-2), which has allowed them to be used in more diverse clinical environments (see Table 14-1).

! ALERT

Flexural strength is the single most important physical property that distinguishes today's ceramics and the best predictor of clinical survival.

The hardness of most glassy or glass-dominated ceramics is substantially higher (>460 kg/mm^2) than human enamel (343 kg/mm^2), and when ceramics occlude against natural teeth, the enamel may wear preferentially. Because of this fact, a denture opposing natural teeth generally will be constructed

TABLE 14-2 Moduli and Strength of Ceramics vs. Teeth and Common Restorative Alloys

Material	Modulus (GPa)	Strength* (MPa)
Ceramics**		
Glassy	65–75	70–90 (Tv)
Glass-dominated	65–75	175–180 (Tv)
Crystalline-dominated	95	300–500 (Tv)
Crystalline	210	600–1100 (Tv)
Common restorative alloys		
TiAl6V (Titanium "Alloy")	100	800 (Te)
Stainless steel (316)	200	650 (Te)
Cobalt–Chromium	230	700 (Te)
Tooth		
Dentin	11	260 (Te)
Enamel	130	10 (Te)

*Te = tensile strength; Tv = transverse strength (flexural strength).
**Typical range for each category.

with polymer rather than porcelain teeth (Chapter 13). Ceramic-induced wear of opposing enamel may be a problem for fixed prosthetic appliances as well, and this potential clinical problem must be anticipated and minimized when planning complex prosthetic treatments, particularly those that involve many restorations. Newer crystalline ceramics have a hardness of 1200 to 1500 kg/mm^2, so the risk of wear of natural teeth is even higher. Current evidence suggests that ceramic-induced wear can be minimized if the restoration surface is very smooth. Therefore, clinical polishing is particularly important for these materials. Furthermore, the newer ceramics (which are hardest) are often used for ceramic cores (see Table 14-1). In this instance, the veneering ceramic, commonly a glassy or glass-dominated type, is the ceramic in potential contact with opposing enamel. However, this situation is changing as full contour zirconia restorations are increasingly common. Long-term clinical evidence is scarce in this area.

Thermal Properties

The coefficient of thermal expansion (CTE) is the degree of expansion or contraction of a material in response to heating or cooling, respectively (Chapter 2). A ceramic with a high coefficient of thermal expansion expands a large amount when heated and contracts a large amount when cooled. The coefficient of thermal expansion is important when a ceramic is bonded to an alloy (ceramic–alloy restoration) or ceramic core (all-ceramic restoration). The expansion of the alloy or core and veneering ceramic must be appropriately matched, or the ceramic will fracture when the restoration cools from firing temperature to room temperature (Figure 14-10). The coefficient of thermal expansion of glassy veneering ceramics for ceramic–alloy restorations is about 12 to 13.5 × 10^{-6}/°C. These CTEs have been designed to be compatible with alloys used for the restorative substructure. The coefficients of veneering ceramics designed to be applied to ceramic core materials or newer unusual alloys such as

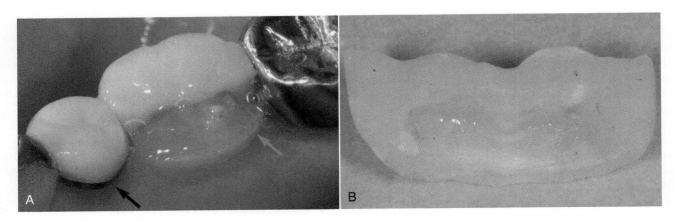

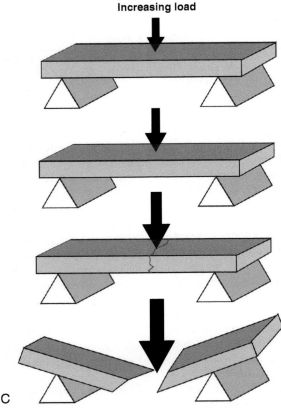

Increasing load

FIG 14-9 Ceramics are inherently more susceptible to fracture in service than alloys or polymers **(A).** For this reason, surgical preparation of the tooth for an all-ceramic restoration attempts to create space for thicker restorations *(blue arrow)*, but fractures sometimes still occur **(A** and **B).** In contrast, in alloy–ceramic restorations *(black arrow)*, the ceramic is supported by an alloy substructure, which reduces (but does not eliminate) the risk of fracture. Note that in the all-ceramic restoration, there is no alloy substructure. The flexural strength test (also known as transverse strength) is used to estimate the ability of dental ceramics to withstand fracture in clinical service. **C,** A beam of ceramic about 1.5 cm long and 2 to 3 mm square is fabricated and suspended on two supports. An increasing load is applied to the top of the bar *(large black arrow)* between the supports. When the maximum strength is reached, the bar fractures, usually abruptly. **(A, B,** Courtesy E. R. Schwedhelm, University of Washington Department of Restorative Dentistry, Seattle, WA.)

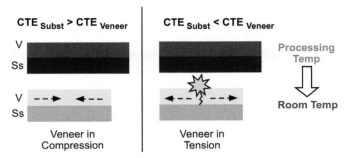

Coefficient of Thermal Expansion (CTE)

Veneer (V): material on the outside of a restoration.
Substructure (Ss): alloy or ceramic material supporting the veneer.

FIG 14-10 Thermal compatibility of a substructure (Ss) and veneering ceramic (V) is critical to the clinical success of all-ceramic or ceramic–alloy restorations. The substructure is an alloy in ceramic–alloy restorations or a ceramic in all-ceramic restorations. The coefficient of thermal expansion (CTE) of a substructure and veneer must be properly matched to lower the risk of failure of the restoration in service. The CTE is a measure of how much a material expands on heating and contracts on cooling. In practice, the CTE of the substructure should be slightly greater than that of the veneer *(left half of diagram)*. In this case, if the substructure and veneer are the same dimension at the processing temperature, the substructure will contract more as the restoration cools to room temperature. Because the veneer is bonded to the substructure, the contraction of the substructure compresses the ceramic *(lower left)*. If the CTE of the veneer is greater than that of the substructure *(right half of diagram)*, then the ceramic will tend to be in tension at room temperature when bonded to the substructure *(lower right)*. Because ceramics are relatively weak in tension (brittle), fracture of the ceramic may occur, either immediately or even years after restoration placement.

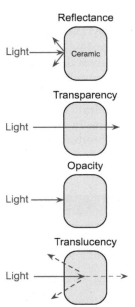

FIG 14-11 Optical properties of dental ceramics. Reflectance is the property of incident light reflecting back toward the source (at several angles) from the surface. Transparent materials allow light to travel through them with little attenuation or net distortion, similar to the glass pane of a window. These types of ceramics do not have significant use in dental restorations. Opaque materials block light transmission altogether. Opacity can be important when undesirable color needs to be masked—for example, when blocking the color of a metal substructure in the ceramic–alloy restoration. Translucent materials allow a limited amount of light to penetrate all the way through a material, but some light is reflected from subsurface layers. Translucency gives the ceramic a depth that is needed to mimic the optical properties of natural teeth.

titanium alloys may be substantially different, however, because the CTEs of these substructures are different from those of traditional casting alloys. The requirement for proper matching of the coefficients of ceramic and alloy implies that not every veneering ceramic will be compatible with every alloy or core ceramic. Given the large number of choices available today, the problem of CTE compatibility is complex, and the laboratory technician must rely on the recommendations of the manufacturer. These constraints also affect the practitioner, who must work within the limits of materials available in a given laboratory and must rely on the laboratory. Good communication among all dental auxiliaries is imperative to assure the best restorative outcomes with these materials.

Glassy ceramics are classified according to their fusing temperature (also called sintering temperature) as follows: 1288° to 1371° C are high fusing; 1093° to 1260° C are medium fusing; and 871° to 1066° C are low fusing. High-fusing types are used to make denture teeth, medium-fusing types are used to fabricate some all-ceramic restorations, and low-fusing types are used for veneering ceramic–alloy and all-ceramic restorations. For ceramic veneers, a fusing temperature must be selected that the alloy or ceramic substructure can withstand without distortion or degradation. The concept of fusing

temperature has less applicability to crystalline-dominated ceramics (which are often pressed or machined) or crystalline ceramics (which are most often machined) (see Figure 14-3).

Optical Properties

When evaluating the optical properties of ceramics, the differences between reflectance, translucency, opacity, and transparency are important (Figure 14-11). When incident light meets the surface of a ceramic, some of the light is reflected from the surface, the amount depending on the structure of the ceramic and the degree of surface roughness. Reflectance is that amount of incident light that is reflected from a surface. The remaining light penetrates the ceramic. If the light's path is unaltered as it passes through the material, the ceramic is transparent; purely amorphous or glassy ceramics tend to be transparent. For example, glasses used for windows are amorphous and allow light to pass through largely unchanged. Transparent ceramics have little use in dentistry. Translucency occurs when the incident light penetrates the surface, but some is transmitted through and some is reflected back out of the material, usually with an altered wavelength. An observer cannot see clearly through a translucent material, and the material appears to have some depth, which results from the light reflected from within the material. In dentistry, glassy and glass-dominated ceramics are translucent (see Figure 14-4); the glassy phase allows light to pass unaltered, whereas the crystalline phase reflects the light, absorbing some wavelengths and reflecting others. It is this differential absorption and reflection of light that gives ceramics the color and depth that make them esthetically useful in dental restorations. In opaque ceramics, incident light is either reflected or absorbed, but little or no light is transmitted. Dental crystalline ceramics are nearly opaque (see Figure 14-4).

> **! ALERT**
>
> Crystalline and crystalline-dominated ceramics are nearly opaque; glassy and glass-dominated ceramics are translucent. Only translucent ceramics are generally useful for esthetic restorations.

The *color* of ceramics obviously is important to the esthetic success of a restoration clinically. Color results when a material reflects light from within, but the wavelength (or color) of the reflected light is changed. The material absorbs some of the light. A complete description of color is complex and beyond the scope of this text. However, one system (called the Munsell system) expresses color in terms of three parameters: hue, value, and chroma. Hue is the basic shade of color, such as green, yellow, or blue. Chroma is the intensity of the color, such as pale blue to brilliant blue. A low chroma indicates grayness. Value is the amount of lightness or darkness. A high value (up to 10) implies lightness, whereas a low value implies darkness. A value of zero is black, regardless of the hue or chroma. Among hue, value, and chroma, value is the most critical parameter for matching the color of ceramics with teeth because the hue and chroma occur within a relatively narrow range for most natural teeth. Experienced ceramicists will evaluate the value closely when matching the shade for a patient. Practically, value can be determined through squinted eyes; the reduced light to the retina diminishes the brain's ability to see color and allows the retinal rods (which are sensitive only to black and white shades) to dominate.

Color matching for ceramic restorations is accomplished using shade tabs, which are constructed of small samples of ceramic. The shade tab is placed adjacent to the tooth to be matched. The light source is critical for proper matching because it has a major influence on how a color appears to an observer (a phenomenon called metamerism). The color of the walls, furniture, and even the patient's dental napkin also may influence shade selection. Thus, the experienced dentist or dental auxiliary will take the shade under lighting and room conditions that do not impede the matching process; some practices even have a special room with special lighting for this purpose. Color matching is an art and requires a great deal of practice to become proficient. Fluorescence and opalescence are other color-related properties of ceramic important to the esthetics of a ceramic dental restoration. However, the detailed discussion of these factors is beyond the scope of this chapter.

Biologic Properties

The biologic response to ceramics is often assumed to be acceptable; ceramics are often reported in the literature or advertising to be inert, biocompatible materials. This assumption stems from the long and positive clinical experience with glassy ceramics, which generally have minimal adverse effects on biologic tissues. However, current evidence suggests that no material is completely inert in the oral cavity, and ceramics are no exception. Some mass loss (corrosion) of glassy ceramics occurs during service, although the amount of mass released is low relative to polymers or alloys that are used in restorative dentistry. Tests *in vitro* and *in vivo* have confirmed the favorable biologic properties of glassy ceramics, and to some extent the glass-dominated ceramics.

The crystalline-dominated and crystalline ceramics have a shorter record of clinical use in dentistry, although some have been used for several years now. *In vitro* (in culture) tests of lithium disilicate ceramics have documented a significant initial toxicity that persists for several weeks in cell culture. The toxic effect diminishes with time, suggesting that an initial corrosion of these ceramics subsides, after which the ceramics are equivalent to the glassy ceramics. Disturbing the surface of these ceramics may temporarily increase the toxicity for some materials.

Crystalline ceramics appear to have good biologic responses in both *in vitro* and *in vivo* tests, although comprehensive long-term studies are not available. These favorable results are consistent with the ability of some ceramics such as zirconia to biointegrate when used as endosseous implants (Chapter 15).

CLINICAL USES OF DENTAL CERAMICS

Ceramic–alloy and all-ceramic types of dental restorations are discussed in the following text. Although both types are still commonplace, there is an ongoing trend of all-ceramic restorations supplanting ceramic–alloy restorations.

Ceramic–Alloy Restorations

Ceramic–alloy restorations (also commonly but inaccurately referred to as porcelain fused-to-metal [PFM] restorations) consist of several layers of ceramic bonded to an alloy substructure (Figure 14-12). The alloy substructure is generally less than 0.5 mm thick in areas that will be covered by the ceramic and is nearly always cast (see Chapters 11 and 12). Ceramic–alloy restorations have sufficient strength to be used in restorations for posterior teeth and long-span bridges (see Table 14-1). In terms of predictability of performance and ability to accommodate diverse clinical situations long term, there is currently no ceramic restoration more proven than the ceramic–alloy restoration. If done properly, ceramic–alloy restorations provide excellent esthetics. However, achieving a good esthetic result depends on careful attention to every detail at every step of the process, including the surgical

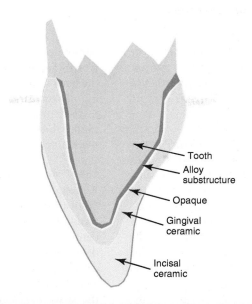

Tooth

Alloy
substructure

Opaque

Gingival
ceramic

Incisal
ceramic

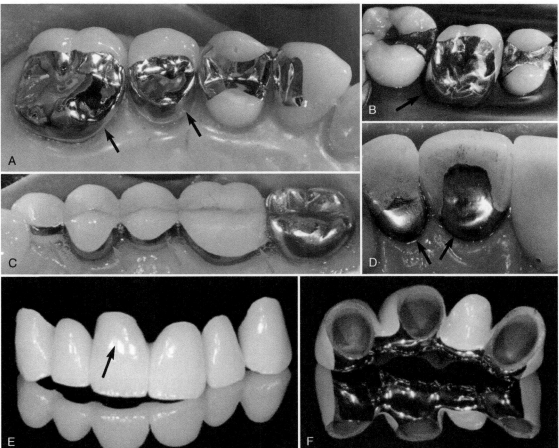

FIG 14-12 *Upper right,* Cross-sectional diagram of a ceramic–alloy restoration on an anterior tooth. The alloy substructure is closest to the prepared tooth. The opaque layer is next, followed by gingival ceramic, then incisal ceramic in appropriate areas. The overlap of gingival and incisal ceramics, combined with the translucent nature of each, gives the restoration a depth of color and a lifelike appearance. The opaquing ceramic blocks the color of the alloy from showing through the other ceramic layers. In some cases, the ceramic does not cover areas of the metal substructure in which esthetics is not as important (e.g., on the lingual). Alloy–ceramic restorations are designed to meet specific esthetic and functional needs of each patient **(A–F).** Ceramic may cover the occluding surface (restorations, *blue arrows*) or may "veneer" the surfaces seen from the facial view (restorations, *black arrows*). (**A, B,** Courtesy Richard D. Tucker, University of Washington Department of Restorative Dentistry, Seattle, WA; **C, D,** courtesy E. R. Schwedhelm, University of Washington Department of Restorative Dentistry, Seattle, WA; **E, F,** courtesy Y-W Chen, University of Washington Department of Restorative Dentistry, Seattle, WA.)

preparation of the tooth. The successful manipulation of ceramics is an art that requires many years of practice to master. Errors in manipulation not only compromise the esthetics of the restoration but its physical integrity as well.

Ceramic–Alloy Bonding

The ceramic–alloy bond is of fundamental importance to the success of ceramic–alloy restorations because the stresses induced in the ceramic by oral forces can be shared and supported by the alloy. Glassy dental ceramics are far too brittle to withstand oral forces by themselves, particularly tensile forces. A testament to this problem is the high failure rate of so-called porcelain jacket crowns. To conserve tooth structure, these all-ceramic crowns were fabricated for upper lateral incisors from glassy ceramics with no alloy substructure. Most of these restorations failed after a short time in service.

> **! ALERT**
>
> Without ceramic–alloy bonding, glassy or glass-dominated ceramics would fracture quickly in service as dental restorations under the stress of oral forces.

Durability of the ceramic–alloy bond is paramount to clinical success of the ceramic–alloy restoration. Any debonding of the ceramic from the alloy after the restoration has been permanently cemented can cause esthetic or functional failure of the restoration. Repair often requires complete replacement, including removal of the old metal substructure and fabrication of a new metal substructure and ceramic veneer. The effects of ceramic–alloy debonding are expensive and traumatic to the patient and should be prevented if at all possible.

The bonding of ceramic to alloy occurs through an oxide on the alloy surface (Chapter 11). Alloys for ceramic–alloy restorations are nearly always specially formulated so that an oxide will form. When ceramic is fired onto the alloy surface, a chemical reaction between the oxide layer of the alloy and the ceramic occurs, which creates the ceramic–alloy bond (see Figure 11-9). Achieving a good bond demands meticulous efforts to limit contamination of the alloy and ceramic and strict adherence to protocols for manipulating the ceramic.

Failures of ceramic–alloy bonds stem from several causes. For example, the alloy may form an inadequate oxide layer, resulting in a weak ceramic–alloy bond. Another cause is formation of an oxide layer that is too thick. Because oxides themselves are brittle ceramic materials, a thick oxide layer increases the risk of ceramic–alloy fracture. However, the most common failure of the ceramic–alloy bond is failure within the ceramic layer itself near the alloy–ceramic interface. Most researchers believe that microscopic cracks occur in areas of high stress, in which an inadequate bond exists between the ceramic and the alloy, or when a mismatch occurs between the coefficients of thermal expansion of the alloy and ceramic (see the previous discussion on properties). When these cracks increase to a critical size, the crack rapidly progresses through the entire ceramic layer, a catastrophic

failure occurs, and the ceramic debonds from the alloy. This type of failure may occur after only a few weeks in service if the flaws in the restoration were severe or might not occur for months or years if the flaws were subtle. It is nearly impossible to detect these flaws reliably during manufacture of the restoration; therefore, adherence to fabrication protocols must be maintained to minimize the introduction of flaws.

Fabrication of Ceramic–Alloy Restorations

Although the technical details of ceramic–alloy restoration fabrication are beyond the scope of this text, a basic understanding of this process helps communication among the dentist, patient, dental auxiliary, insurance company, and dental laboratory. Fabrication of these restorations starts with casting and recontouring the alloy substructure (Chapter 11). The alloy thickness is generally less than 0.5 mm to maximize the space available for the ceramic, which promotes more esthetic optical properties of the ceramic. The substructure is then "degassed" in a ceramic oven (Figures 14-6 and 14-13). Degassing removes impurities from the alloy surface and promotes the formation of an oxide layer on the alloy. The term *degassing* is really a misnomer because there is no evolution or removal of gas in this step.

After the alloy has been degassed, an opaquing ceramic is applied to hide the color of the alloy substructure (see Figures 14-13 and 14-14). The opaque ceramic is condensed and sintered onto the alloy (see the previous discussion). If successfully applied, the opaque layer forms a bond with the alloy and blocks the alloy color from being transmitted through the ceramic. Different types of alloys have different oxide shades that may be harder or easier to mask; for example, nickel- and cobalt-based alloys have dark gray oxides that require thicker opaque layers to mask compared to the light yellow oxides of gold-based alloys (see Figure 11-10).

> **! ALERT**
>
> Esthetic success with ceramic–alloy restorations requires careful attention to detail at each step in the fabrication process.

After opaquing, the gingival and incisal ceramics are applied over the opaque layer (see Figures 14-13 and 14-14). The gingival ceramic is applied first to the gingival half of the crown. It is yellower and less translucent than the incisal ceramic and mimics the dentin of the tooth. This ceramic is applied in the same manner as the opaque (in a paste with condensation), is fired onto the opaque, and bonds to it by the sintering mechanism previously described. The incisal ceramic is added primarily to the incisal third of the crowns (see Figure 14-14). Its higher translucency mimics natural tooth structure well. Finally, a glaze layer, which is a thin, nearly transparent, low-fusing ceramic, is applied. The glaze seals the ceramic surface and provides a high luster to the surface. Metal oxide "stains," which have hues appropriate for teeth, are sometimes applied over or under the glaze to provide individual characterization of the crown and improve the color match with the

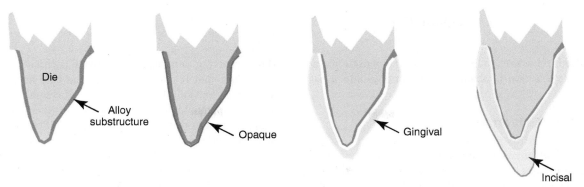

FIG 14-13 Steps involved in the fabrication of a ceramic–alloy crown. The alloy substructure (also called a "coping," *left diagram at arrow*) is first heated to create an oxide layer and remove organic impurities (degassing, not shown). Next, one or more layers of opaque ceramic are applied to mask the color of the metallic oxide (shown in blue to delineate here). Then, the gingival ceramic, which has a more yellow hue, is added, followed by incisal ceramic. (Opaque is the white layer in the two right diagrams.) Finally, stains may be added to characterize the shade of the ceramic, and a glaze is applied to provide a smooth surface finish. Staining and glazing place extremely thin films of ceramic on the restoration and are not shown in this diagram.

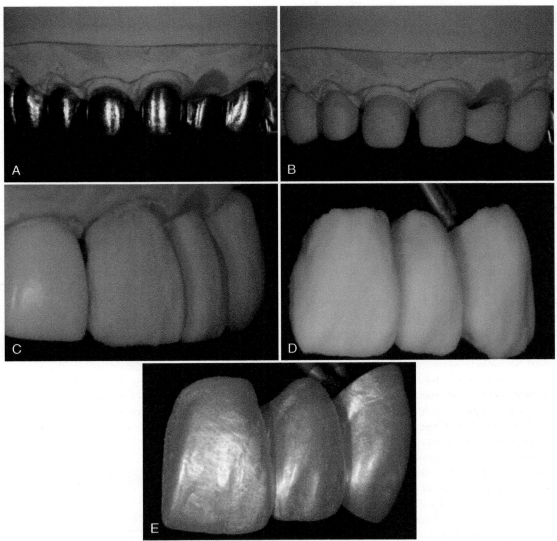

FIG 14-14 Fabrication of ceramic–alloy restorations by stacking. Castings **(A)** are contoured and fired (degassed) to prepare surfaces for application of the ceramic. Opaquing ceramic is applied to mask the gray color of the metal oxide on the metal substructures **(B)**. The dentinal ceramic is applied first **(C)**, followed by the enamel ceramic to full contour **(D)**. Once the ceramic is "stacked" to full contour, it is fired in the ceramic oven for 10 to 12 minutes **(E)**. Additional ceramic may be added at this point, or stains and glaze may be applied to finish the restoration. (Courtesy Y-W Chen, University of Washington Department of Restorative Dentistry, Seattle, WA.)

adjacent teeth. However, staining cannot compensate for an inappropriate selection of shades for the gingival and incisal layers.

All-Ceramic Restorations

All-Ceramic Crowns and Fixed Partial Dentures

The principal advantage of any all-ceramic restoration is the potential for better esthetics. Because all-ceramic restorations do not use an alloy substructure, all of the thickness of the restoration is ceramic, which allows the laboratory technician to create a more lifelike esthetic result. Furthermore, all-ceramic restorations have no alloy oxide color to mask. However, the ceramic must survive stresses from oral forces in the absence of an alloy substructure. Furthermore, any unnatural colors of the tooth, as well as the color of the cement, must be accommodated.

> **! ALERT**
>
> An all-ceramic crown is often composed of a high-strength opaque ceramic core with a bonded veneer of a weaker but translucent glassy or glass-dominated ceramic. Newer designs have only high-strength crystalline or crystalline-dominated ceramics.

Today's all-ceramic crowns take advantage of fabrication technologies that have improved ceramic strength and are reliable in anterior applications (see Table 14-1). All-ceramics also are used for posterior crowns, and some practitioners have extended the use of these materials to fixed partial dentures of three units or more, although prospective, randomized, long-term clinical data are sparse to support such uses.

A few current all-ceramic crowns are made entirely of glass-dominated ceramics (see Table 14-1). The improved strength of these materials over glassy ceramics makes them plausible alternatives for some anterior restorations and a few posterior restorations (see Table 14-2). An important consideration with these translucent restorations is the color and overall condition of the tooth. For example, amalgam cores will show through the final restoration. The shade of the cement also must be considered.

Many all-ceramic restorations use a high-strength ceramic core covered with a veneering ceramic (Figure 14-15). For this type of restoration, the high-strength core replaces the alloy substructure in its role to support and strengthen the veneering layers. The core materials are crystalline or crystalline-dominated ceramics formed by pressing or machining, less often these days by infusion (see the previous section on fabrication techniques and Figure 14-4). The core ceramics have not been traditionally used for the entire restoration because they are opaque (because of their high crystalline content; see the previous discussion on optical properties, Figure 14-11). The esthetic nature of these all ceramic restorations has traditionally been created using a glassy or glass-dominated veneering ceramic. Veneering layers are commonly custom-stacked onto the core in a manner similar to that used for ceramic–alloy restorations (see the ceramic–alloys section), but they also may be pressed or milled.

The veneering ceramic must have a coefficient of thermal expansion that is compatible with the core as well (see the properties section, Figure 14-10). All-ceramic restorations with an opaque high-strength core may be cemented without concern about the cement shade because of the opacity of the core. Increasingly, doped zirconia ceramics and, to a more limited extent, lithium disilicate ceramics are being used for the entire all-ceramic restoration in the posterior teeth (so-called monolithic design). These restorations are strong, may require less tooth reduction than ceramic–alloy or layered all-ceramic restorations, and are opaque enough to mask tooth defects. They also take advantage of CAD-CAM fabrication techniques with a digital impression. However, these restorations lack high esthetic qualities. Moreover, the high hardness of zirconia relative to tooth structure increases the risk of inappropriate wear of opposing teeth or restorations, particularly if the ceramic surface is not smooth enough. Long-term clinical data on performance of these restorations are lacking at present.

The decision to use an all-ceramic or a ceramic–alloy restoration is complex, particularly for posterior restorations and especially for posterior bridges (see Table 14-1). Although all-ceramic restorations have improved tremendously in strength since the days of porcelain-jacket crowns, they are still relatively brittle materials that will fracture in service more often than ceramic–alloy restorations. In some cases, layered all-ceramic restorations require the removal of more tooth structure to maximize the thickness of the restoration (and reduce fracture risk), which increases the risk of tooth pulpal pathology in some individuals. This requirement for greater thickness has become less important as the core ceramics have become stronger. The cementation of all-ceramic restorations may be more complex, and they are more difficult to adjust in service for occlusion. The use of all-ceramic restorations has been increasing on the presumption of superior esthetics versus ceramic–alloy restorations, and this presumption is true in some clinical situations. However, a well-constructed ceramic–alloy restoration may be just as esthetic in many clinical situations, without the complications, costs, and clinical risks of the all-ceramic material. The key to an appropriate choice of material lies in careful consideration of all dimensions of the patient's restorative needs and oral conditions, with emphasis placed on long-term preservation of oral health and tissue. As experience with all-ceramics improves and long-term data become available, these restorations seem likely to dominate restorations requiring ceramics.

> **! ALERT**
>
> The clinical choice between ceramic–alloy and all-ceramic restoration should consider many aspects of the patient's oral condition as well as restorative material properties and currently available clinical evidence on material performance.

Ceramic veneers (also referred to as ceramic or porcelain laminates) are made from traditional or newer ceramics and are intended to replace only the facial and incisal portions of anterior teeth (Figure 14-16). Veneers are most often used on

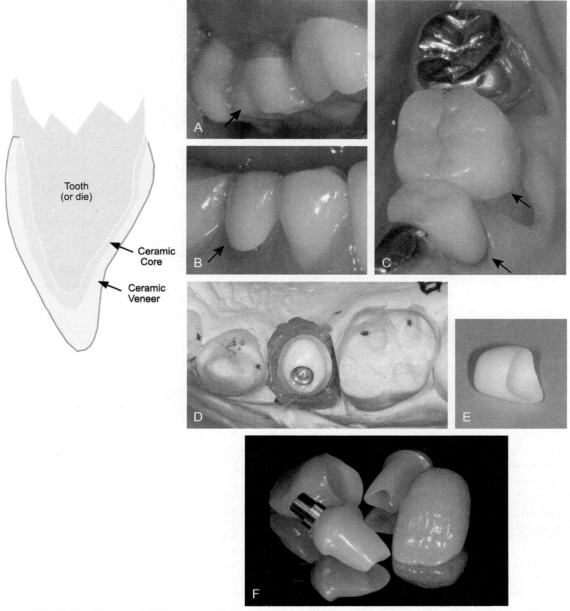

FIG 14-15 *(Diagram left)* Cross-sectional diagram of an all-ceramic restoration on an anterior tooth. Unlike ceramic–alloy restorations (see Figure 14-12), there is no alloy substructure; rather, a high-strength ceramic core material is fabricated to fit onto the prepared tooth by either pressing or milling. Because the core, composed of crystalline-dominated or crystalline ceramic, is often opaque, an opaque layer is not needed in most cases to mask any colors from the tooth. The ceramic veneering layer (shown in the diagram as a single layer) is added next and must completely cover the core (see also Figure 14-8). All-ceramic restorations (**A–F,** *black arrows*) are increasingly common for crowns and for bridges. Furthermore, crystalline ceramics are being used for all-ceramic cores and implant abutments onto which the high-strength substructure is placed **(D–F).** (**A–E,** courtesy E. R. Schwedhelm, University of Washington Department of Restorative Dentistry, Seattle, WA; **F,** courtesy Y-W Chen, University of Washington Department of Restorative Dentistry, Seattle, WA.)

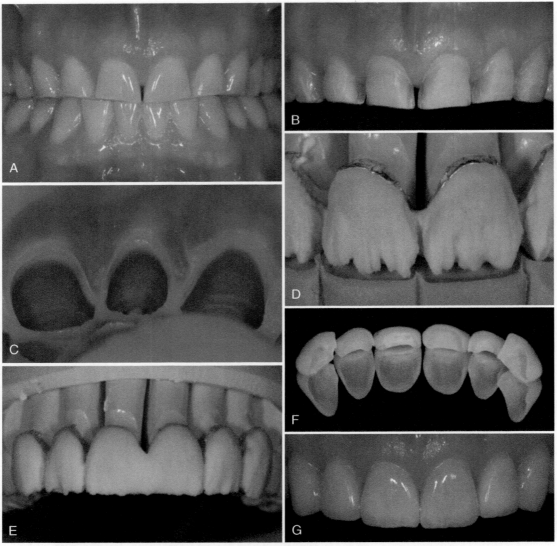

FIG 14-16 Ceramic veneers have no high-strength substructure but are bonded to enamel and sometimes dentin to obtain the strength needed to avoid fracture of the glassy or glass-dominated ceramic. Veneers are used when a more aggressive restoration is not needed. The original tooth shapes **(A)** are prepared for the veneers **(B)**; then an impression is taken. The dentinal porcelain is stacked on the working dies (**C,** here using the platinum foil technique rather than a refractory die) using an index of the final tooth contour as a guide (gray material in **D**). The enamel ceramic is added **(E),** and the restorations are fired **(F).** Resin cements are used to bond the ceramic into place **(G).** Because veneers are translucent (not opaque), the shade of the cement is critical to an appropriate esthetic result. (**A–G,** Y-W Chen, University of Washington Department of Restorative Dentistry, Seattle, WA.)

maxillary anterior teeth. The preparation of the tooth may require only a fraction of a millimeter of tooth reduction in some areas. Because of this minimal preparation, veneers are exquisitely fragile restorations before they are bonded to the tooth. Veneers are fabricated from glassy or glass-dominated ceramics (see Table 14-1), and the surface of the veneer that contacts the tooth must be treated using a strong acid (hydrofluoric acid gel) to facilitate bonding of the veneer to the tooth. Thus, when these delicate restorations are returned from the laboratory, extreme care must be taken not to break them. Veneers are bonded to the tooth using specialized resin-based, shade-controlled, light-activated cements and acid-etching techniques. Despite their fragile nature in the unbonded state, veneer restorations are quite durable once bonded to the tooth and reinforced by the enamel and dentin, provided that the bonding process has been successful. Veneers are clinically most successful if bonded to enamel (compared to dentin).

Ceramic onlays are intracoronal (inside the tooth, Chapter 1), posterior restorations and are used in clinical situations in which amalgam, composite, or gold inlays were prescribed previously (Figure 14-17). Ceramic onlays are composed of crystalline or crystalline-dominated ceramics. The opacity of these ceramics is generally not a liability in the posterior intracoronal restoration. Ceramic onlays are generally machined. The newest technologies do not use a traditional impression of the tooth but capture a digital image of the cavity preparation using a small intraoral camera (a so-called digital impression). This image is then fed into a computer, is adjusted by the operator, and then is used to direct the computer to machine the appropriate shape. In some practices, the restoration may be prepared while the patient is present, eliminating the need for an additional appointment. Whether formed by an impression and refractory die or by CAD-CAM, ceramic onlays are generally cemented using resin-based cements. Because ceramic onlays are used for intracoronal lesions in the posterior teeth, the shade and opacity properties of the cement are less important than for all-ceramic crowns or veneers. However, the bonding of the cement is critical to prevent secondary caries.

The choice between ceramic onlay and composite to esthetically restore small posterior lesions remains controversial. Ceramic onlays use a more aggressive and less customizable tooth preparation but require less manipulation of materials by the practitioner and less chair time. Composites require much more clinical finesse and chair time but are more customizable in terms of shade, shape, and restoration design for good retention and longevity. Many practitioners feel that the long-term marginal seal of ceramic onlays is inferior to that of composites. If CAD-CAM is to be used to make "while you wait" restorations, then ceramic onlays require the practitioner to purchase expensive equipment.

> **! ALERT**
>
> Ceramics are now being used for implant abutments, and ceramic endosseous implants are becoming more commonplace.

Ceramic Implant Abutments and Implants

Perhaps the most recent application of ceramics is in the area of implantology. Crystalline ceramic implant abutments (Figure 14-18) are being used instead of titanium alloy, particularly in anterior restorations in which the gray color of the titanium alloy is a liability. Ceramic abutments are almost always formed by machining in combination with a digital image captured by a computer-driven scanner. The bright white, opaque color of most crystalline ceramics is itself an esthetic liability, and shaded ceramics have been recently introduced to reduce this problem. Ceramic implant abutments are commonly restored with an all-ceramic restoration, itself consisting of a crystalline ceramic core veneered with a glassy or glass-dominated ceramic (see Figure 14-18). Most recently, crystalline endosseous implants, composed of zirconia, have been introduced. These materials are discussed in Chapter 15.

New Problems with All-Ceramic Restorations

All-ceramic techniques and materials continue to revolutionize clinical dentistry, but along with new materials and technologies have emerged several unanticipated clinical challenges. One such problem is the bonding of veneering ceramics to core ceramics (Figure 14-19). Because ceramics are all fundamentally similar in atomic structure (Figure 14-1), many initially assumed that bonding ceramic veneer to ceramic core bonding would not be a major clinical concern. Clinically, this assumption has not been supported: debonding of veneering ceramics from core ceramics has emerged as a significant clinical problem. In principle, the stresses between ceramics that develop as they bonded are regulated by the CTEs of both materials, just as they are in ceramic–alloy bonding. An appropriate "match" between the CTEs of the veneer and core appears to be important, if incompletely defined. However, a lack of awareness of the requirement for a compatible CTE match between veneer and core, coupled with more complex cooling management of the fired restoration (because ceramics are inherently insulating) has made ceramic–ceramic debonding a significant clinical issue. Time will likely provide clarity on the appropriate management of this and other clinical problems associated with all-ceramic restorations.

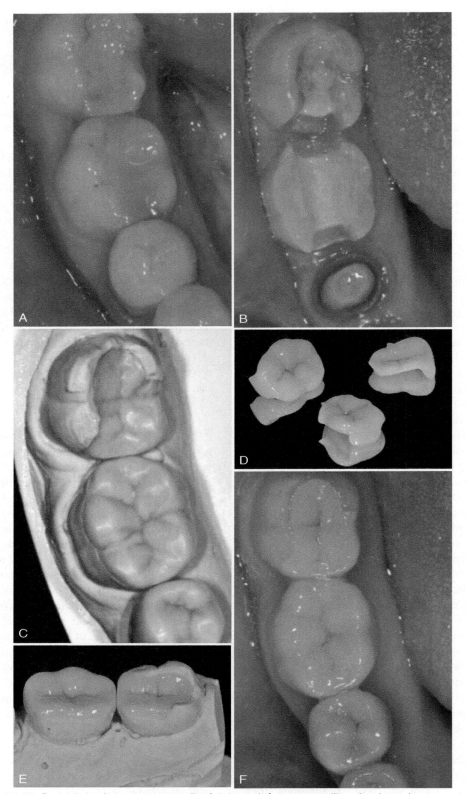

FIG 14-17 Ceramic onlays are generally fabricated from crystalline-dominated or crystalline ceramics. The higher strength ceramics are necessary for onlays to minimize the risk of fracture in service. The original restoration (**A,** teeth #30, 31) is removed and the tooth is prepared for an intracoronal onlay restoration **(B).** After an impression and fabrication of a working die, the restoration is waxed to full contour **(C);** then a crystalline-dominated ceramic (lithium disilicate here) is pressed to form the restorations **(D).** The restorations are adjusted on the working die **(E)** and then cemented into place **(F).** Ceramic onlays are generally cemented with resin-based cements. Fabrication of ceramic onlays today is also accomplished by computer-aided machining and a digital impression. (Courtesy Satoshi Go, private practice, Seattle, WA.)

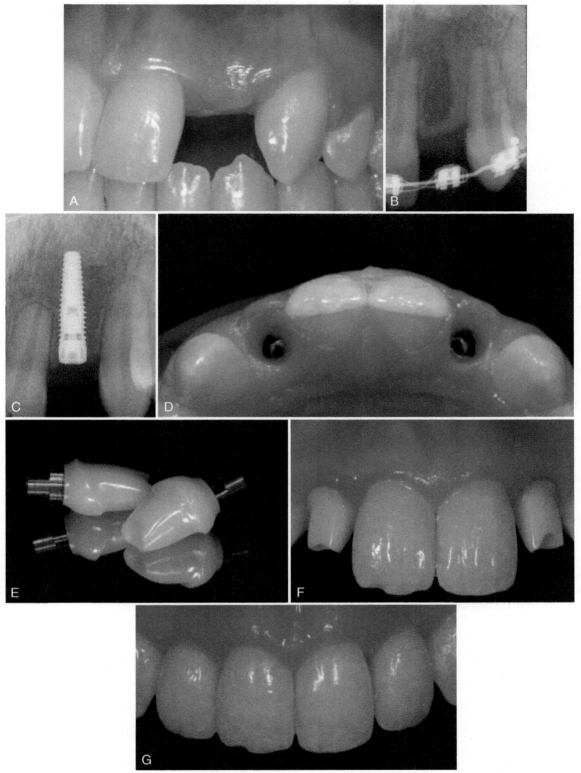

FIG 14-18 Fabrication of an all-ceramic restoration on a ceramic implant abutment using digital impressions and CAD-CAM techniques. The space for a congenitally missing tooth #10 (**A** #10 shown, #7 also missing) is first optimized using orthodontics **(B),** followed by placement of an endosseous implant **(C).** Temporaries are used to contour the anterior tissues **(D),** which is critical to the esthetic result in this area. A digital impression (using a special impression coping) is obtained, and all-ceramic custom abutments with titanium alloy fixture interfaces are milled from zirconia using a CAD-CAM process **(E).** Once the abutments are seated in the mouth **(F),** all-ceramic restorations are fabricated from crystalline ceramics (core) with glassy or glass-dominated ceramics as a veneer. The final restorations are cemented in the mouth **(G).** (Courtesy Y-W Chen, University of Washington Department of Restorative Dentistry, Seattle, WA.)

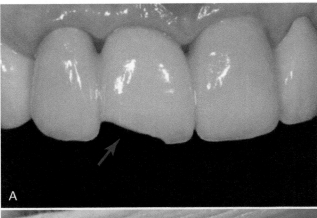

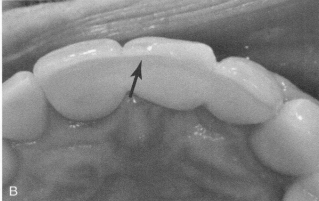

FIG 14-19 Although debonding of ceramics from alloy sub-structures is a well-known clinical problem (see Figure 11-11), debonding of veneer ceramics from core ceramics in all-ceramic restoration is emerging as a significant clinical problem as well. Here **(A, B),** the veneering glassy ceramic has debonded from the zirconia crystalline core *(blue arrows)*. Failures of this nature may result from incompatible coefficients of thermal expansion of the veneering and core ceramics (see Figure 14-10), inappropriate cooling of the restoration during firing of the glassy ceramic, or contamination of the core surface during glassy ceramic application. In any case, as with ceramic–alloy failures, ceramic–ceramic bonding failures are difficult to repair and often must be redone completely. (Courtesy Y-W Chen, University of Washington Department of Restorative Dentistry, Seattle, WA.)

QUICK REVIEW

Ceramics play a central and increasing role in esthetic dental restorations. Early dental ceramics were amorphous glasses (so-called glassy or feldspathic ceramics) with embedded crystals of leucite for strength and esthetics. These ceramics are still used in the fabrication of ceramic–alloy restorations in which ceramic is chemically bonded to and supported by an alloy substructure. The ceramic–alloy restoration is the ceramic restoration with the longest clinical track record. Meticulous techniques and a compatible ceramic and alloy are essential to obtain a strong bond between the ceramic and alloy. In contrast, all-ceramic restorations have no alloy substructure. Core ceramics for these restorations are either dominated by a crystalline phase or are entirely crystalline. These restorations may be fabricated using several different techniques, including pressing, machining, or to a lesser extent today, infusion. All-ceramic crowns can be remarkably esthetic, and it is this quality that has driven their clinical use. Veneers of glassy or glass-dominated ceramics are used to mask the facial surfaces of deformed or defective enamel, and crystalline ceramic onlays may be made for intracoronal dental restorations. Most recently, crystalline ceramics such as doped zirconia have been used for full-contour crowns, implant abutments, and implants themselves. For any ceramic restoration, intraoral failure, usually via fracture, remains a significant clinical problem, but appropriate manipulation and case selection now minimize this difficulty. Newer clinical problems such as veneer-core debonding have emerged, but these will likely be managed as experience with these materials increases.

SELF-TEST QUESTIONS

Test your knowledge by answering the following questions. For multiple-choice questions, one or more responses may be correct.

1. The raw materials used to make feldspathic dental ceramics include:
   a. Zinc oxide
   b. Alumina
   c. Silica
   d. Feldspar
   e. Oxides or carbonates of sodium or potassium
   f. Fluxes
2. During the sintering of ceramics, what occur(s)?
   a. The ceramic completely liquefies.
   b. Shrinkage occurs.
   c. Adjacent particles fuse at points of contact.
   d. Infusion occurs.
3. Which of the following statements is/are true regarding the strength of ceramics?
   a. Ceramics are strong in compression but weak in tension and bending.
   b. Alumina addition strengthens ceramic.
   c. Surface scratches strengthen ceramic.
   d. Flexural strength is commonly used to assess ceramic strength.
   e. Most ceramics fail in clinical service by fracturing.

4. Factor(s) that promote strong ceramic-to-alloy bonds is/are:
   a. An oxide layer on the alloy surface
   b. A gold coating on the alloy surface
   c. A coefficient of thermal expansion of the alloy slightly greater than that of the ceramic
   d. A rough alloy surface

Use short statements to answer the following questions.

5. A dentist takes a shade for a ceramic restoration using the dental light to illuminate the teeth. What do you predict about the match of the crown when the patient is at home?

6. A lab technician has successfully used a certain brand of ceramic for years with a high-noble casting alloy. The technician changes alloys and continues to use the same ceramic but notices cracking of the ceramic and debonding of the ceramic from the alloy. What may the problem be?

7. After degassing the metal substructure of a ceramic–alloy crown, a lab technician adjusts the thickness of the alloy and then fires the opaque and ceramic onto the alloy. One year after the crown is cemented in the mouth, the ceramic debonds. Why?

8. Ceramic veneers have no opaque layer. What problems do you think this might pose for managing the shade after final cementation?

For the following statements, select true or false.

9. In feldspathic ceramics, leucite is a glassy phase in a crystalline matrix.
   a. True
   b. False

10. Crystalline ceramics are the weakest type of ceramic among today's dental ceramics.
    a. True
    b. False

11. Degassing of an alloy during the fabrication of a ceramic–alloy restoration is done to clean the alloy surface and form an oxide layer on the alloy.
    a. True
    b. False

12. In a ceramic–alloy restoration, the ceramic is designed to have a coefficient of thermal expansion larger than the alloy to place the ceramic in compression.
    a. True
    b. False

13. Sintering is a process during which particles of ceramic fuse at points of contact.
    a. True
    b. False

14. In spite of its high strength, a crystalline ceramic cannot be used for the entire restoration because of its opacity.
    a. True
    b. False

15. Crystalline-dominated ceramics must be veneered to provide an esthetic restoration.
    a. True
    b. False

Use a term or a phrase to fill in the following blanks.

16. Feldspathic dental ceramics are characterized as being _____.

17. The property that describes the linear expansion of ceramic per °C is _____.

18. _____ is the intensity of a color, whereas _____ identifies the lightness or darkness.

19. In ceramic–alloy restorations, the bond between the ceramic and alloy is _____ in nature.

20. The core ceramic in a restoration is more _____ than the gingival or incisal ceramic.

SUGGESTED SUPPLEMENTARY READINGS

Denry IL, Kelly JR: State of the art of zirconia for dental applications, *Dent Mater* 24:299, 2008.

Kelly JR, Denry IL: Stabilized zirconia as a structural ceramic: an overview, *Dent Mater* 24:289, 2008.

Kim J-W, Covel NS, Guess PC, et al: Concerns of hydrothermal degradation in CAD/CAM zirconia, *J Dent Res* 89(1):91, 2010.

Miyazaki T, Nakamura T, Matsumura H, Ban S, Kobayashi T: Current status of zirconia restoration, *J Pros Res* 57:236, 2013.

evolve Please visit *http://evolve.elsevier.com/Powers/dentalmaterials* for additional practice and study support tools.

15

Dental Implants

OBJECTIVES

After reading this chapter, the reader should be able to:

1. List the types of materials that have been used for endosseous implants, and explain which osseointegrate or biointegrate with bone.
2. Compare and contrast biointegration and osseointegration.
3. Explain how oral forces applied to an endosseous implant stress bone differently than natural teeth do.
4. Describe the clinical treatment sequences used to place endosseous implants and the advantages and disadvantages of each sequence.
5. Describe what instrumentation is needed to clean endosseous implants at the gingival level and why special instruments are needed.
6. Describe the alloys of titanium that are used for endosseous implants in terms of composition, physical properties, and surface properties.
7. Explain why ceramic coatings are applied to endosseous implants.
8. Explain the advantages and disadvantages of zirconia as an endosseous implant material, and compare these characteristics with titanium-based implants.
9. Describe how digital imaging is used for placement and restoration of endosseous implants.

> **! ALERT**
>
> Endosseous implants are placed directly into bone; most dental implants used today are endosseous implants.

Attempts to implant a material into bone to replace a tooth date back thousands of years, yet modern dental implantology is less than 45 years old. Implant placement into the maxilla or mandible creates complex interfaces between the implant material and the oral tissues. At these interfaces, the implant material must not harm the hard or soft tissues and must withstand the physical and chemical environment of the oral cavity over a service life that may span decades. The tissues must remain viable and functional to retain the implant when it is placed under loads during chewing, brushing, speaking, and other oral functions.

This chapter focuses on the endosseous implant, which is the most common type of dental implant used today (Figure 15-1). Endosseous implants are placed into bone, as opposed to other types of implants that might be placed external to the bone. Today, the endosseous implant is used to solve complex clinical problems in an increasing number of individuals. The role of endosseous implants will expand as more practitioners master placement techniques and new materials and strategies are developed to predictably treat complex clinical situations. Dental auxiliaries must understand the nature of implant materials and clinical manipulation of implants to provide appropriate care in a contemporary dental practice.

IMPORTANT PRINCIPLES

Implant Surgery

The successful placement of an endosseous implant relies on a series of strategic surgical and restorative decisions (Figures 15-2, 15-3, 15-4). The goals are to maximize bony support for the implant, impart minimal trauma and inflammation that might impede healing, and provide a restorative foundation that supports optimal esthetics and function while minimizing destructive intraoral forces.

In the traditional surgical (two-stage, delayed restoration) method, the extraction socket of a tooth is allowed to fill in with bone for 3 to 6 months before the implant is placed. Once healing is complete, the bone is prepared with special metallic burs driven at slow speeds (<2000 rpm) to specific depths with special handpieces and copious water cooling. Many times, the location of bony preparation (osteotomy) is guided by an acrylic stent, which is often constructed with the aid of traditional radiographs or computed tomography (CT) scans. During preparation of the osteotomy, the objective is to avoid temperatures in the bone above 37° C that will damage tissues, cause protein coagulation, and trigger inflammation. The osteotomy burs are composed of special alloys of titanium to avoid deposition of trace metal contaminants that may themselves cause adverse biologic reactions. The water coolant is sterile to avoid contamination of the placement site with bacteria or other microorganisms. The amount of bone removed is controlled carefully in a series of steps to coincide with the diameter and length of implant to ensure the bone and implant heal in close proximity to each other.

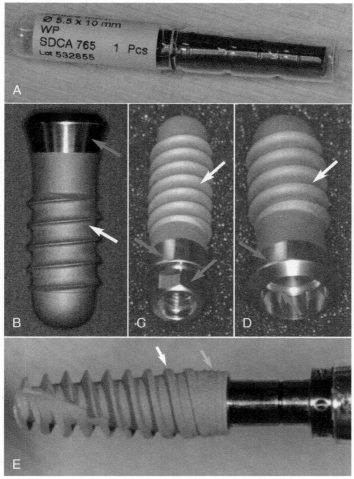

FIG 15-1 Endosseous implants are placed into the maxilla or mandible, but they protrude through the gingiva to serve as surrogates for teeth. Today's implants are primarily alloys of titanium and oxygen; relatively few are all-ceramic (zirconia). Before placement, the implant must be protected from both chemical and biologic contamination and is therefore encased in special containers that are opened only at the time of surgery **(A)**. Endosseous implants are commonly threaded **(B–E)** to facilitate precise placement and initial retention and stability in bone. Surfaces that contact bone have special treatments that promote osseointegration (*white arrows* in **B–E**). Implants placed to the soft tissue level have a smooth surface to promote soft tissue adaptation (*red arrows* in **B, C,** and **D**); those that are placed to the bone level have no smooth surface (*blue arrow* in **E**). The attachment between the implant and implant restoration occurs via an external (*green arrow* in **C**) or internal (*green arrow* in **D**) union that prevents rotation of the final restoration. Today's endosseous implants are made in a wide variety of diameters, tapers, and lengths. Parallel-sided implants **(B, C, D)** or tapered implants **(E)** are used in different clinical situations. Different diameters, lengths, and styles are now available through many manufacturers. (**A,** Courtesy Dr. Regina Messer, Georgia Regents University, Augusta, GA.; **B–D,** courtesy Dr. Mats Kronström, University of Washington, Department of Restorative Dentistry, Seattle, WA; **E,** courtesy Y-W Chen, University of Washington, Department of Restorative Dentistry, Seattle, WA.)

Once the implant site is prepared in the bone, implants may be placed to the bone level or tissue level. The screw-type implant (compared to friction fit) is the most common style used today (see Figure 15-1) because it allows a snug fit of the implant into the socket *and* controlled application of force to final position of placement. As with the surgical preparation, special instruments are used in an atraumatic manner to ensure preservation of the bone and minimal contamination of the wound site. The implant itself is meticulously handled to avoid chemical or microbial contamination.

Depending on the type of implant placed, several strategies are used when the implant is placed (see Figures 15-2 and 15-3). For tissue-level implants, the soft tissue may be sutured around the implant, which will be left protruding through the tissue, and a small cap will be placed to prevent contamination of the internal parts of the implant. This strategy is called a one-stage restoration; it is important to understand that the

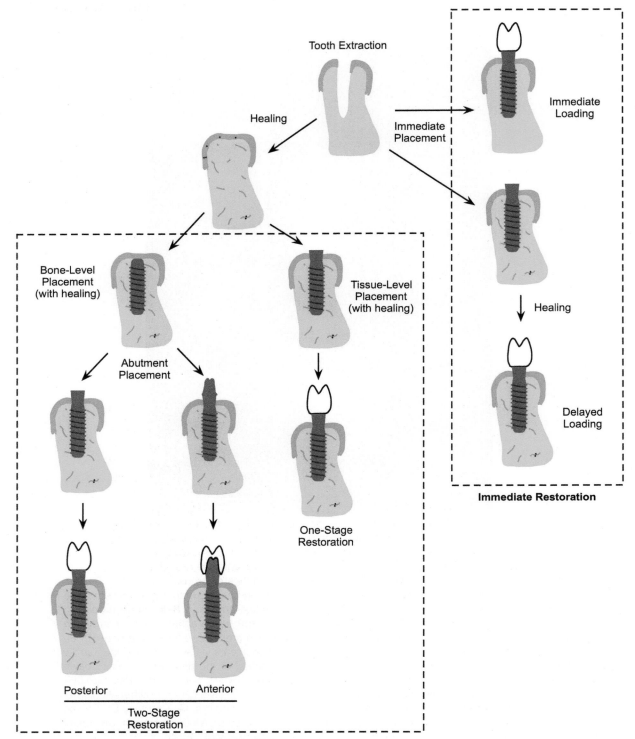

FIG 15-2 Sequence of implant placement. Several strategies are used to place implants today. Most implants are placed into healed bone in one- or two-stage procedures. Care must be taken to ensure that adequate bone exists to support the dental prosthesis. In two-stage restorations, the implant is placed to the level of the bone; then it is allowed to heal for approximately 3 months. At a second surgery, one of several types of abutments is placed, and the soft tissue is allowed to heal. Posterior teeth sometimes receive a platform implant that receives a screw-retained crown; anterior implants receive a tooth-shaped (custom) abutment onto which a crown is either cemented or screwed. In one-stage restorations, the implant with a built-in abutment is placed at the tissue level. After a period of healing, the crown is placed. Today, several other techniques are sometimes used. The implant may be placed immediately after tooth extraction (immediate restoration). Although placement may be at the bone or tissue level, only the tissue level is shown here. After placement, the practitioner has the option of loading the implant into occlusal function immediately or after healing. Most experts today generally consider immediate placement and immediate loading to be higher-risk strategies.

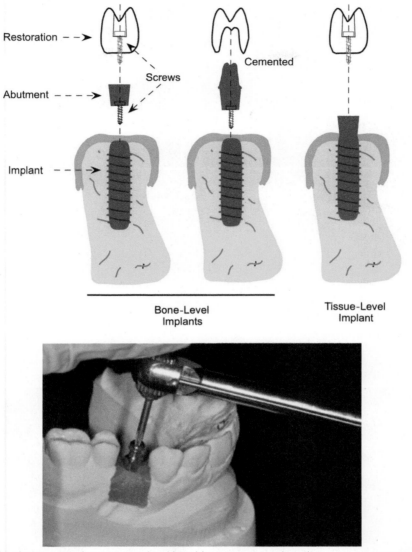

FIG 15-3 Implant restorations are retained by either screws or dental cements or some combination of these two. For bone-level implants, a screw is used to retain the abutment to the implant itself. If the abutment is of the platform type *(left diagram)*, the restoration will be retained with a second screw *(red)* that is accessed through a hole in the restoration. If the abutment is of the custom type *(middle diagram)*, the restoration will be retained by a traditional cement. For tissue-level implants *(right diagram)*, the restoration may be retained by a single screw. Screws for implants are precisely engineered of specific materials that limit loosening or fracture. They are torqued to specific tightness using a torque wrench intraorally *(lower photo)*. Failure to use the appropriate torque may lead to early failure of the restoration. Implant screws are designed to be used only once. For screw-retained restorations, the hole in the occlusal part of the restoration is generally covered with resin composite material. (Photo courtesy Dr. Y-W Chen, University of Washington, Department of Restorative Dentistry, Seattle, WA.)

implant is generally not in occlusion during the healing. For bone-level implants, two strategies may be used. In a one-stage surgery, a healing abutment with a cap is placed immediately after the implant, and the tissue is managed around the abutment as with the tissue-level implant. In a two-stage surgery, a healing cap is placed on the implant and the tissue is positioned over the cap to allow healing with the implant submerged. In this case, a second surgery is needed to place the abutment through the soft tissue. Two-stage surgeries may be used when there are questions about the likelihood of osseointegration or when other procedures such as bone grafting are done at the time of the initial implant. In all cases, the implant is allowed to heal for at least 6 weeks (generally 2 to 3 months) without occlusal loading. The avoidance of any movement (<100 μm) is imperative to successful integration of the implant with the bone.

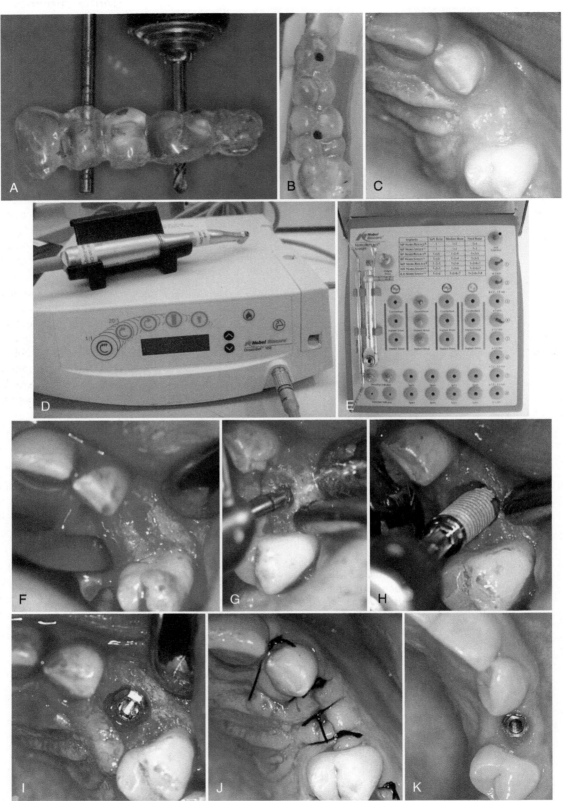

FIG 15-4 Clinical sequence of two-stage implant placement. After careful treatment planning to determine the final position of the implant **(A, B, C)**, an acrylic surgical stent **(A and B)** is made that will guide the position and angulation for the osteotomy. Special handpieces **(D)** and burs **(E)** are used that minimize trauma to the bone during the osteotomy and maximize changes of successful osseointegration. A gingival flap is retracted **(F)**, and the osteotomy is performed in several stages **(G)** under copious water irrigation. The implant is screwed into place to the appropriate depth **(H and I)**, and then the flap is repositioned with sutures **(J)**. After healing (2 to 3 months), a second minor surgery is used to expose the implant prior to abutment placement **(K)**. (Courtesy Dr. Mats Kronström, University of Washington, Department of Restorative Dentistry, Seattle, WA.)

The ability to satisfactorily restore the teeth is determined, to a large extent, on the position of the implants. Thus, advanced planning by the dentist and good communication with the surgeon are essential to ensure that the restoration will be able to be appropriately constructed and placed. The dental auxiliary is a critical link in this chain of communication. Several types of final abutments are possible (see Figures 15-2 and 15-3). In posterior teeth, a platform abutment is common; this type of abutment is a relatively flat junction onto which the posterior implant crown is fabricated and secured with a screw (see Figures 1-9 and 15-3). In anterior teeth, a tapered abutment, either with a standard shape or custom made, is most often used. Once the final abutments are in place, the prosthesis is constructed in much the same manner as for natural teeth. The prosthesis may be cemented permanently or screwed into place with a small screw that penetrates the top of the crowns and threads into the abutments (Figure 15-3). The use of screws allows the prosthesis to be removed if necessary to permit reevaluation or cleaning of the implants. The hole for the screw is often filled with a small composite to obscure the opening. The torque applied to abutment or restorative screws is a critical factor; overtorqueing may lead to screw failure or distortion of the implant fixture, abutment, or restoration. For this reason, torque wrenches are always used to assure an appropriate level of torque of screws (Figure 15-3).

The placement strategies described in the previous paragraphs are currently the most common and reliable methods of ensuring a successful result. However, some clinicians have advocated the placement of an implant into the extraction socket of a tooth immediately after extraction (see Figure 15-2). Furthermore, some clinicians promote the immediate loading of an implant after its placement at an extraction site by placing the restoration at the time of the surgery. The restoration may be permanent or temporary in these cases. However, all of these ideas are controversial and far less common than the two-stage, no-loading procedure previously described. Success rates with immediate loading or immediate placement are generally lower.

Osseointegration and Biointegration

For dental implants made of titanium alloy, the interface between the alloy and bone must be nearly direct with no intervening fibrous tissue and as little space as possible. This special interfacial condition is called osseointegration and occurs when the bone grows to within 100 Å (1 angstrom $= 10^{-10}$ meters) of the titanium surface (Figure 15-5). Within the 100 Å, there is only extracellular matrix and no collagen or fibrous tissue. This degree of proximity is an extremely rigorous requirement achieved only if the surgical technique is atraumatic (see the previous discussion on surgical techniques) and the material does not have adverse biologic effects. To date, only a few materials, including commercially pure titanium, titanium–aluminum–vanadium alloy, tantalum, and several ceramic materials such as zirconia, are known to permit osseointegration (see the later discussion on implant materials). When the implant is osseointegrated, virtually no mobility of the implant in the bone is clinically detectable, and to the clinician it feels similar to the pathologic condition of natural tooth ankylosis. For an implant to be deemed successful, osseointegration must be maintained throughout its lifetime.

> **! ALERT**
>
> Osseointegration is the occurrence of extremely close proximity between a titanium alloy and supporting bone with no intervening fibrous tissue or collagen. Biointegration is the occurrence of continuity of ceramic implant to bone without intervening space. In both osseointegration and biointegration, the supporting bone must remain vital.

For ceramic implant materials (primarily made of zirconia at present), the integration of the ceramic with the bone has no intervening space (see Figure 15-5). Rather, continuity exists from the implant to the bone. This interfacial condition is

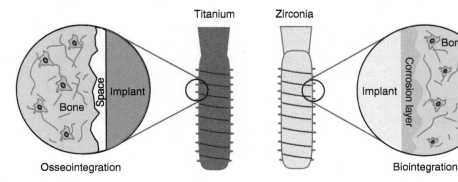

FIG 15-5 Osseointegration versus biointegration. For titanium-alloy implants, the goal is to achieve an osseointegrated interface *(left)*. At the osseointegrated interface, the bony tissue grows to within 100 Å of the implant surface, with no intervening collagen or fibrous tissue. For all-ceramic implants, often zirconia *(right)*, the bony tissue should merge with the ceramic, and no intervening space will be present. Most research indicates that some sort of corrosion or dissolution of the ceramic occurs to mediate biointegration of the bony tissue and the implant surface.

called **biointegration**. Biointegration is thought to require a chemical degradation of the ceramic implant that favors bone formation and is able to integrate with the surrounding bone, which itself has a significant ceramic component. The nature of the biointegrative interface and material characteristics that promote and maintain it are not fully understood. Furthermore, the advantages of biointegration over osseointegration are not known, particularly over the long term. Both interfaces are similar to the clinical ankylosis of natural teeth. Metallic implants coated with a ceramic initially promote a biointegrated interface, but long term, the stability of the interface is less clear because coatings tend to degrade with time.

Implants and Force

> **! ALERT**
>
> Bony support for endosseous implants may be compromised by excessive compressive forces or peri-implantitis.

Although endosseous implants provide an esthetic substitute for a lost or missing tooth, they also are placed to restore lost masticatory function. Thus, the interface between the bone and the implant must withstand the forces generated during chewing and other oral habits for up 40 years. Research has shown definitively that excessive force will compromise osseointegration or biointegration, but the degree of force and the clinical conditions that lead to deterioration of bony support (versus forces that bone can tolerate) are not fully understood. Presumably, a prime consideration is the fundamental difference between the *implant*–bone interface and the *tooth*–bone interface. These two interfaces transmit occlusal forces quite differently (Figure 15-6). In the natural state, occlusal forces are transferred from tooth to bone via the periodontal ligament as tensile forces. Therefore, a downward (apical) force on the tooth results in a tensile force on the bone. These tensile forces stimulate bone deposition, limit bone resorption, and favor the maintenance of the bony support. Thus, unless the forces are excessive or grossly misdirected, occlusal loads on natural teeth favor bone maintenance. However, in the dental implant, no periodontal ligament exists, and occlusal loads are transmitted to the bone mostly by compressive forces. These compressive forces tend to cause resorption of bone. Thus, the design of implant-supported dental prostheses must limit the magnitude of compressive force and stress transmitted to bone to levels below that which causes bone resorption. Limiting compressive stress in bone is one area of active investigation in implantology research. Of particular interest is how much compressive stress may be tolerated without resorptive consequences for alveolar bone. To limit compressive stresses, clinicians will adapt the design of the dental prosthesis, the number of implants supporting a prosthesis, the type of implant, or the diameter and length of the implant. Patient characteristics must also be considered, including occlusal habits (clenching/bruxism) and the quality of bone in the jaw.

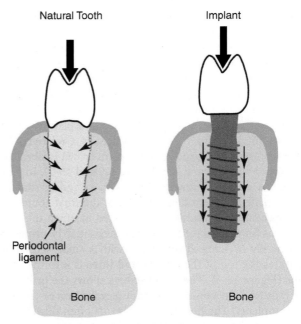

FIG 15-6 Transduction of occlusal force to bone in natural teeth versus implants. Natural teeth are retained by the periodontal ligament (PDL), which is a collagenous tissue extending from the alveolar bone into the cementum of the tooth *(left)*. When occlusal forces are placed on the tooth *(large arrows)*, the PDL transduces these forces into tensile forces on the alveolar bone *(small arrows)*. Tensile forces tend to stimulate bone formation, preserving bone density around the natural tooth over time. In the osseointegrated or biointegrated implant *(right)*, there is no PDL, and occlusal forces are transduced into compressive forces in the alveolar bone. Because compression generally leads to bone resorption, excessive occlusal forces destroy the implant–bone interface.

CLINICAL ISSUES

Types and Uses of Implants

Early in modern-day implantology, most dental implants were not endosseous but were either placed between the gingiva and bone (subperiosteal implants) or designed to "sandwich" the mandible (transosseous implants). These early strategies were painful, required aggressive surgical interventions, carried high risks of postoperative infection, and were not functionally successful in the long term. Early attempts to place endosseous implants failed because the surgical techniques and materials did not promote osseointegration or biointegration. Various geometries, including screws, cylinders, meshes, hollow cylinders, and large blades, were used to try to find a geometry that would maintain long-term osseointegration during oral function. When materials that promoted an osseointegrated or biointegrated interface were discovered and surgical techniques developed to reliably obtain those interfaces, the endosseous implant became a viable treatment option. Today, the screw type of endosseous implant has virtually supplanted all other types of implants (see Figure 15-1); subperiosteal and transosseous strategies are nearly unknown.

Initially, endosseous implants were used only to support complete dentures, primarily in the mandible. One early strategy used four to six implants to retain a mandibular complete denture prosthesis (implant-retained complete denture) (Figure 15-7). The mandibular edentulous condition was a natural initial focus because of the difficulties patients often have with adapting to traditional complete dentures for an edentulous lower arch. However, as techniques and materials have improved, implant-retained maxillary dentures also have become commonplace. The number of required implants has declined, and implants have been used to support, rather than retain, complete dentures. In this supportive strategy, the implant has a ball or other device as the intraoral component, a so-called locator abutment or locator attachment (see Figure 15-7). The denture has an elastomeric or magnetic component embedded into the tissue side of the denture, which engages the locator. Locator attachments help prevent the denture from dislodging during function and support the edentulous ridge during chewing or biting. Implant-supported dentures may be constructed primarily or as a second step after fabrication of the traditional complete denture. Locator implants are most common in the mandible. More recently, one to two small implants (called mini-implants) have been used as locator implants to support lower dentures. These smaller implants may be sufficient to support a complete denture, particularly in the mandible.

Since the 1990s, single or multiple mandibular or maxillary endosseous implants also have become commonplace as alternatives to bridges or partial dentures in the partially edentulous mouth. Today, the placement of a single endosseous implant is a viable treatment alternative for a tooth requiring endodontic therapy, a buildup, and a crown, particularly in the posterior. The choice between endodontic therapy and implant placement is complex and beyond the scope of this discussion. Cemented prostheses that connect endosseous implants to natural teeth are not common because they have high failure rates. Failure is likely a result of the normal small movement of the natural tooth, which transmits too much force to the endosseous implant, leading to destruction of the osseointegrated interface.

Definition of Clinical Success of Implant Therapy

The technical definitions of success for endosseous implants are extremely rigorous compared with standards in use as recently as the mid-1980s. Today, clinical success is defined as an osseointegrated or biointegrated implant with no measurable clinical mobility of the implant under occlusal function. Clinically, tapping the implant with an instrument elicits a high-pitched, sharp sound that is distinct from natural teeth. For most clinical situations, success rates are greater than 95% at 10 years as long as an implant osseointegrates initially and the clinical environment is not extreme (i.e., occlusal forces are not too high or directed in inappropriate directions, or patients fail to remove plaque). Success rates decrease if the density or quantity of bone is less or if the implants are loaded immediately. Generally, the maintenance of bony support around the implant is a key factor in its longevity. Some ongoing horizontal loss of bone (less than 0.5 mm/year) is common, but rates of horizontal loss greater than 0.5 mm/year or the appearance of vertical bony defects are signs of a failing implant. In any case, the criteria for the clinical success of endosseous implants are far more rigorous today than in 1979, when the National Institutes of Health defined an endosseous implant as successful if it had less than 0.5 mm of mobility in any direction, with a 5-year retention rate of 75%.

Clinical Maintenance

The increase in the use of endosseous implants in edentulous and partially dentulous patients has raised questions of what inflammatory processes might contribute to loss of bony support and how clinicians might limit bone loss. These questions stem from the established role of inflammation in loss of natural teeth (see Chapter 1). Most clinicians agree that although the original periodontal anatomy is absent around an implant, a plaque-mediated inflammatory process similar to periodontal inflammation occurs. This process is peri-implantitis, and current evidence indicates that it is caused by microorganisms similar to those responsible for periodontitis. Peri-implantitis causes a similar progression of loss of soft tissue attachment and erosion of supporting bone that are hallmarks of periodontitis. The goals for the clinician are therefore to maintain soft and hard tissue integration of the implant by limiting plaque accumulation and maturation. This goal may be difficult to achieve in patients who initially lost natural teeth through poor oral hygiene; thus patient motivation for postplacement care should be a primary consideration in planning implant treatment.

The patient may clean dental implants with traditional devices, including toothbrushes, proxy brushes, toothpastes, floss, floss threaders, and other oral hygiene aids (Figure 15-8). The regimen for cleaning must be customized to each patient because the numbers and types of implants and associated prostheses are different in each patient. Access to surfaces of the implants near the gingiva may be more difficult to achieve than with the normal dentition, so special care must be taken to ensure that the patient is properly instructed. Dental auxiliaries should consider that oral hygiene skills and priorities for an implant patient may not be ideal and may have led to the loss of the natural teeth in the first place.

For the dental team, traditional instrumentation with metallic scalers and curettes is not appropriate for cleaning the implant, because these instruments damage the surface of the implants and may compromise the integration of the implant or increase the retention of plaque. Sonic and ultrasonic cleaners also are contraindicated, as are aggressive abrasives. Plastic or Teflon scalers (see Figure 15-8) are commonly used to clean the implant surface.

IMPLANT MATERIALS

Early Materials: Polymers, Ceramics, and Metals

Historically, many polymers, ceramics, and metals have been used for endosseous dental implants. Polymers have not been

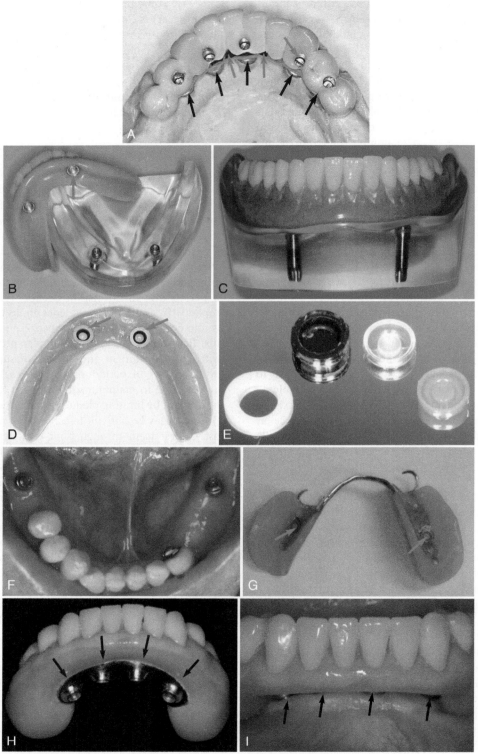

FIG 15-7 Implant-retained and implant-supported dentures. Implants are used to support and retain complete arch fixed prostheses **(A, H, I).** In these prostheses, multiple implants *(black arrows)* are connected to an alloy substructure *(blue arrows)* onto which ceramic or acrylic polymer is added. The entire prosthesis is stabilized with screws (e.g., *red arrow* in **A,** not visible in **H, I),** which allows removal of the prosthesis if necessary. Implants are also used to support (in combination with the edentulous ridge) a complete denture **(B** and **C).** These implant-supported dentures are often retained by locators *(green arrows)* that do not hold the prosthesis rigidly but prevent inadvertent displacement when the prosthesis is in function such as chewing. The locators **(D** and **E)** are generally silicone rings that snap onto a special implant abutment and can be replaced as they wear. Implant-supported partial dentures with locators also are possible **(F** and **G),** particularly in distal extension partials (where no posterior teeth remain). (**A–G,** Courtesy Dr. Mats Kronström, University of Washington, Department of Restorative Dentistry, Seattle, WA; **H** and **I,** courtesy Dr. Y-W Chen, University of Washington, Department of Restorative Dentistry, Seattle, WA.)

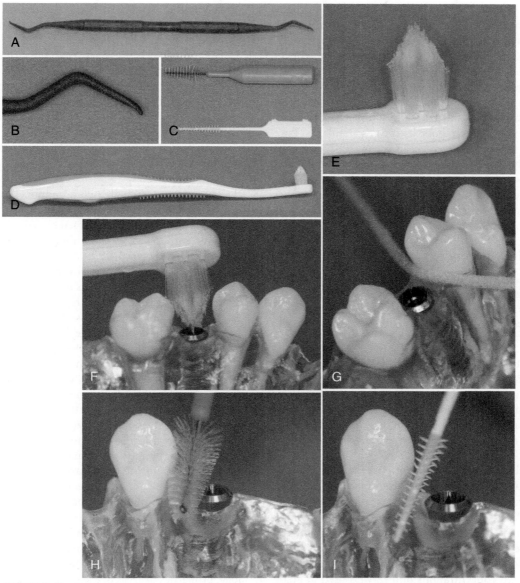

FIG 15-8 Devices and instruments used to clean implants and tissues adjacent to implants. Special plastic scalers (**A;** detail in **B**) are used to clean the implant surfaces in contact with tissues. The plastic spares the relatively soft titanium alloy and prevents gradual alloy degradation. Other devices such as brushes are appropriate to clean the implants or teeth adjacent to implants (**C, D,** and **E**). Super-floss (**F**) also may be used. These devices are able to gently remove plaque and food debris from areas around the implant and remaining adjacent natural teeth (**F, G, H,** and **I**). Effective removal of plaque is imperative to prevent the chronic inflammatory processes of periodontitis in adjacent natural teeth and peri-implantitis around implants, both of which lead to loss of alveolar bone and restoration failure. (Courtesy Dr. Mats Kronström, University of Washington, Department of Restorative Dentistry, Seattle, WA.)

successful because of their lack of strength and inability to osseointegrate or biointegrate. A variety of polymer types have been tried, including poly (methyl methacrylate) (denture-base resin), polytetrafluoroethylene (Teflon), polyethylene, polysulfone, and polyurethane. However, none of these materials has been successful clinically, and none is used today for endosseous implants.

Ceramic materials have been more successful than polymers as endosseous implants. Several forms of carbon have been used,

including vitreous (or amorphous) carbon, carbon silicates, and crystalline carbon. Although the carbon materials have low corrosion rates, they are not suitable for endosseous implants by today's standards because they do not stably osseointegrate. Alumina, hydroxyapatite, and tricalcium phosphates were introduced in the 1960s and 1970s, and use of these materials has persisted because they promoted either biointegration or osseointegration. However, these ceramics were brittle and tended to fracture when subjected to oral forces. For these reasons, these ceramics are used only as coatings on alloy implants, a strategy that continues to wane. In recent years, newer ceramics have emerged that biointegrate and have sufficient strength to reduce fracture risks (see the subsequent discussion).

Metals and alloys were probably the first materials used for endosseous implants. Until about 1970, the use of stainless steel, cobalt–chromium, and tantalum alloys was common, although success rates were poor by today's standards. Pure gold and gold alloys also were used during this time, but not successfully. In this era, only tantalum alloys showed any ability to osseointegrate in endosseous applications. However, tantalum alloys induce an osseointegrative response that is inferior compared with titanium alloys, and titanium alloys have supplanted tantalum alloys.

Titanium Alloys for Endosseous Implants

> **! ALERT**
>
> Titanium alloys are the most successful material for endosseous dental implants and have the longest clinical track record.

The discovery that titanium alloys predictably promote long-term osseointegration with bone revolutionized the use of endosseous implants in dentistry. Two types of titanium alloys are commonly used today: commercially pure (cp) titanium and titanium alloy. These terms are unfortunate because both are technically incorrect but their usage is commonplace.

Commercially pure titanium is not pure titanium. Rather, it is an alloy of approximately 99 wt% titanium and small amounts (from 0.18 to 0.40 wt%) of oxygen and trace amounts (less than 0.25%) of iron, carbon, hydrogen, and nitrogen (see Table 15-1). These trace elements must be carefully controlled and are included by design to promote favorable alloy properties. The amount of oxygen determines the grade of the alloy, with oxygen concentrations of 0.18 wt% used in grade 1 alloys and 0.40% in grade 4 alloys. Increasing amounts of oxygen increase the strength and decrease the ductility of these alloys, leaving the modulus, density, and melting range unaffected (see Table 15-1). Despite concentrations of less than 0.25%, the other trace elements are critical to the strength,

phase structure, and corrosion resistance of these alloys. As far as is known, all of these alloys are equivalent in their ability to osseointegrate with bone.

Titanium alloy is the other commonly used implant material in dentistry. The term *titanium alloy* is not accurate because all metallic endosseous materials are alloys, yet this term has been commonly applied to an alloy similar to commercially pure titanium but with 6 wt% aluminum and 4 wt% vanadium added. The addition of aluminum and vanadium doubles the tensile strength of this alloy relative to grade 4 titanium but also reduces its ductility (see Table 15-1). The modulus and melting range of titanium alloy are essentially the same as commercially pure titanium. Titanium alloy also osseointegrates with bone, but some research has reported minor differences in the character of the bone around the implant, with traces of aluminum and vanadium present. The consequences of these trace elements are not clear.

The surface of commercially pure titanium or titanium alloy is covered with a complex mixture of adherent titanium oxides (Figure 15-9). Multiple types of oxides exist at the surface, and their presence is essential to the osseointegrative properties of these alloys. The thickness of the oxide layer varies but is generally 20 to 100 Å, with oxides rich in oxygen closer to the surface and those poor in oxygen nearer the alloy. Titanium alloys spontaneously re-form these oxides extremely quickly (less than 1 millisecond) after any damage to the alloy surface removed them because titanium is too reactive to exist unoxidized in an oxygen atmosphere. Yet during manufacturing, oxides must be formed in a controlled environment, because contaminants from the air will be incorporated into the oxide layer and may adversely affect the ability of the alloy to osseointegrate. Thus, scratches or other disruption of the original manufacturer's oxide layer are discouraged, and any perturbation or contamination of the original surface will increase the risk of failure of the implant (Figure 15-10). Clinically, cleaning of these surfaces should not disrupt the oxide layer to avoid changing the biologic properties of areas of the implant that are exposed to the oral cavity. For this reason, special instruments are used to clean implants (see the previous discussion).

The surface treatment and surface morphology of titanium alloys also influence osseointegrative responses. The objective of surface modification is to maximize the amount of implant

TABLE 15-1	**Composition and Important Properties of Common Titanium-Based Alloys for Endosseous Dental Implants (wt%)**					
	O (wt%)	Ti (wt%)	Modulus (GPa)	Tensile strength (MPa)	Elongation (%)	Density
Cp* Titanium alloys						
Grade 1	0.18	>99	100	240	24	4.5
Grade 2	0.25	>99	100	345	20	4.5
Grade 3	0.35	>99	100	450	18	4.5
Grade 4	0.40	>99	100	550	15	4.5
Ti-Al-V alloy						
	0.13	>89	110	900	12	4.5

*Cp: Commercially pure.

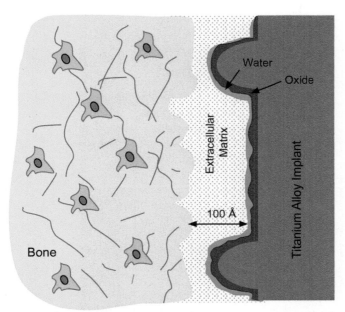

FIG 15-9 The bone–titanium-alloy interface in osseointegration. In an osseointegrated interface, the bone does not contact the implant alloy directly. The oxide layer on the alloy (20 to 100 Å thick) allows a deposition of water (only one or two molecular layers) and extracellular matrix (ECM) components onto itself that permit osteoblasts to produce a mineralized matrix to within 100 Å of the oxide. The collagenous fibers of the bone integrate with components of the ECM, but there is no organized collagen per se in the 100-Å space. The exact biochemical organization within the 100-Å space is not known. The presence of the oxide is required for osseointegration. The ability of alloy oxides to encourage or permit an extracellular matrix organization that favors bone approximation is not common and is thought to be a key attribute of titanium alloys that makes them clinically usable as endosseous implants.

surface with good bony approximation (somewhat inappropriately called bone–implant "contact"). A variety of strategies have been used to create surfaces that maximize bone–implant contact, including acid etching, sandblasting, plasma spraying, oxidization, and various electropolishing techniques. These treatments may increase the surface area of the implant available for osseointegration, may change the chemistry of the surface to promote better osseointegration, or both. In general, rougher surfaces and those with greater surface areas promote the greatest amounts of bone–implant contact. Sandblasting or acid-etching treatments that increase the oxide formation on the implant also promote good bone–implant contact. The manufacturer is responsible for creating the implant surface, but the dental team must take meticulous measures to ensure that the surface is not altered or contaminated prior to surgery.

The low corrosion of commercially pure titanium or titanium alloy in bone, soft tissues, or the oral cavity is one of its greatest assets from biologic and restorative perspectives. Although studies have shown that trace levels of elements are released from these alloys into bone, the levels are low (less than 1 part per billion in most cases), and the effects of these trace levels appear to be minimal. Similarly, trace levels of the implant metals can be found distributed into various body tissues, including lung, liver, spleen, and kidney. However, no ill effects of these elements in these tissues are known at these low levels. The reason that the surface oxide of these alloys promotes osseointegration is not well understood, but the low degradation of the alloy components is undoubtedly a favorable factor.

Ceramic Coatings

> **! ALERT**
>
> Ceramic coatings improve bone–implant bond strengths, but their long-term stability in service is uncertain, and their use has waned considerably.

Because some ceramics promote biointegration and strong bone–implant bonds, titanium alloys have been coated with thin layers of these ceramics to try to combine the high strength of the alloy with the favorable integrative characteristics of these ceramics. Until recently, ceramics by themselves have proven too brittle to serve as dental implants. The thickness of most ceramic coatings ranges from 50 to 100 μm and generally is deposited onto the metal alloy with a plasma spraying technique. The ceramic coating may have several characteristics that influence its solubility, strength, and biologic properties, including its porosity, crystallinity, composition, strength, and thickness. The bond strength of the ceramic to the alloy is also a significant concern. The effectiveness and longevity of ceramic coatings are controversial, although studies support that these coatings promote a stronger bone–implant bond more quickly than alloy alone and promote biointegration rather than osseointegration. *In vivo*, degradation of the coatings with time is a significant issue, and the consequences of this degradation on the long-term integration of the implant with bone are not known. Debonding of the coating from the base alloy also remains a significant concern that has as yet undetermined effects of long-term implant performance. To a large extent, it appears that all-ceramic zirconia implants will supplant ceramic-coated titanium implants or that titanium-alloy implants will remain the mainstay of endosseous dental implantology.

Ceramic Implants

Improved manufacturing technologies and research have yielded ceramics that may be strong enough to serve long-term roles as endosseous implants and implant abutments. Historically, the risk of catastrophic fracture was a major barrier to such usage. The most common all-ceramic implants are currently of zirconia (see Chapter 14). As implants, these ceramics promote biointegration when compared to osseointegration, yet they do not have the technical difficulties or liabilities that are inherent to ceramic-coated titanium. For example, all-ceramic zirconia has a well-controlled crystal structure, surface morphology, and composition; control of these properties in coatings is problematic. Zirconia also does not rely on a ceramic–metal bond, and degradation over time is likely to be less than for coatings. Several companies

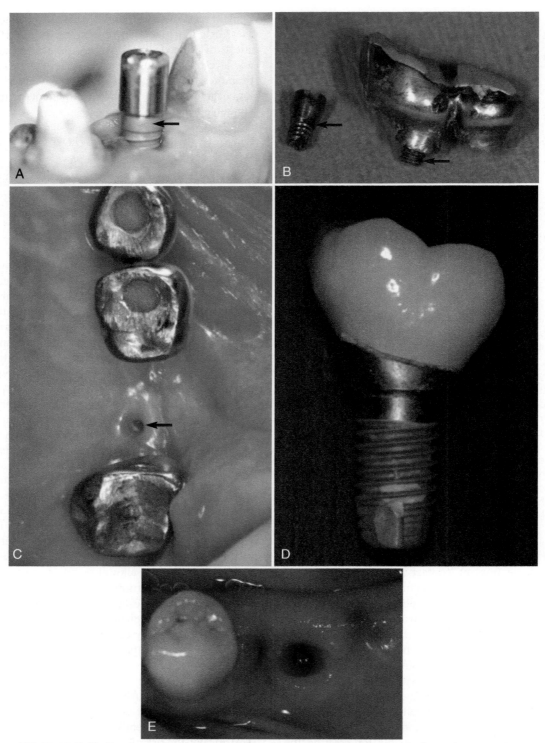

FIG 15-10 Failed implants. The exposed threads of an implant (*arrow* in **A**) indicate that osseointegration has not fully occurred or has regressed since placement. The implant will not be stable to support a prosthesis and must be removed and replaced, probably after bone grafting. In other cases, the implants remain stable, but the retaining screw fractures (*arrows* in **B**). The screws can generally be replaced. Occasionally, an implant does not osseointegrate after placement (*arrow* in **C**). The incomplete tissue healing suggests inflammation, soft tissue down-growth, and lack of bone integration. If the osseointegration is initially stable but is lost over time, the implant will be shed **(D, E).** In **D,** note that there is no bone adhered to the implant, suggesting complete loss of integration. (**A,** Courtesy Dr. Mats Kronström, University of Washington, Department of Restorative Dentistry, Seattle, WA; **B–E,** courtesy Dr. Y-W Chen, University of Washington, Department of Restorative Dentistry, Seattle, WA.)

currently sell zirconia implants in the United States; more will likely emerge in the coming years. However, given the long-term data available and excellent record of success with titanium alloy endosseous implants, zirconia implants will be closely scrutinized in the near term to ensure comparable results.

All-ceramic materials also are becoming more common for implant abutments (Figure 15-11). These devices may be made from several types of ceramics (see Chapter 14), but zirconia is the most common because of its strength. The driving forces behind the use of all-ceramic abutments are the esthetics and favorable biologic properties of these materials, which are in intimate contact with bone, gingival tissues, and the oral cavity. A white abutment may be more esthetic for implant restorations in the "esthetic zone." Ironically, the extremely white, opaque nature of zirconia is sometimes an esthetic liability as well. In response, companies have developed shaded zirconia for abutments, although the long-term physical and biologic performances of these modified materials are not clear at present. One can anticipate rapid changes in this area of dental materials in the coming years.

Digital imaging has been increasingly used to plan treatment for implant patients as well as guide implant placement. Today, digital imaging combined with CAD-CAM technologies are being used to manufacture restorations (Figure 15-12). Using commonly available digital intraoral scanners, a restoration can be fabricated today without a traditional impression and, in some cases, without a laboratory model. As techniques improve, interest in their use will increase in the coming years as they reduce the time and materials needed to fabricate implant restorations, improve patient comfort, and improve the fit clinical compatibility of restorations.

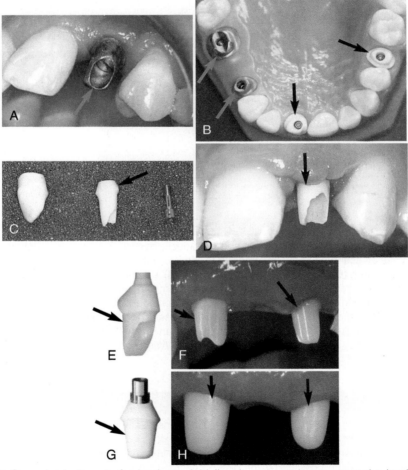

FIG 15-11 Ceramic abutments for implants. Initially, abutments that connect the implant to the restoration were made only of alloy (*red arrows* in **A** and **B**). In the anterior area where esthetic concerns dominate, the alloy color may be difficult to mask or may darken the color of the gingiva. In these esthetic situations, ceramic abutments have been developed (*black arrows* in **B, C, D–H**). Some ceramic abutments are a hybrid of titanium alloy and zirconia (**G**). This hybrid maximizes esthetics in the tissues and mitigates risks of wear between the zirconia and much softer titanium implant in the bone. The ceramic abutment is retained with a screw (**B** and **C**) and is typically restored with an all-ceramic crown (**C,** *left*). The ceramic abutment has just been placed (**D, F**); in **F,** the soft tissue is poorly contoured but will remodel around a temporary restoration that will be added next (**H**). (**A–D,** Courtesy Dr. Mats Kronström, University of Washington, Department of Restorative Dentistry, Seattle, WA; **E–H,** courtesy Dr. Y-W Chen, University of Washington, Department of Restorative Dentistry, Seattle, WA.)

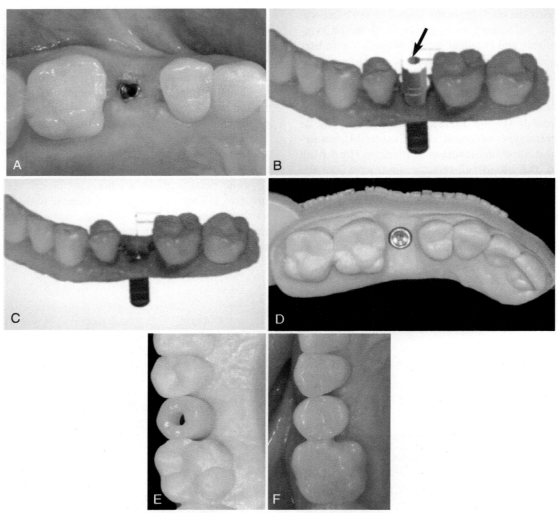

FIG 15-12 Digital implantology. Digital imaging is gradually becoming common in dental implantology. In this case a "scanning body" is attached to the implant in **A,** and a digital image is captured in the patient's mouth **(B).** The scanning body (*arrow* in **B**) is removed virtually from the image **(C),** providing a virtual image of the relationship between the implant and the adjacent teeth. A model is digitally printed **(D),** and the abutment and implant are fabricated **(E).** The implant is then delivered to the patient **(F)** without having ever taken an impression of the patient. If the construction of the restoration is straightforward, the restoration can be milled without the printed model in **E** and **F.** (Courtesy Dr. Y-W Chen, University of Washington Department of Restorative Dentistry, Seattle, WA.).

QUICK REVIEW

Today, the restoration of endosseous dental implants is a routine part of dental practice. The ability of an implant to osseointegrate with bone has revolutionized the placement of these implants. Reliable osseointegration has been made possible by the discovery of atraumatic surgical techniques and the development of titanium alloys, combined with empirical knowledge of the appropriate clinical applications. By far, the most successful materials for endosseous implants have been the titanium alloys. These alloys can be subdivided generally into commercially pure titanium and titanium–aluminum–vanadium alloys, and both are used in dental practice today. The effectiveness of ceramic coatings on implants remains controversial, and although all-ceramic implants were not successful historically because of their brittleness, newer, stronger all-ceramic materials such as zirconia show promise as implants and implant abutments. The use of digital imaging and CAD-CAM technologies will increase as they become more reliable and simpler. The bone around endosseous implants may suffer from a chronic, progressive inflammation similar to periodontal inflammation. This inflammation is called peri-implantitis and results in loss of bony support for the implant and inflammation of the gingival tissues. Peri-implantitis can be limited by appropriate plaque-reduction measures similar to those used to treat periodontal disease, although special techniques and instruments are necessary to avoid damage of the implant surfaces when patients or dental professionals clean the implants.

❓ SELF-TEST QUESTIONS

Test your knowledge by answering the following questions. For multiple-choice questions, one or more responses may be correct.

1. In osseointegration, a layer of fibrous tissue remains between the implant and the bone.
   a. True
   b. False
2. Osseointegration and biointegration both result in which condition(s)?
   a. Clinical ankylosis of the implant
   b. Formation of a periodontal-like ligament
   c. A defined space between the implant and the bone
   d. A clinically unacceptable result
3. In placement of endosseous implants, the surgical techniques maximize the speed of bone removal.
   a. True
   b. False
4. Grade 1 and grade 4 of commercially pure titanium alloys differ primarily in their amount of which elements?
   a. Nitrogen
   b. Helium
   c. Oxygen
   d. Nickel
5. The tensile strength of which materials is the greatest?
   a. Grade 1 titanium alloy
   b. Grade 4 titanium alloy
   c. Titanium–aluminum–vanadium alloy
   d. Alumina ceramic
6. Which method is the most clinically proven method of surgically placing endosseous implants?
   a. Two-stage placement with no immediate loading
   b. Two-stage placement with immediate loading at the second stage
   c. One-stage placement with no immediate loading
   d. One-stage placement with immediate loading
7. Compressive forces tend to cause what in bony tissues?
   a. Deposition
   b. Ankylosis
   c. Increases in density
   d. Resorption
8. Today, restorations bridging natural teeth and endosseous implants are not common.
   a. True
   b. False
9. Clinically successful endosseous implants have which attribute(s)?
   a. Less than 0.5 mm of mobility in any direction
   b. Less than 1 mm of mobility in any direction
   c. No clinically detectable mobility
   d. No mobility for the first 1 year after placement, followed by less than 0.5 mm of mobility in any direction in subsequent years

10. Which instrument(s) should the hygienist use to clean implants?
    a. Traditional curettes and scalers
    b. Sonic scalers
    c. Ultrasonic scalers
    d. Plastic scalers
11. Commercially pure titanium is 100% titanium.
    a. True
    b. False
12. Only titanium alloys have shown the ability to osseointegrate or biointegrate into bone.
    a. True
    b. False
13. The thickness of most ceramic coatings on implants is approximately:
    a. 100 Å
    b. 100 µm
    c. 1 mm
    d. None of the above
14. The release of elements from titanium alloys into the body is:
    a. Not detectable
    b. Detectable but at apparently insignificant levels
    c. Significant and a trigger of bone resorption
15. Ceramic coatings on endosseous implants are always crystalline and porous.
    a. True
    b. False
16. Zirconia implants do not promote biointegration or osseointegration.
    a. True
    b. False
17. Zirconia is a(n):
    a. Polymer
    b. Composite
    c. Alloy
    d. Ceramic
18. Implant abutments may be:
    a. Custom fabricated
    b. Made of titanium alloy or zirconia
    c. In the shape of a crown preparation or platform
    d. Cemented to the implant
19. Occlusal force on an endosseous implant results in
    a. Compressive forces in bone
    b. Tensile forces in bone
    c. Tensile forces in the implant
    d. Compressive forces in the implant

SUGGESTED SUPPLEMENTARY READINGS

Al-Amieh B, Lyons K, Swain M: Clinical trials in zirconia: a systematic review, *J Oral Rehabilitation* 37:641, 2010.

Albrektsson T: Direct bone anchorage of dental implants, *J Prosthet Dent* 50:255, 1983.

Kronström M, Davis B, Loney R, Gerrow J, Hollender L: A prospective randomized study on the immediate loading of manibular overdentures supported by one or two implants; a 3 year follow-up report, *Clin Implant Dent Relat Res* 16:323, 2014.

Thalji G, Bryington M, DeKok IJ, Cooper LF: Prosthodontic management of implant therapy, *Dent Clin North Am* 58:207, 2014.

Wataha JC: Materials for endosseous dental implants, *J Oral Rehabil* 23:79, 1996.

evolve Please visit *http://evolve.elsevier.com/Powers/dentalmaterials* for additional practice and study support tools.

abfraction area Such an area may result from repeated bending of a tooth, which causes the enamel to flake away from the cervical region of the tooth.

abrasion Process of wear whereby a hard, rough surface or hard, irregularly shaped particles plow grooves in a softer material and cause material from such grooves to be removed from the surface.

abrasion resistance A property of a material that describes its ability to resist scratching or loss of mass during manipulation.

abutment teeth Teeth adjacent to the edentulous space where a fixed partial denture (bridge) is being placed.

acrylic polymer Polymer formed through free-radical polymerization.

addition polymerization Type of free-radical polymerization distinctive because it produces no reaction by-products.

addition silicone Impression materials (also known as vinyl polysiloxanes [VPS]) developed as an alternative to polysulfides and condensation silicones.

admixed amalgam Amalgam alloy that contains silver–tin particles and silver–copper particles.

agar A reversible hydrocolloid derived from seaweed.

alginate Flexible impression material in which the alginate in water (sol) reacts chemically with calcium ions to form insoluble calcium alginate (gel).

all-ceramic Esthetic restoration made from special ceramics with no metal substructure.

alloy A mixture of two or more metals or nonmetals.

alumina Al_2O_3, aluminum oxide.

amalgam The mixture of a metal or alloy with liquid mercury. In dentistry, amalgam refers to the mixture of a silver-based alloy with mercury to form a silver-colored restorative material.

amalgamation Reaction that occurs between mercury and amalgam alloy.

amine Organic molecule that contains nitrogen and is used as an accelerator in polymerization reactions.

amorphous (glassy) phase Increased transparency of a ceramic; occurs when the continuity of the crystalline array is interrupted by fluxes.

base Layer of material that acts as an insulator and protective barrier beneath restorations.

base metal A metal that is not noble. In pure form, base metals have a greater tendency to corrode in the oral environment than noble metals.

bending moment Force × distance in bending.

binder Material that holds an investment or other ceramic together.

biofilm A community of different species of bacteria that adheres to a surface like enamel, the soft tissues, or a restorative material.

biointegration Integration of the implant with the bone with no intervening spaces.

bisphenol A-glycidyl methacrylate (Bis-GMA) A polymer formed by the reaction of bisphenol A and glycidyl methacrylate that, when reacted with diacrylates, forms the polymer used in pit and fissure sealants and in composite restorative materials.

brazing Process in dentistry by which special alloys are used to join other alloys.

bridge Prosthetic device that consists of artificial teeth suspended between and cemented to abutment teeth; now commonly referred to as a fixed partial denture.

burnout Process of wax elimination by thermal decomposition.

calcium sulfate dihydrate Composition of a gypsum product such as plaster once it has been mixed with water; $CaSO_4 \cdot 2H_2O$.

calcium sulfate hemihydrate Composition of unreacted particles of a gypsum product such as plaster; $CaSO_4 \cdot \frac{1}{2}H_2O$.

camphorquinone Chemical light-cured in order to generate free radicals for polymerization of acrylics.

caries Tooth decay.

cast A replica of a patient's teeth and adjacent oral structures made by pouring an impression of the mouth with a gypsum material.

casting A process by which a wax pattern of a shape is converted into metal.

casting ring A metal ring used to support the investment during the casting process.

catalyst Material that initiates a chemical reaction but is not consumed in the reaction.

ceramic A material that contains various amounts of silica, feldspar, and alumina or other metal oxides.

ceramic bonding alloy A dental casting alloy designed to accept the chemical bonding of a ceramic veneer. These alloys are used for ceramic (porcelain)-fused-to-metal (PFM) restorations.

ceramic coating Coating applied to titanium implants to try to combine the high strength of the alloy with the favorable integrative characteristics of these ceramics.

ceramic onlays An intracoronal restoration made entirely of ceramic that replaces one or more tooth cusps.

ceramic veneers An extra-coronal restoration made entirely of ceramic that covers the facial and sometimes the incisal surface of anterior teeth. Veneers are constructed to improve esthetics and are more conservative than crowns.

chelate Complex compound formed from an organic molecule with two functional groups that are so arranged that a metal may become

part of a ring structure with the organic molecule.

chroma Relative intensity of the color of an object.

cleansing abrasive Soft, fine particles intended to remove soft materials that adhere to teeth or restorative materials.

coefficient of thermal expansion (CTE) A thermal property of a material that quantifies how much a material will expand when it is heated and contract when it cools. The linear coefficient is the change in length per unit length per degree Celsius.

commercially pure titanium A metal containing approximately 99% Ti with small amounts of O_2 and trace amounts of Fe, C, H, and N.

complete denture A prosthesis for an edentulous arch designed to restore occlusion, esthetics, and speech.

compomer A polyacid-modified composite that polymerizes and also undergoes an acid–base reaction when exposed to moisture from the oral environment.

composite Material composed of two or more physically homogeneous portions that has properties intermediate to the two portions.

compressive strength Stress required to rupture a material when it is pressed together (forces applied opposite but toward each other).

compule A form of unit-dose packaging for light-cured composites and compomers.

computer-aided design/computer-aided milling (CAD/CAM) Practice of using computers to produce restorations directly from the digital impression data.

condensation Process of adapting plastic amalgam to prepared cavity walls and margins to develop a uniform mass with minimum voids and minimum excess mercury.

condensation silicone Flexible impression material that gives off a by-product during polymerization.

copolymer A polymer that consists of two or more types of "mers" or units.

corrosion An electrochemical reaction of a material, usually metallic, that results in the release of ions and electrons from the material, the surface or internal destruction of the material, and the formation of new reaction products.

creep The gradual dimensional change of a material under a load or stress. In dentistry, creep occurs to some materials (especially some amalgam) as a result of the occlusal load over a long period of time.

cross-linked polymer Polymers that are three-dimensional network molecules.

cross-linking Process of linking chemically unbonded polymer strands by adding a cross-linking agent.

crown Restoration that makes up the entire portion of a tooth normally covered with enamel.

crystalline phase   The component of a ceramic material that is composed of regular arrays of metal oxides.

curing   Initiation of the polymerization of acrylic polymers.

D

degassing   A process used during the fabrication of ceramic–metal restorations. High heat is applied to the alloy substructure to clean the alloy and cause formation of an oxide layer to which the porcelain will bond.

density   The mass of a substance divided by its volume.

dental casting alloy   An alloy that is melted and cast into the shape of the wax model of a restoration, usuallly for all alloy restorations.

dentinal tubules   Microscopic channels that extend from the pulp through the dentin.

denture base   Material used to contact the oral tissues and support artificial teeth.

die   A stone, epoxy, or metallic replicate of a tooth prepared for a restoration.

dihydrate   Dihydrate form of calcium sulfate ($CaSO_4 \cdot 2H_2O$).

dimensional change   Shrinkage or expansion of a material; usually expressed as a percentage of an original length or volume.

dimethacrylate   Methacrylate monomer with a reactive, or polymerizable, group on each end.

ductility   Ability of a material to be stretched without rupturing.

E

elastic modulus   Ratio of the stress to the strain of a material within its elastic limit.

elastomeric   Impression materials that are flexible polymers when set.

endosseous dental implant   An implant (usually Ti or Ti alloy) implanted directly into the bone of the mandible or maxilla, used to support a prosthesis.

epoxy   Organic compound containing two terminal groups, such as that react with an organic diamine to form an epoxy resin.

ester wax   Wax that contains carbon, hydrogen, and oxygen atoms that is typically obtained from insects (e.g., beeswax) or from trees (e.g., carnauba wax).

extracoronal restoration   Restorations used to restore teeth with extensive damage that cannot be managed with intracoronal restorations.

F

feldspathic ceramic   Term used for "porcelain" in dentistry; most esthetic, but weakest of the ceramics.

filler   Solid particles added to polymers to change their optical or physical properties.

finishing abrasive   Hard, coarse particles used primarily for developing desired contours of a restoration or tooth preparation and for removing gross irregularities on the surface.

fixed partial denture   Also referred to as a "bridge"; prosthetic device that consists of artificial teeth suspended between and cemented to abutment teeth.

flexural strength (transverse strength)   A strength of a material in which a bar of the material is placed on two supports and a force is applied opposite the supports and between them until the bar fractures. Flexural strength is a combination of tensile and compressive strength.

flux   A chemical used to dissolve the oxide on the surface of an alloy and allow a melted solder to flow and bond to the alloy; also a substance used to lower the fusing temperature of a ceramic.

forces   Application of energy to a substance that causes a change in the substance.

free radical polymerization   Process by which acrylic polymers are formed, using monomers that have a carbon–carbon double bond as their reactive group.

fusing temperature   The temperature at which a material (usually a ceramic or an alloy) changes from a liquid to a solid.

G

galvanism   Effect of electric potentials in the mouth as a result of the use of dissimilar metals as restorative materials.

gamma (γ) phase   Silver-tin compound that composes the original particles of most amalgam alloys and that exists in the hardened dental amalgam.

gamma-1 (γ₁) phase   Silver–mercury compound that is a reaction product in dental amalgam.

gamma-2 (γ₂) phase   Tin–mercury compound that is a reaction product in dental amalgam.

gel   Flexible colloidal system (solid) in which the solid and the liquid phases are continuous. Agar and alginate impressions are hydrogels in which one phase is water and the other phase is agar or alginate.

glass   A noncrystalline or semi-crystalline brittle solid that is often present in dental ceramic materials.

glass ionomer   Restorative material characterized by soluble glass particles in a glass-acid matrix.

gloss   Measure of the reflection of light from a surface.

grain boundaries   Boundaries between crystals in ceramics or alloys.

grains   Microscopic crystals that make up cast alloys or ceramics.

greening   Discoloration of ceramic that occurs when some of the metals in the alloy vaporize and contaminate the ceramic.

gypsum   A chemical, calcium sulfate hemihydrate, which converts to calcium sulfate dihydrate when mixed with water. It is available in three common forms: plaster, stone, and high-strength die stone.

H

hardness   The ability of a material to resist indentation or scratching or, to some extent, wear.

hemihydrate   Hemihydrate form of calcium sulfate ($CaSO_4 \cdot 1/2H_2O$).

high-noble alloys   An alloy that, by definition of the American Dental Association, has $\geq$ 60 wt% noble metal and $\geq$ 40 wt% gold.

homopolymer   Acrylics in which the polymer strands contain only one type of monomer.

hue   Color of an object.

humectant   Chemical used in dentifrices that keeps the paste from drying out.

hybrid ionomer   A resin-modified glass ionomer that undergoes both polymerization and an acid–base reaction.

hydrocarbon   Wax composed only of carbon and hydrogen atoms and typically made from petroleum (e.g., paraffin wax).

hydrocolloid   Two-phase (physically distinguishable) dispersed system in which one of the phases is water.

hydrophilic   Surface that is readily wetted by water as indicated by a low contact angle of water on the surface.

hydrophobic   Surface not readily wetted by water with a contact angle greater than 90 degrees.

hygroscopic   Tending to absorb water from the air.

hygroscopic expansion   The greater increase in volume of a gypsum investment found when it sets in contact with water.

hysteresis   In agar impression materials, the phenomenon of the agar gel melting to form a sol at a temperature higher than that at which the agar sol solidifies to the gel.

I

implant abutment   The part of an implant that acts as a connection between the implant and the restorative prosthesis.

implant-retained denture   A mandibular complete denture prosthesis retained by four to six implants.

implant-supported denture   Constructed after fabrication of the traditional complete denture; locator attachments help prevent the denture from dislodging during function and support the edentulous ridge during chewing or biting.

impression compound   An older thermoplastic impression material.

indirect technique   Shaping of a wax pattern on a model of the prepared tooth (die).

initiator   Reactive material that starts a chemical reaction.

inlay   Intracoronal restoration prepared outside the mouth and cemented to a tapered cavity preparation.

intracoronal restoration   Used to repair damage that is restricted to the internal parts of the tooth.

investment   A mixture of silica and a binder (such as gypsum) used to invest a wax pattern during the casting process.

ionic bond   Chemical bond formed when electrons are transferred completely from on atom (usually a metal) to another atom (usually a non-metal).

K

Knoop hardness   Unit of measure of hardness of dental materials.

L

leach Extraction of a soluble substance from a material by a liquid.

leucite One type of crystalline phase in ceramics.

liner Materials used in thin layers in cavity preparations to protect the dental pulp.

locator abutment A device that attaches to an endosseous implant to help position and retain a removable prosthesis such as a complete denture, which itself houses a complementary receptacle to the locator.

lost-wax technique A technique in which a wax pattern of an object is embedded in a stonelike investment, the pattern is eliminated, and then the space is cast into metal or another material.

luting Bonding of a restoration to tooth structure with a dental cement.

M

malleability Ability of a material to be rolled into a sheet without fracture.

Maryland bridge A term used to describe a resin-retained fixed partial denture; it is unique in that the fixed partial denture does not have crowns for abutments; rather it attaches via an alloy bonded to enamel.

matrix A phase of a material that is formed by reactants (versus unreacted starting products); common in cements, composite materials, and other materials.

melting range Reflects the melting points of the constituents of an alloy.

mercaptan Low-molecular-weight polymer with reactive sulfur-hydrogen groups (–SH).

metamerism Phenomenon in which the light source is critical for proper matching because it influences how a color appears to an observer.

methyl methacrylate Monomer used in denture base resins and in some esthetic restorative materials. In many cases, it is polymerized to form the polymer, poly(methyl methacrylate).

milling A manufacturing process whereby the product is created by cutting from a larger block of starting material. In contemporary milling, the cutting is often computer-directed from a digital file.

mini implants Small implants used as locator implants to support lower dentures.

model plaster Gypsum product; used for study models that do not require abrasion resistance.

model Replica typically made of a gypsum product used primarily for observation.

modulus The resistance of a material to strain, or its stiffness.

monomer A single organic molecule used to prepare a high-molecular-weight polymer.

monophase In dentistry, an elastomeric impression material with a high viscosity under low shear stress and low viscosity under high shear stress.

N

nanofilled Class of composites used in dentistry with nano-scale fillers.

Newton Unit of measurement of force; used in dentistry to measure the magnitude of biting forces.

noble alloy An alloy that, by definition of the American Dental Association, has ≥ 25 wt% noble metal but <60 wt% noble metal.

noble metals Metals that are highly resistant to oxidation, tarnish, and corrosion.

O

obtundent The quality of reducing discomfort that may be related to caries and its removal.

oligomer A moderate-molecular-weight organic molecule made from two or more organic molecules.

onlay Indirect restoration consisting of a solid substance fitted to a cavity in a tooth and cemented into place; extends to replace a cusp.

opacity The degree to which light is not allowed to travel through a material.

opaque A special porcelain with low translucency used to block the color of the metal substructure from showing through in a PFM restoration.

opaquing ceramic Material applied to hide the color of an alloy substructure; the opaque layer forms a bond with the alloy and blocks the alloy color from being transmitted through the ceramic.

osseointegration Interface condition when bone grows to within 100 Å of the surface of the implant with no intervening fibrous tissue.

P

palatal area Area involving the palate or roof of the mouth.

pattern wax A type of wax used to fabricate a model of a dental restoration. In dentistry, pattern waxes include inlay wax, casting wax, and baseplate wax.

percent elongation The amount of deformation that a material can withstand under tensile stress before rupture.

percolation Penetration and forcing out of oral fluids between a dental restoration and the tooth as a result of differences in thermal coefficients of expansion of the materials.

peri-implantitis A chronic, progressive inflammation of the gingival tissues around the implant that can result in loss of bony support.

perlite Volcanic glass used for polishing that becomes finer during use.

pickling A process of submerging a cast restoration in a hot acid to remove surface oxides formed during the casting process.

plasticizer Compound added to a polymer to reduce its hardness.

polishing abrasive Fine particles used to smooth surfaces that have been roughened typically by finishing abrasives or by a wear process in the mouth.

polyether Elastomeric impression material that has ether groups along the main molecule.

polymers Organic molecules of high molecular weight made up of many repeating units.

polymerization Process of preparing large molecules (polymers) from small ones (monomers).

poly(methyl methacrylate) (PMMA) Polymer produced from methyl methacrylate.

polysulfide rubber Elastomeric impression material formed by the reaction of a low-molecular-weight polymer with reactive mercaptan (–SH) groups.

polyurethane Polymer that is formed by the reaction of a polyalcohol (HO–R–OH) and a diisocyanate (O=C=N–R–N=C=O) and that has been used for maxillofacial appliances.

polyvinyl acetate-polyethylene Thermoplastic polymer used to form custom-made mouth protectors.

pontic Artificial replacement teeth used in a fixed partial denture.

porcelain A ceramic material that, in dentistry, is made up of a glass with an embedded crystalline phase called leucite.

porosity Voids in a material that reduce the apparent density.

precapsulated Method of using sealed disposable hard plastic capsules of silver alloy powder and mercury to prepare dental amalgam that provides the proper ratio of alloy powder to mercury, limits handling of pure mercury by the dental team, produces amalgams with consistent physical properties, and keeps the mercury clean.

predominantly base-metal alloy An alloy that, by definition of the American Dental Association, has <25 wt% noble metal.

primer/adhesive A multifunctional monomer with a hydrophilic end that wets and bonds to tooth structure and a hydrophobic end that reacts with the carbon double bonds of the restorative resin, such as composite or compomer.

processing wax A type of wax used in an auxiliary role in the fabrication of a dental restoration. Examples include beading wax, boxing wax, and sticky wax.

proportional limit Minimum stress at which the ratio of stress to strain of a material is no longer constant.

pulp capping Application of a material to a cavity preparation that has exposed or nearly exposed the dental pulp.

R

record base Made from unfilled PMMA; used as a component of record base-wax rim combinations that serve as trial dentures used to determine jaw relations and tooth position for the final denture.

reflectance The amount of incident light that is reflected from a surface.

removable partial denture Used to replace multiple missing teeth; also common in situations in which there is no distal abutment tooth available to anchor a fixed bridge.

residual monomer Monomer that remains unreacted after a polymerization reaction and that can be released into the oral cavity.

residual stress Stress that remains in a material as a result of manipulation; when released by the action of time and temperature, distortion of the material results.

resilience The energy required to stress a material up to the point of permanent deformation.

resin-modified glass ionomer Composite restorative material that contains a polymer binding and dispersed ceramic particles.

retarder Chemical that decreases the rate of a chemical reaction to allow for a longer working time.

rouge Form of iron oxide used for polishing gold alloys.

S

setting time The time it takes for model plaster to set; can be influenced by a variety of factors.

shear strength Stress required to rupture a material when one portion is forced to slide over another portion.

silane coupling agent A bifunctional, silicon-organic compound that couples the inorganic filler particles and resin matrix.

silicon carbide Second hardest of the dental abrasives and is usually applied to paper or plastic disks.

silicone Polymer used as an elastomeric impression material in which the main portion of the molecule consists of silicon-oxygen bonds as, for example, the following.

silver alloy Powder comprised mostly of silver, copper, and tin, that is mixed with mercury to produce dental amalgam.

sintering The process used during fabrication of ceramic restorations in which particles of the ceramic are heated until they fuse (melt) together at their edges.

soft liner Soft polymer used as a thin layer on the tissue-bearing surface of a denture.

sol Colloidal system (liquid) in which the dispersed phase is solid and the continuous phase is liquid; for example, in agar sol the agar is the dispersed solid, and water is the liquid.

solder A special alloy used to join other alloys together in a heating operation known as soldering or brazing.

sorption Nonspecific term that includes both absorption (internal) and adsorption (surface) of liquids by a solid.

spatulation A term used to describe the mixing (by hand or mechanically) of a material.

spherical amalgam Dental amalgam containing spherical alloy particles that requires less mercury and sets somewhat faster than standard amalgam.

sprue Channel through which molten metal is fed to the mold cavity.

stacking Technique used to form ceramic dental restoration; used to apply ceramics to alloys or high-strength ceramic substructures, or to fabricate laminate veneers.

stereolithography Die preparation technique in which a laser polymerizes the die from a vat of monomer.

strain Deformation per unit length.

strength The resistance of a material to fracture when placed under stress.

stress Force per unit area.

substrate alloy Joined alloy created by use of solders.

syneresis Formation of an exudate, or film of liquid, on the surface of hydrocolloid gels.

T

tarnish Corrosion of a material restricted to its surface, usually resulting in a discoloration of the surface. The effects of tarnish can be removed by polishing.

temporary filling Material used to fill a tooth until cavity preparation or placement of a final restoration.

tensile strength Stress required to rupture a material when it is pulled apart (forces applied opposite and away from each other).

tensile stresses Force per unit area that tends to stretch, or elongate, an object.

thermal conductivity Quantity of heat transferred per second across a unit area (cm^2) and a unit length (cm) when the temperature difference along the length is 1° C/cm.

thermal expansion Increase in volume of a material caused by a temperature increase.

thermoplastic Property of becoming softer on heating and harder on cooling; a reversible process.

thixotropic The property of a material that results in low flow under low load but flows readily when placed under load.

3-D printing An additive layering process used to make an object from a digital file.

titanium alloy A metal that contains approximately 90% Ti, 6% Al, and 4% V.

toughness Amount of energy required to stress a material to fracture.

translucency Relative amount of light transmitted through an object.

transparent Having the property of transmitting light through its substance without appreciable scattering.

transverse strength (flexural strength) The strength of a material when tested by placing a small beam onto two supports at each end of the beam and then applying stress to the center of the beam until the material fractures. Commonly used to test ceramic materials.

trituration A term used to describe the process of mixing silver alloy with liquid mercury to form a dental amalgam.

twisting moment Force × distance in twisting.

U

ultimate strength Maximum stress a material sustains before it fractures.

V

value The lightness of or relative amount of light reflected from a color.

varnish Resin surface coating formed by evaporation of a solvent.

veneer Thin covering over another surface; in dentistry a restorative material placed over a tooth surface, either to improve the aesthetics of a tooth or to protect a damaged tooth surface.

W

water–powder ratio The ratio of the amount of water (volume) to the amount of powder (mass) used when mixing a material such as gypsum.

wax rim Used as a component of record base–wax rim combinations that serve as trial dentures used to determine jaw relations and tooth position for the final denture.

welding A process of joining two alloys in which no secondary alloy (or solder) is involved; the alloys join by fusing directly with one another.

wettability Wettability is a measure of the affinity of a liquid for a solid as indicated by spreading of a drop.

wetting Spreading of a liquid over a solid surface.

wrought alloy A cast alloy that has been worked (rolled, drawn, etc.) mechanically into another form.

Y

yield strength Stress at which an arbitrary amount of permanent strain occurs in a material.

Z

zirconia Crystalline ceramic that is composed of zirconium and oxygen, is exceptionally strong, and has no glassy phase.

Note: Page numbers followed by "*f*" indicate figures, "*t*" indicate tables, and "*b*" indicate boxes.